Mental Health Primary Care in Prison

Adapted for Prisons and Young Offenders Institutions, with permission, from the *WHO Guide to Mental Health in Primary Care*

Publisher's note

Please note that throughout this book the symbol 💾 is used to denote additional resource material (see p. ix) that was originally provided on disks — this material is now available online only at http://www.rsmpress.co.uk/bkwho4.htm.

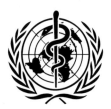

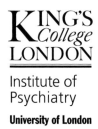

King's College London
Institute of Psychiatry
University of London

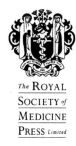

The ROYAL SOCIETY *of* MEDICINE PRESS *Limited*

World Health Organization Collaborating Centre for Research and Training for Mental Health

Mental Health Primary Care in Prison

A guide to mental ill health in adults and adolescents in prison and Young Offender Institutions

Edited by:
Jo Paton and Rachel Jenkins

The WHO Collaborating Centre for Research and Training for Mental Health gratefully acknowledges financial support from the NHS Forensic Mental Health R&D Programme who funded the development of the Guide, the Prison Service Health Task Force who funded the printing of copies for Prison Service staff and the Department of Health who funded the printing of copies for prison leads in Primary Care Trusts and the Health Services Research Directorate, Institute of Psychiatry, King's College London, for support in kind.

UK Edition

World Health Organization Collaborating centre for Research and Training for Mental Health

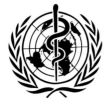

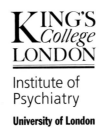

KING'S College LONDON

Institute of Psychiatry

University of London

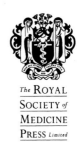

The ROYAL SOCIETY *of* MEDICINE PRESS *Limited*

Adapted with permission from the *WHO Guide to Mental Health in Primary Care*, published on behalf of the World Health Organization by the Royal Society of Medicine Press Limited, 1 Wimpole Street, London, W1G 0AE. ISBN 1 85315 451 2

© 2002 WHO Collaborating Centre for Research and Training for Mental Health, the Institute of Psychiatry, Kings College London

Reprinted 2009

This edition published by the Royal Society of Medicine Press Ltd, 1 Wimpole Street, London W1G 0AE, UK. Tel: +44 (0)20 7290 2921; Fax: +44 (0)20 7290 2929; Email: publishing@rsm.ac.uk; Website: www.rsmpress.co.uk

The authors have worked to ensure that all the information in the book containing drug dosages, schedules and routes of administration is accurate at the time of publication and consistent with the standards set by the World Health Organization (WHO) and the general medical community. As medical research and practice advance, however, therapeutic standards may change. For this reason, and because human and mechanical errors sometimes occur, we recommend that readers follow the advice of a physician who is directly involved in their care or the care of a member of their family.

Reference this book as: Paton J and Jenkins R (eds) *Mental Health Primary Care in Prison*. London, Royal Society of Medicine, 2002.

British Library Cataloguing in Publication Data
A catalogue record for this book is available from the British Library

ISBN: 978-1-85315-523-9

Distribution in Europe and Rest of World:
Marston Book Services Ltd
PO Box 269
Abingdon
Oxon OX14 4YN, UK
Tel: +44 (0)1235 465500
Fax: +44 (0)1235 465555
Email: direct.order@marston.co.uk

Distribution in Australia and New Zealand:
Elsevier Australia
30–52 Smidmore Street
Marrickville NSW 2204, Australia
Tel: +61 2 9517 8999
Fax: +61 2 9517 2249
Email: service@elsevier.com.au

Distribution in the USA and Canada:
Royal Society of Medicine Press Ltd
c/o BookMasters Inc
30 Amberwood Parkway
Ashland, OH 44805, USA
Tel: +1 800 247 6553/+1 800 266 5564
Fax: +1 419 281 6883
Email: orders@bookmasters.com

Typeset by Phoenix Photosetting, Chatham, Kent
Printed and bound by Marston Digital, Oxon, UK

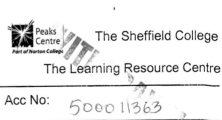

Contents

Prevalence of mental and personality disorders in prisoners

Managing specific mental disorders

Mental disorders in young people

Mental disorders in women who are mothers

Managing mental disorders — general skills

Mental Health Act and Common Law

For general nurses and healthcare officers

Comorbidity

Suicide and self-injury

Groups with particular needs

Dealing with difficult behaviours

Ethical issues   300

Voluntary and community agencies

Interactive summary cards — for discussion by the professional and patient together

Stress Reactions for Detainees

1. Arabic
2. Farsi
3. Tamil
4. Turkish

For other information leaflets for patients see Contents of Disks   ix

Contents of the disks*

* Please note that the following resource material is now available online only at http://www.rsmpress.co.uk/bkwho4.htm

Information for use with patients

Most patient leaflets are on the disk 🖫.
Stress and stress reactions — in Arabic, Tamil, Turkish and Farsee are in hard copy at the end of the book because they cannot be printed easily using a standard printer: (see the disk for English language and other language versions 🖫)

Note: the following are available on an accompanying disk only — for printing out as required or adapting and producing in another format 🖫.

DISK 1

For use with patients: information and self-help leaflets

Coping with anxiety
Coping with depression
Getting a good night's sleep.
Traumatic stress: learning to cope
Stress and stress reactions — for immigration detainees (in English, Albanian, French, Portuguese, Russian, Somali, Spanish and Lingala). Arabic, Tamil, Turkish and Farsee versions in hard copy in the book.
Harm minimisation advice — for drug users
Coping with the side-effects of medication
Manic depression (bipolar disorder)
Lithium toxicity
Domestic violence. Home Office leaflet
Just imprisoned? NACRO leaflet

DISK 2

Information for prison officers and other staff

Checklist for managers — keeping mental-health problems to a minimum on your unit
Working with a prisoner who has a severe mental illness
Coping with difficult behaviours (behavioural disorders)
Suicide prevention
Suicide – ideas for support
Immediate management on discovery of an incident of self-injury
Mothers and babies — psychological issues
Understanding self harm
Learning disability
For information on anxiety, depression, sleep problems and traumatic stress (for both patients and staff) see 'Information for use with patients'

Resources for use by professionals

Mental State Examination form
Nurse initial assessment form

Brief risk indicator check list
AUDIT questionnaire — screen for alcohol misuse
Severity of Alcohol Dependence Questionnaire (SADQ)
Severity of Opiate Dependence Questionnaire (SODQ)
Drug-use diary
Edinburgh Postnatal Depression Scale
Abbreviated mental test score — screen for dementia
Food and behaviour diary — use in bulimia nervosa
Early warning signs (of relapse) form — use in severe mental illness

Other information

Offending behaviour programmes — what are they?
Types of temporary release from prison
Template confidentiality agreement with a patient
Example of a communication-sharing proforma used in the Scottish Prison Service
Executive letter about sharing information and confidentiality
Connections between ICD 10 and ICD10–PHC

Foreword

The Prison Service in the UK has under its care one of the most vulnerable and mentally unhealthy populations anywhere. Epidemiological studies agree that the prevalence of serious personality disorders, drug and alcohol dependence, suicidal and self-harming behaviour, and all forms of mental illness (both psychotic and neurotic) is alarmingly high — much higher than in the general population. The most seriously ill prisoners need in-patient hospital treatment and should be moved to a more appropriate setting at the earliest opportunity. But for most, the aim is for care equivalent to that available in the community to be provided within the prison setting.

Prisons require mental-health services that are abundant and of high quality. The partnership between the Prison Service and the National Health Service (NHS) aims to introduce these and, over time, to achieve an equivalence of care. Even should this aim become a reality, however, prison healthcare staff (doctors, nurses, healthcare officers) will still need good mental-health skills and knowledge to carry out their primary-care role. This Guide is designed to support them in doing that in collaboration with others — which, in the prison context, may include chaplains, probation officers, psychologists and prison officers, as well as mental-health specialists. The Guide is an adaptation of a guide for primary-care professionals working in the community. As such, it provides a directly equivalent resource and supports the process of achieving equivalence. Although it is not intended to be viewed as Prison Service policy, it has been developed with the active participation of many people — especially prison healthcare staff and NHS mental-health workers. Thus, it is an example of partnership between the Prison Service and the NHS. I commend this Guide and hope it is a useful resource in the years to come.

Mr Martin Narey
Director General, HM Prison Service

Dame Lesley Southgate
President, Royal College of General Practitioners

Professor John Gunn
Chair Faculty of Forensic Psychiatry, Royal College of Psychiatrists

Dr Beverly Malone
General Secretary, Royal College of Nursing

Mr John Mahoney
Head Mental Health Branch, Department of Health

Professor Sian Griffiths OBE
President, Faculty of Public Health Medicine

Dr Felicity Harvey
Head Health Policy Unit, HM Prison Service

International foreword

Mental and behavioural disorders are a major public health problem. They are frequently found in all societies and cultures, are more disabling than many chronic and severe physical diseases, and do not easily get better or limit themselves without treatment. Yet, although simple, effective and acceptable treatments are available, they are not utilised sufficiently. There is a need to improve the identification and management of mental disorders at the primary-care level.

In all societies, the prevalence of mental disorders in prisons is high, but access to services to treat them is often very low. Prison healthcare staff face a particularly difficult job in providing good-quality care within this environment. In addition, especially in countries where the conditions that their prisoner-patients are held in are poor, prison healthcare staff face the practical and ethical challenge of advocating for change.

The World Health Organization (WHO) has developed a range of clinical tools to assist primary-care practitioners (even without psychiatric training) and community health workers (even without advanced medical training) to deal appropriately with the mentally ill people with whom they come into contact. The latest of these tools is this book. It is a further development of the primary-care version of the state-of-the-art classification of mental disorders for use in clinical practice and research (ICD-10 Chapter V, Primary Care Version). It is the first guide to mental health for primary-care workers in prisons throughout the world. Although developed initially in the UK, a future development will adapt it to form a 'generic' international version that can be adapted in turn to local needs in different countries.

The WHO would be pleased to see this primary-care prison version of the mental disorders classification become part of all medical and nursing curricula for prison practitioners, since it sets out precisely what a general practitioner should know in diagnosing and treating mental-health problems.

Dr Bedirhan Ustun
World Health Organization

Introduction

Up to 200,000 people flow in and out of prison each year, many staying only a few months. Prisoners have both an extremely high prevalence and complexity of mental disorders, often combining vulnerability factors (such as homelessness or a history of abuse) with multiple disorders and substance abuse. They include some of the most disturbed, disturbing and socially excluded members of our society. They present a tremendous challenge to those charged with their care.

As in the community, most care for mental-health problems in prisons is provided by doctors, nurses and others who are not mental-health specialists. This book has been written to help the generalists carry out the mental health aspects of their role and to help those in Primary Care Trusts and Health Authorities who are their partners. It assumes that generalist staff will have access to specialist advice and treatment and does not attempt to be a guide to secondary- or tertiary-level psychiatry. Nevertheless, it recognises that the role of primary care within prisons is a particularly demanding one.

What is in the Guide?

This book is divided into five main sections:

- Section 1 contains information about the diagnosis and management of specific mental disorders, in adults, young people and women who are mothers. The primary-care management of people with personality disorder forms part of this section.
- Section 2 focuses on core management issues and skills that are relevant to a number of mental disorders — for example, assessment, referral, resettlement, managing patients who are at risk of suicide and those who have self-harmed.
- Section 3 contains information about the mental-health needs of particular groups of prisoners (eg detained asylum seekers and those with Learning Disability). It also gives advice about how to respond to the needs of prisoners who have had particular life experiences (such as sexual assault, abuse in childhood or domestic violence) that put them at increased risk of developing a mental disorder.
- Section 4 looks at possible responses to prisoners who behave in ways that are difficult to manage, such as those who are aggressive or who refuse food. Many of these prisoners will not have a mental disorder, but mental disorder is a factor that must be considered.
- Section 5 considers important related matters, such as legal and ethical issues and working with voluntary organisations.

What is the role of primary-care staff in mental health in prison?

Prison healthcare staff and governors are now working in collaboration with Primary Care Trusts and Health Authorities to jointly provide health services of an equivalent standard to services outside prison. In mental health, this means working to meet the standards set out in the National Service Framework. Thus, the role of primary-care staff in prisons can be summarised as:

- Supporting the governor and other staff to develop an environment that supports mental health and well-being (Standard 1).

1

- Identifying prisoners with mental and substance abuse disorders (Standard 2).
- Managing prisoners with common mental disorders eg depression (Standard 2).
- Referring appropriately for assessment, advice or treatment (Standard 2).
- Working with diverse groups of patients from many different cultures.
- Providing information and guidance for those who provide regular and substantial care for prisoners with mental-health problems — in prison, often staff as well as family members (Standard 6).
- Contributing to the multidisciplinary work to prevent suicide (Standard 7).

The Guide provides information that supports all the activities listed above.
However, health services in prisons are currently in transition. This is reflected in the Guide which includes information:

- about psychological therapies that have been shown to be effective for certain conditions, even though some (perhaps many) prison healthcare staff may not have access to these at the moment
- for generalists to help them in roles that go beyond those expected of primary-care staff outside prisons — for example, advice for generalist nurses working with acutely mentally ill patients in an in-patient setting. We have not, however, included information about running an in-patient Mental Health Unit, even though there are, at the moment, still some such units in prisons that are managed on a day-to-day basis by generalist healthcare staff.

What sort of Guide is it?

Advice and information for individual clinicians

This Guide is aimed at individual clinicians — nurses, doctors or healthcare officers in the prison health centre. It is not a guide for managers about service development, nor should its advice and suggestions be viewed as mandatory Prison Service policy. However, as we recognise that services are at different stages of development in different establishments, we have included, where appropriate, brief suggestions for how services for particular conditions might be further developed.

Multidisciplinary — including disciplines other than health

The Guide emphasises throughout the contribution that staff from disciplines other than health can and do make to the management of patients with mental disorders. The management advice for each condition includes information and advice for healthcare workers to give, with patient permission, to prison officers and other staff involved in the care of the prisoner. The purpose is to ensure that the management of the patient supports rather than undermines recovery, whether the patient is on the wings, in education or workshops. The related information sheets for other staff are also aimed at that goal. Of course, on occasion patients may withhold permission for information to be shared. However, many will agree if asked, to at least certain information being shared in order that they may receive the most appropriate treatment on ordinary location.

This multidisciplinary approach is in line with standard 6 of the National Service Framework for Mental Health, which requires that healthcare workers provide information and guidance for those who provide regular and substantial care for people with mental-health problems. In the prison context, 'those who provide regular and substantial care' will vary. This is reflected in the wording used in the

Guide. In the Guide for primary-care workers in the community, we use the phrase 'Essential Information for the Patient and Family'. In this Guide, we have substituted the phrase 'Essential Information for the Patient and Primary Support Group'. The primary support group might include family members, residential staff, workshop supervisors, chaplains or others as appropriate. Informing and supporting those who care for the patient, whether family members or prison officers, has to be done with patient permission (except where there is a risk of serious harm to the patient or others).

Voluntary and community agencies

The Guide emphasises throughout the contribution that can be made by self-help, voluntary and community agencies. These agencies can help augment and support healthcare treatment, addressing the practical and social problems that cause or exacerbate illness and which healthcare professionals may be untrained or too busy to deal with. Poor access to such forms of community support makes the life of both prisoners and primary healthcare staff much more difficult.

Comorbidity

The Guide attempts, as much as is possible, to give advice about dealing with the huge comorbidity which is the norm in prisons. Clinicians need to be aware of comorbidity of all kinds — between behavioural disorders, mental disorders and substance misuse disorders. Dichotomous thinking has no place in prison healthcare, eg that an inmate is either ill or dependent on substances, or that an inmate is either genuinely mentally ill or personality-disordered. It is essential to think multi-axially — to be aware of physical, social and psychological dimensions and also to be aware of multimorbidity.

Broader prison environment

Although this book is aimed at the individual clinician, it is important to recognise the crucial importance of the broader institutional context within which healthcare takes place. Mental health, in particular, is affected by environmental factors such as access to exercise, fresh air, constructive activities, time out of cell and contact with family and friends outside the prison. It is important for healthcare staff to actively promote health, including mental health, at both the individual and establishment level. How this may be done is set out in the World Health Organization (Regional Office for Europe) Health in Prisons Project Consensus Statement on Mental Health Promotion in Prisons (www.hipp-europe.org). This highlights the following practical and effective ways of enhancing mental health and reducing mental ill-health:

- regular physical exercise
- access to the arts
- antibullying strategies
- depression prevention:
  - cognitive-behavioural therapies
  - spiritual reflection, eg religion, meditation or yoga
- skills acquisition
- utilising prisoners' resources, eg for peer support.

3

A Management Checklist of prison procedures which can promote mental health within the prison is contained in the Consensus Statement (it is provided on the disk 💾).

How the Guide was developed

The World Health Organisation (WHO) developed a state of the art classification of mental disorders for use in clinical practice and research: the 'Tenth Revision of the International Classification of Diseases (ICD-10). To extend this development into primary care, it published in 1996 the 'Diagnostic and Management Guidelines for Mental Disorders in Primary Care (ICD-10 Chapter V, Primary Care Version). These guidelines were developed by an international group of general practitioners, family physicians, mental-health workers, public health experts, social workers, psychiatrists and psychologists with a special interest in mental-health problems in primary care, using a consensus approach. The WHO guidelines were extensively field-tested in over 40 countries by 500 primary-care physicians to assess their relevance, ease of use and reliability.[1,2]

These guidelines and other WHO primary-care resources were adapted for the UK by a national editorial team, coordinated by the WHO Collaborating Centre at the Institute of Psychiatry. The evidence base was reviewed, information on psychological therapies added, the views of primary-care nurses, counsellors and patient groups were consulted and the text agreed, following several rounds of consensus and a conference. This UK version 'The WHO Guide to Mental Health in Primary Care' was published in 2000.

This subsequent version for prison staff was developed following a survey of prison healthcare staff about whether a version tailored specifically to their needs would be useful, and if so, what should be in it. This has resulted in a guide covering a considerably broader range of topics and including material specifically written for prison nurses and healthcare officers as well as doctors; and with information sheets for prison officers as well as patients. The process followed was a consensus one similar to that followed for the community primary-care guide. The number and range of different professions and groups involved was larger — a reflection of the complexity of the prison environment. A list of all involved can be found in the Acknowledgements section page 351.

Evidence on which the specific mental disorder guidelines are based

The diagnosis sections are based on the ICD-10 classification of mental disorders. ICD-10 is itself a consensus document, tested for reliability. The ICD-10 diagnostic criteria presented here have been tested among primary-care professionals to check for face validity and usefulness.

References supporting evidence have been given in line with the principles set out below.

Treatments (medication and psychotherapies)

The recommendations about medication are all in line with the *British National Formulary (BNF)*. Where recommendations about medication are unexceptional and in line with both the *BNF* and established practice for many years, references have not been given.

References have been reserved for key statements about medication and about particular psychotherapies or for statements about which evidence and opinion are divided. Where possible, evidence has been given from Cochrane reviews, high quality published reviews and meta-analyses or randomised controlled trials (RCTs). Discussions have been held with experts and authors of key areas of research. The evidence has been graded as follows:

Strength of the evidence supporting the recommendation

A = Good evidence to support

B = Fair evidence to support

C = Preliminary evidence to support

Quality of the evidence supporting the statement

I = Evidence obtained from a meta-analysis of trials, including one or more well-designed RCTs

II = Evidence obtained from one well-designed RCT

III = Evidence obtained from one or more controlled trials, without randomisation

IV = Evidence obtained from one or more uncontrolled studies

V = Opinions of respected authorities, based on clinical experience, descriptive studies or reports of expert committees. Occasionally the 'respected authorities' comprise collective patient experience. Where this is the case, it is clearly stated.

Where a qualitative review of previously published literature without a quantitative synthesis of the data is referenced, it has been graded in accordance with the type of studies the review includes. Where a reference is marked 'N', this means that the note contains additional information or a discussion of the issues, as well as the reference.

Information and advice

The sections on 'Essential information for the patient and primary support group' and 'Advice and support for the patient and primary support group' are primarily the result of consensus. There are no trials comparing the outcome of patients given different sorts of advice by their general practitioner. The advice itself is based on a mixture of evidence and consensus of professionals and patients.

Referral

The referral recommendations are based on consensus and will vary from place to place, depending on services available in all care sectors.

Please note that throughout this book the symbol 💾 is used to denote additional resource material that was originally provided on disks — this material is now available online only at http://www.rsmpress.co.uk/bkwho4.htm.

References

1 Goldberg D, Sharp D, Nanayakkara K. The field trial of the mental disorders section of ICD-10 designed for primary care (ICD-10-PHC) in England. *Family Practice* 1995; 12(4).

2 Ustun B, Goldberg D, Cooper J, Simon G, Sartorius N. A new classification of mental disorders based on management for use in primary care (ICD-10-PHC). *British Journal of General Practice* 1995; 45: 211–215.

Prevalence of mental and personality disorders in prisoners

Prevalence of psychiatric disorder and self-harm in sentenced prisoners

Study 1: Gunn J, Maden A, Swinton M. Treatment needs of prisoners with psychiatric disorders. *British Medical Journal* 1991; 303: 338–341
Aimed to identify those prisoners with psychiatric disorders needing treatment

Disorder or condition	Population	Prevalence of men (%)
Psychosis (including schizophrenia)	studied 1365 men at five local, 10 training and two open prisons	2.4
Affective psychosis		0.5
Neurotic disorders		5.2
Personality disorder		7.3
Alcohol dependence		8.6
Drug dependence		10.1

Study 2: Singleton N, Meltzer H, Gatward R, Coid J, Deasy D. *Psychiatric Morbidity of Prisoners in England and Wales.* London: ONS, 1998
Aimed to provide baseline information about the prevalence of psychiatric disorders in prisons in order to inform policy decisions about services

Disorder or condition	Population	Prevalence of men (%)	Prevalence of women (%)[b]
Any schizophrenic or delusional disorder	studied 1121 men and 584 women aged 16–64 years in a random, national sample of all prisons	6	13
Affective psychosis		1	2
Neurotic disorders		40	63
Personality disorder		64	50
Alcohol dependence[a]		30	19
Drug dependence (opiates, stimulants or both)		34	36
Suicide attempt in the last year		7	16
Self-harm (not a suicide attempt) in the current prison term		7	10

[a]Measured as AUDIT ≥ 30.
[b]Prevalence of schizophrenic or delusional disorders, affective psychosis and personality disorder was made from a combined sentenced and remand female sample.

Prevalence of psychiatric disorder and self-harm in remand prisoners

Study 1: Maden A, Taylor CJA, Brooke D, Gunn J. *Mental Disorders in Remand Prisoners.* London: Department of Forensic Psychiatry, Institute of Psychiatry, 1995

Disorder or condition	Population	Prevalence of men and women combined (%)
Schizophrenia, psychosis or a delusional disorder	studied 544 men, 206 young offenders and 245 women in a random national sample	5.5
Neurotic disorder		19.1
Personality disorder		11.0
Substance misuse		39.0

Study 2: Singleton N, Meltzer H, Gatward R, Coid J, Deasy D. *Psychiatric Morbidity of Prisoners in England and Wales.* London: ONS, 1998

Disorder or condition	Population	Prevalence of men (%)	Prevalence of women (%)[b]
Any schizophrenic or delusional disorder	studied 1250 men and 187 women aged 16–64 years in a random national sample of all prisons	9	13
Affective psychosis		2	2
Neurotic disorder		59	76
Personality disorder		78	50
Alcohol dependence[a]		30	20
Drug dependence (opiates, stimulants or both)		43	52
Suicide attempt in the last year		15	27
Self-harm (not a suicide attempt) in the current prison term		5	9

[a]: Measured as AUDIT ≥ 30.
[b]: Prevalence of schizophrenic or delusional disorders, affective psychosis and personality disorder was made from a combined sentenced and remand female sample.

Prevalence of selected risk factors for mental disorder: Singleton et al. 1998

Experience	Men sentenced (%)	Men remand (%)	Women sentenced (%)	Women remand (%)
In Local Authority care as child	26	33	25	29
Victim of violence in the home at any time in the past	25	28	48	51
Victim of sexual abuse at any time in the past	8	9	31	34

Prevalence of mental disorders among community and delinquent samples of adolescents

Disorder or condition	Community samples (%)	Delinquent samples (%)
Conduct disorder	2–10	41–90
Attention deficit disorders	2–10	19–46
Substance abuse and dependence	2–5	25–50
Mental retardation	1–3	7–15
Learning and academic disabilities	2–10	17–53
Mood disorders	2–8	19–78
Anxiety disorders	3–13	6–41
Post-traumatic stress disorders	1–3	32
Psychosis and autism	0.2–2	1–6
Any disorder present	18–22	80

Source: Kazdin AE. Adolescent development, mental disorders and decision making of delinquent youths. In Grisso T, Schwartz RG (eds), *Youth on Trial: A Developmental Perspective on Juvenile Justice*. Chicago: University of Chicago Press, 2000, vol. 2, pp. 33–64.
Evidence is summarised from a range of studies. The levels of disorders in adolescents held in detention centres or prisons tend to be towards the higher end of the range.

Acute psychotic disorders — F23

Includes acute schizophrenia-like psychosis, acute delusional psychosis, and other acute and transient psychotic disorders

Presenting complaints

Patients may experience:

- hallucinations, eg hearing voices when no one is around
- strange beliefs or fears
- apprehension, confusion
- perceptual disturbances
- aggression, frequent adjudications
- self-harm
- food refusal (they may suspect that food is being poisoned).

Staff or relatives may ask for help with behaviour changes that cannot be explained, including strange or frightening behaviour, eg withdrawal, suspiciousness and threats.

A 'first-onset psychosis' may present at first as persistent changes in functioning, behaviour or personality (eg withdrawal), but without florid psychotic symptoms.[N1] The first episode of psychosis most commonly occurs in the late teens and early 20s (see **First-onset psychosis**, page 131).

Diagnostic features

Recent onset of:

- hallucinations: false or imagined perceptions, eg hearing voices when no one is around
- delusions: firmly held ideas that are false and not shared by others in the patient's social, cultural or ethnic group, eg patients believe they are being poisoned by neighbours, receiving messages from the television or being looked at by others in some special way
- disorganised or strange speech
- agitation or bizarre behaviour
- extreme and labile emotional states.

Differential diagnosis

- Physical disorders that can cause psychotic symptoms include:
  — drug-induced psychosis and
  — alcoholic hallucinosis

It is not possible to tell from the symptoms alone whether psychiatric symptoms are substance-induced, whether the patient has a psychotic disorder, or both a substance misuse and a psychotic disorder. Check their psychiatric history, keep an open mind (eg in a teenager or young adult, a 'substance-induced psychosis' might be the early stages of schizophrenia) and chart symptoms over time (see **Comorbidity**, page 191). Also:

— infectious or febrile illness and

— epilepsy.

- See **Delirium—F05** for other potential causes (page 41).
- **Chronic psychotic disorders — F20#**: if psychotic symptoms are recurrent or chronic.
- **Bipolar disorder — F31**: if the symptoms of mania, eg elevated mood, racing speech or thoughts, exaggerated self-worth, are prominent.
- **Depression** (depressive psychosis) — **F32#**, if depressive delusions are prominent.

Essential information for the patient and primary support group

- Agitation and strange behaviour can be symptoms of a mental illness.
- Acute episodes often have a good prognosis,[N2] but the long-term course of the illness is difficult to predict from an acute episode.
- Advise the patient and members of the primary support group about the importance of medication, how it works and the possible side-effects.
- Continued treatment may be needed for several months after symptoms resolve.

If the patient requires treatment under the Mental Health Act 1983, advise the family, if possible, about the related legal issues (see Use of the Mental Health Act**, page 163).**

Advice and support of the patient and primary support group

- Assess the risks and consider whether a move to the healthcare centre (or establishment with a healthcare centre) is indicated. If there is a significant risk of suicide, violence or neglect, close observation in a secure place or transfer to an NHS hospital may be required. Consider the use of the Mental Health Act for transfer especially, but not solely, if the patient refuses treatment.
- Order a urine drug screen for medical (not disciplinary) purposes (see **Comorbidity**, page 191).
- If it is decided that it is safe for the patient to live on an ordinary location, seek patient permission to involve the residential manager and other relevant staff (eg workshop manager, teacher, chaplain) in implementing a management plan, including the location, activities, the early response to signs of relapse and the monitoring of medication. Discuss the following:
  — Ensure the safety of the patient and those caring for him/her:
    — Staff, listeners/buddies, family or friends should be available for the patient if possible.
    — Ensure that the patient's basic needs (eg food, drink, accommodation) are met.
  — Minimise stress and stimulation, eg reducing noise, shouting, bullying, teasing.
  — Do not argue with psychotic thinking (you may disagree with the patient's beliefs, but do not try to argue that they are wrong).
  — Avoid confrontation or criticism, unless it is necessary to prevent harmful or disruptive behaviour.[N3] Respond gently and with reassurance to slow responses to orders (eg slowness in going into cell). Use of control and restraint should be a last resort.
  — Encourage resumption of normal activities after symptoms improve.

— The information sheet on managing difficult behaviour (psychosis) on the disk may be helpful to staff 💾.

- Especially if the patient becomes depressed, consider options for support, education and reassurance about their psychotic illness, including possible relapse and their future life chances. Mental-health staff may be able to provide individual counselling, goal planning and monitoring of early warning signs of relapse.

Referral and throughcare

Referral to the secondary mental-health services should be made under the following conditions:

- as an emergency, if the risk of suicide, violence or neglect is considered significant
- urgently for **all** first episodes to confirm the diagnosis and to arrange care planning and the appointment of a key-worker. Specific interventions for people experiencing their first episode of psychosis, including specific psycho-education of the patient and primary support group, should be developed[5]
- for **all** relapses, to review the effectiveness of the care plan, unless there is an established previous response to treatment and it is safe to manage the patient in the establishment
- if there is non-compliance with treatment, problematic side-effects, failure of community treatment or concerns about comorbid drug and alcohol misuse.

Particularly on relapse, referral may be to the community mental-health team or to a member of it, such as a community psychiatric nurse (CPN), as well as to a psychiatrist (for more details, see **Managing the interface with the NHS and other agencies**, page 149).

If there is fever, altered consciousness, rigidity and/or labile blood pressure, stop the antipsychotic medication and refer immediately to the on-call physician for investigation of neuroleptic malignant syndrome.

If release is planned, work cooperatively with probation or the throughcare planning officers to ensure that appointments with a general practitioner and specialist in mental healthcare are arranged and that housing, money for food, clothes and heating are arranged.

If release is not planned, inform the local mental-health services that the patient may present to A&E in the area and advise them to look out for him/her (for more information on referral and throughcare, see **Managing the interface with the NHS and other agencies**, page 149).

Medication

- Antipsychotic medication can reduce psychotic symptoms over 10–14 days. Where access to a specialist is speedy and symptoms relatively mild, especially for a first referral, the specialist may prefer to see the patient unmedicated.
- Examples of drugs you may wish to use before the patient sees a specialist include an atypical antipsychotic[N6] (eg olanzapine, 5–10 mg day^{-1}, or risperidone, 4–6 mg day^{-1}) or a typical drug (eg haloperidol, 1.5–4 mg up to three times per day) (see *BNF*, Section 4.2.1). Patients experiencing a first episode of psychosis require lower doses of medication and may benefit from an atypical drug.[N7] In a case of relapse where the patient has previously responded to a drug, restart that drug. The dose should be the lowest possible for the relief of symptoms.[8]

- Anti-anxiety medication may also be used for the short term in conjunction with neuroleptics to control acute agitation and disturbance (see *BNF*, Section 4.1.2). (Examples include diazepam, 5–10 mg up to four times per day, or lorazepam, 1–2 mg up to four times per day.) If required, diazepam can be given rectally or lorazepam IM (though this must be kept refrigerated).
- Monitor compliance (eg call up for a review if more than two doses are missed) and check that the patient is not being pressured or bullied into giving the medication to someone else.
- Continue antipsychotic medication for at least 6 months after symptoms resolve.[9] Close supervision is usually needed to encourage patient agreement.
- Be alert to the risk of comorbid use of street drugs (eg opiates, cannabis, benzodiazepines).
- Monitor for side-effects of the medication:
  — Acute dystonias or spasms may be managed with oral or injectable anti-Parkinsonian drugs (see *BNF*, Section 4.9.2) (eg procyclidine, 5 mg three times per day, or orphenadrine, 50 mg three times per day).
  — Parkinsonian symptoms (eg tremor, akinesia) may be managed with oral anti-Parkinsonian drugs (see *BNF*, Section 4.9.2) (eg procyclidine, 5 mg three times per day, or orphenadrine, 50 mg three times per day).
  — Withdrawal of anti-Parkinsonian drugs should be attempted after 2–3 months without symptoms as these drugs are liable to misuse and may impair memory.
  — Akathisia (severe motor restlessness) may be managed with dosage reduction or β-blockers (eg propranolol, 30–80 mg day^{-1}) (see *BNF*, Section 2.4). Switching to an atypical antipsychotic (eg olanzapine or quetiapine) may help.
  — Other side-effects, eg weight gain and sexual dysfunction.

For more detail on antipsychotic drugs and their differing side-effect profiles, see *Maudsley Prescribing Guidelines*[10]. The 2001 edition (ISBN 1-853-17963-9) is available from: ITPS. Tel: 01264 332424.

Resources for patients and primary support groups

Manic Depression Fellowship: 020 7793 2600
(Support and information for people with manic depression and their families and friends)

MIND Infoline: 08457 660163 (outside Greater London): 020 8522 1728 (Greater London)
(National telephone information service on mental health issues)

National Schizophrenia Fellowship: 020 8974 6814 (adviceline: Monday–Friday, 10:30 am–3 pm)
(Advice and information for people suffering from schizophrenia, and their families and carers)

SANEline: 08457 678000 (7 nights a week, 12 pm–2 am)
(National helpline for mental-health information and support to anyone coping with mental illness)

Resource leaflets:
Coping with the Side-effects of Medication
Working with a prisoner who has a severe mental illness

Adjustment disorder — F43.2

Including acute stress reaction

Presenting complaints

- Patients feel overwhelmed or unable to cope.
- There may be stress-related physical symptoms such as insomnia, headache, abdominal pain, chest pain and palpitations.
- Patients may report symptoms of acute anxiety or depression.
- Patients may seek drugs to help them deal with their feelings.
- Alcohol use may increase.

Diagnostic features

- Acute reaction to a recent stressful or traumatic event.
- Extreme distress resulting from a recent event, or preoccupation with the event.
- Symptoms may be primarily somatic.
- Other symptoms may include:
  — low or sad mood
  — anxiety
  — worry
  — feeling unable to cope.

An acute reaction usually lasts from a few days to several weeks.

Differential diagnosis

Acute symptoms may persist or evolve over time. If significant symptoms persist for more than 1 month, consider an alternative diagnosis.

- If significant symptoms of depression persist, see **Depression — F32#** (page 47).
- If significant symptoms of anxiety persist, see **Generalised anxiety — F41.1** (page 64).
- If significant symptoms of both depression and anxiety persist, see **Chronic mixed anxiety and depression — F41.2** (page 33).
- If stress-related somatic symptoms persist, see **Unexplained somatic complaints — F45** (page 94).
- If symptoms are due to a loss, see **Bereavement — Z63** (page 23).
- If anxiety is long-lasting and focused on memories of a previous traumatic event, see **Post-traumatic stress disorder — F43.1** (page 82).
- If dissociative symptoms (sudden onset of unusual or dramatic somatic symptoms) are present, see **Dissociative (conversion) disorder — F44** (page 15).

Essential information for the patient and primary support group

- Stressful events often have mental and physical effects. The acute state is a natural reaction to events.
- Adjustment to imprisonment is commonly stressful (especially if the patient is in prison for the first time, has a high public profile or is a sexual offender) with understandable concerns about their family and the case.

- Stress-related symptoms usually last only a few days or weeks.
- All people are affected by their environment. Symptoms are likely to be fewer and less persistent if the environment can be improved (eg a reduction in the fear of bullying/assault, more time out of the cell, contact with family, access to work and opportunities to be creative).

Advice and support of the patient and primary support group[N11]

- Review and reinforce the positive steps the patient has taken to deal with the stress.
- Identify the steps the patient can take to modify the situation that produced the stress. There is a problem-solving sheet on the disk 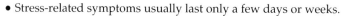. If the situation is within the prison (eg bullying), support the patient in dealing with it (eg discuss the problem with residential manager, with patient permission).
- If the situation cannot be changed, discuss coping strategies. Explore whether the patient is using destructive strategies (eg drugs, aggression, self-injury). Encourage exercise, art, reading, work and contact with others. Consider acting as the patient's advocate to increase access to, for example, suitable work placements that involve contact with supportive people, art materials and exercise.
- If the stressor is recent imprisonment itself, ensure the patient has copy of the *Prisoners' Information Book*. See the disk for a copy of the *Just Imprisoned?* leaflet and the **Resource directory** (page 316) for agencies that offer support. If the patient cannot read, advise him/her to approach the personal officer or listener/buddy with questions.
- Identify relatives, friends, staff and helplines able to offer support, eg listener/buddy, Samaritans, chaplain and personal officer.
- Short-term rest and relief from stress may help the patient. Encourage a return to usual activities within a few weeks.
- Encourage the patient to acknowledge the personal significance of the stressful event.
- Offering a further consultation with a member of the primary-care team to see how the situation develops can be valuable in helping the patient through the episode.

Medication

Most acute stress reactions will resolve without the use of medication. Skilled general practitioner advice and reassurance is as effective as benzodiazepines.[N12] However, if severe anxiety symptoms occur, consider using anti-anxiety drugs for up to 3 days. If the patient has severe insomnia, use hypnotic drugs for up to 3 days. Doses should be as low as possible (see *BNF*, Sections 4.1.1 and 4.1.2).

Referral

See **Referral criteria for non-urgent referral** (page 152). It is usually self-limiting. Routine referral to the secondary mental-health services is advised if:

- symptoms persist and general referral criteria are met and
- you are unsure of the diagnosis.

Consider recommending a counsellor, if available, or voluntary/non-statutory counselling[13] services, if available, in all other cases where symptoms persist.

Resources for patients and primary support groups

Childline: 0800 1111 (24-hour freephone helpline)
(For children and young people in trouble or danger)

Citizens Advice Bureau (see the local telephone directory)
(Free advice and information on Social Security benefits, housing, family and
personal matters, money advice, and other issues)

Relate: 01788 573241
(Counselling and psychosexual therapy for adults with relationship difficulties.
For agencies that provide opportunities for creative activity in prisons, see the
Resource directory, page 316)

Samaritans Helpline: 08457 909090 (24 hours, 7 days per week)
(Support by listening for those feeling lonely, despairing or suicidal)

Victim Support: 0845 3030900 (supportline: Monday–Friday, 9 am–9 pm;
Saturday and Sunday, 9 am–7 pm; Bank Holidays, 9 am–5 pm)
(Emotional and practical support for victims of crime)

UK Register of Counsellors: 08704 435232
(Provides the names and addresses of BACP-accredited counsellors)

Resource leaflets:
Reactions to Traumatic Stress: What To Expect
Getting a Good Night's Sleep

Alcohol misuse — F10

Presenting complaints

Patients may present with:

- a depressed mood
- nervousness
- insomnia
- physical complications of alcohol use (eg ulcer, gastritis, liver disease, hypertension)
- accidents or injuries due to alcohol use
- aggression, frequent adjudications
- poor memory or concentration
- evidence of self-neglect (eg poor hygiene)
- failed treatment for depression.

There may also be:

- legal and social problems due to alcohol use, eg drink-drive charges, driving when previously disqualified because of alcohol use, assault, marital problems, domestic violence, child abuse or neglect, and
- signs of alcohol withdrawal, eg sweating, tremors, retching, hallucinations, seizures.

Patients may sometimes deny or be unaware of alcohol problems. Imprisonment may bring their first experience of withdrawal. Staff may request help before the patient does. Problems may also be identified during routine reception screening or 2–3 days following reception.

Diagnostic features

- Harmful alcohol use:
  — heavy alcohol use (eg > 28 units per week for men, > 21 units per week for women)
  — overuse of alcohol has caused physical harm (eg liver disease, gastrointestinal bleeding), psychological harm (eg depression or anxiety due to alcohol) or has led to **harmful legal consequences** (eg imprisonment).
- Alcohol dependence: present when three or more of the following are present:
  — A strong desire or compulsion to use alcohol.
  — Difficulty controlling alcohol use.
  — Withdrawal symptoms (eg agitation, tremors, sweating, nausea, headache) even when drinking is ceased.
  — Tolerance, eg drinks large amounts of alcohol without appearing intoxicated.
  — Continued alcohol use despite harmful consequences.

Blood tests such as γ-glutamyl transferase (GGT) and mean corpuscular volume (MCV) can help identify heavy drinkers. Administering the AUDIT questionnaire may also help diagnosis. If AUDIT > 8, use of the Severity of Alcohol Dependence Questionnaire (SADQ) can help identify the severity of dependence. Copies of the AUDIT and SADQ are on the disk 💾.

Differential diagnosis

Symptoms of anxiety or depression may occur with heavy alcohol use. Alcohol use can also mask other disorders, eg social phobia and generalised anxiety disorder. Assess and manage symptoms of depression or anxiety if the symptoms continue after a period of abstinence (see **Depression — F32#** or **Anxiety — F41.1**, pages 47 and 33).

Drug misuse may also coexist with these conditions.

Essential information for the patient and primary support group

- Alcohol dependence is an illness with serious consequences.
- Ceasing or reducing alcohol use will bring mental and physical benefits.
- Drinking during pregnancy may harm the baby.
- For most patients with alcohol dependence, the physical complications of alcohol abuse or a psychiatric disorder, abstinence from alcohol is the preferred goal.[14] Sometimes, abstinence is also necessary for social crises, to regain control over drinking or because of failed attempts at reducing drinking. Because abrupt abstinence occurs upon reception into prison and causes withdrawal symptoms in people dependent upon alcohol, detoxification under medical supervision in a Detoxification Unit is necessary.
- In some cases of harmful alcohol use without dependence or where the patient is unwilling to quit, controlled or reduced drinking is a reasonable goal but may only be pursued after release.
- Relapses are common. Controlling or ceasing drinking often requires several attempts. The outcome depends on many factors, including the motivation and confidence of the patient, the offending behaviour, polydrug use, their mood or other mental disorder.

Advice and support to the patient and primary support group[15]

For all patients:
- Discuss the benefits and costs of drinking (including the links between drinking and offending) from the patient's perspective.
- Give feedback information about the health risks, including the results of GGT and MCV.
- Emphasise the personal responsibility for change.
- Give clear advice to change.
- Assess and manage any physical health problems and nutritional deficiencies (eg vitamin B, thiamine).
- Consider the options for problem-solving or targeted counselling to deal with life problems related to alcohol use.
- If there is no evidence of physical harm due to drinking or if the patient is unwilling to quit, a controlled drinking programme is a reasonable goal if the patient is about to be released:
  — Negotiate a clear goal for decreased use (eg no more than a certain number of drinks per day, with a certain number of alcohol-free days per week).
  — Discuss strategies to avoid or cope with high-risk situations (eg release, social situations and stressful events).
  — Introduce self-monitoring procedures (eg a drinking diary) and a safer drinking behaviour (eg time restrictions, deceleration of drinking).

For patients with physical illness and/or dependency or failed attempts at controlled drinking, an abstinence programme is indicated.

For patients willing to stop now:

- Discuss the symptoms, risks of detoxification and management of alcohol withdrawal (especially if they have no previous experience of detoxification).
- Discuss the strategies to avoid or cope with high-risk situations (eg release, social situations and stressful events).
- Make specific plans to avoid drinking (eg ways to face stressful events without alcohol, ways to respond to friends who still drink).
- Help patients to identify family members or friends who will support ceasing alcohol use.
- Consider options for support after withdrawal.

For patients not willing to stop or reduce now and who are about to be released, a harm-reduction programme is indicated:

- Do not reject or blame.
- Clearly point out the medical, legal and social problems caused by alcohol.
- Consider thiamine preparations.
- Make a future appointment with the general practitioner/primary care to reassess their health and alcohol use.

For patients who do not succeed or who relapse or transfer to using a different drug while in prison:

- Identify and give credit for any success.
- Discuss the situations that led to relapse.
- Return to earlier steps above.

Self-help organisations (eg Alcoholics Anonymous), voluntary and non-statutory agencies are often helpful.[16]

Medication

- In prison, it is often difficult to confirm a patient's history of previous substance use. Therefore, detoxification should always be undertaken in a supervised in-patient setting (see **Prison Service Order 3550: Clinical Services for Substance Misusers**).
- For patients with mild withdrawal symptoms, frequent monitoring, support, reassurance, adequate hydration and nutrition are sufficient treatment without medication.[17]
- Patients with a moderate withdrawal syndrome require benzodiazepines in addition to frequent monitoring, support, reassurance, adequate hydration and nutrition. Detoxification should only be undertaken by practitioners with appropriate training and supervision.
- Patients at risk of a complicated withdrawal syndrome (eg with a history of fits or delirium tremens, a history of very heavy use and high tolerance, significant polydrug use, severe comorbid medical or psychiatric disorder) or are a significant suicide risk may require a transfer to an NHS hospital.
- Chlordiazepoxide (Librium), 10 mg, is recommended. The initial dose should be titrated against withdrawal symptoms, within a range of 5–40 mg four times per day. (See *BNF* section 4.10.) This requires close, skilled supervision.

- The following regimen is commonly used, although the dose level and length of treatment will depend on the severity of alcohol dependence and individual patient factors (eg weight, sex, liver function):
  — Days 1 and 2:   20–30 mg QDS
  — Days 3 and 4:   15 mg QDS
  — Day 5:   10 mg QDS
  — Day 6:   10 mg BD
  — Day 7:   10 mg nocte
- Chlormethiazole is not recommended for craving or detoxification under any circumstances.[18]
- Dispensing should be dose by dose and supervised to prevent the risk of misuse or overdose.
- Thiamine (150 mg day^{-1} in divided doses) should be given orally for 1 month.[19] As oral thiamine is poorly absorbed, transfer the patient immediately to A&E for parenteral supplementation if any **one** of the following is present: ataxia, confusion, memory disturbance, delirium tremens, hypothermia and hypotension, opthalmoplegia, or unconsciousness. These may indicate the onset of Wernicke's encephalopathy.
- Daily observation is essential in the first few days, then it is advisable thereafter to adjust the dose of the medication, to check for serious withdrawal symptoms and to maintain support.
- Anxiety and depression often co-occur with alcohol misuse. The patient may have been using alcohol to self-medicate. If symptoms of anxiety or depression increase or remain after an abstinence of more than 1 month, see **Depression — F32#** or **Generalised anxiety — F41.1** (pages 47 and 64). Selective serotonin re-uptake inhibitor (SSRI) antidepressants are preferred to tricyclics (TCAs) because of the risk of tricyclic–alcohol interactions (fluoxetine, paroxetine and citalopram do not interact with alcohol) (see *BNF*, Section 4.3.3). For anxiety, benzodiazepines should be avoided because of their high potential for abuse[20] (see *BNF*, Section 4.1.2).

For further information on alcohol detoxification, see *Drug Misuse and Dependence — Guidelines on Clinical Management*.[21]

For information on brief interventions for people whose drinking behaviour puts them at risk of becoming dependent, see *Brief Intervention Guidelines*.[22]

Referral

Consider referral:

- to the Detoxification Unit if the patient is dependent upon alcohol
- to involve the in-house or secondary mental-health services in addition if the patient has an associated major psychiatric disorder, or if the symptoms of mental illness persist after detoxification and abstinence
- for counselling targeted at problems associated with/triggering drinking and relapse prevention work, if available.

Before release:

- If possible, arrange for on-going rehabilitation support in the community. If it is available, specific social skills training[N23] (which aims to improve, for example, relationship skills and assertiveness) and community-based treatment packages[N24] (which provide help with finding a job and social life) both may be effective in reducing drinking.

- Refer patients with a mental illness who are misusing alcohol and who express some motivation to reduce their use to a specialist NHS alcohol service, a mental-health service or both. Ideally, care will be provided by a team skilled in treating both mental illness and substance abuse.[25] If either the psychiatric or substance misuse problem appears to predominate, refer initially to that service. Make the rationale clear in the letter/fax. If both types of disorder are of equal significance, then negotiate with both agencies about the preferred initial referral route. It may be that the individual will require support and input by both agencies. Some agencies can provide services jointly. Liaise with the service to ensure continued prescription of psychotropic medication, if appropriate.
- Stress to the patient that relapses are to be expected, are not signs of failure and will not mean a loss of your support and respect.

See **Comorbidity** (page 191).

Resources for patients and primary support groups

Al-Anon Family Groups UK and Eire: 020 7403 0888 (helpline: Monday–Friday, 10 am–10 pm); 0141 2217356
(Support for families and friends of alcoholics whether still drinking or not). Also:

Alateen: for young people aged 12–20 affected by others' drinking

Alcoholics Anonymous: 08457 697555 (24-hour helpline)
(Helpline refers to telephone support numbers and self-help groups across the UK, for men and women trying to achieve and maintain sobriety)

Drinkline: 0800 917 8282 (freephone national alcohol helpline: Monday–Friday, 9 am–11 pm; Saturday and Sunday, 6 pm–11 pm)

The following organisations provide leaflets to support brief interventions for people at risk of becoming dependent on alcohol:

Alcohol Focus Scotland: 0141 5726700

Health Education Board for Scotland: 0131 536 5500

Health Promotion England: 020 7725 9030

Northern Ireland Community Addiction Service: 02890 664 434

Secular Organisations for Sobriety (SOS): 020 8698 9332
(Non-religious self-help group)

Bereavement — Z63

Presenting complaints

An acute grief reaction is a normal, understandable reaction to loss. The patient:
- feels overwhelmed by loss
- is preoccupied with the lost loved one and
- may present with somatic symptoms following loss.

Grief may be experienced on the loss of a loved one and also with other significant losses (eg the loss of a child taken into care, a job, lifestyle or limb, the breakdown of a relationship). It may precipitate or exacerbate other psychiatric conditions and may be complicated, delayed or incomplete, leading to seemingly unrelated problems years after the loss.

Diagnostic features

Normal grief includes preoccupation with the loss of the loved one. However, this may be accompanied by symptoms resembling depression, such as:
- low or sad mood
- disturbed sleep
- loss of interest
- guilt or self-criticism
- restlessness
- guilt about actions not taken by the person before the death of the loved one
- seeing the deceased person or hearing their voice
- thoughts of joining the deceased.

The patient may:
- withdraw from their usual activities and social contacts
- find it difficult to think of the future and
- increase their use of drugs.

Differential diagnosis

Depression — F32#. Bereavement is a process. A helpful model is to think of four tasks to be completed by the bereaved person:
- accepting the reality of the loss — the patient may feel numb
- experiencing the pain of grief
- adapting to the world without the deceased and
- 'letting go' of the deceased and moving on.

Consider depression if:
- the person becomes stuck at any point in the process
- a full picture of depression is still present 2 months after the loss or
- there are signs that the grief is becoming abnormal (severe depressive symptoms of retardation, guilt, feelings of worthlessness, hopelessness or suicidal ideation of a severity or duration that significantly interferes with daily living).

There is a higher risk of an abnormal grief reaction under the following circumstances: where the bereaved person is socially isolated or has a history of depression or anxiety; where the bereaved killed the dead person or their relationship was ambivalent in other ways; where the dead person was a child; and where the death was violent, occurred by suicide or occurred suddenly in traumatic circumstances (especially if the body is not present).

Essential information for the patient and primary support group

- Important losses are often followed by intense sadness, crying, anger, disbelief, anxiety, guilt or irritability.
- Bereavement typically includes a preoccupation with the deceased (including hearing or seeing the person).
- A desire to discuss the loss is normal.
- Inform patients, especially those at greater risk of developing an abnormal grief reaction, of local agencies, such as Cruse Bereavement Care, which offer bereavement counselling and aim to help guide people through their normal grief.[26]
- Inform patients who have lost or fear losing a child to the care system of agencies that offer advice and support (see **Resources** below). Inform them that they can still be part of their children's lives, eg by exchanging news in letters or talking face to face. If children are in care, an application can be made for children to visit in private conditions or, if this is not desired, application can be made to visit the children at their home. Visiting orders need not be surrendered for this purpose.

Advice and support to the patient and primary support group

- Enable the bereaved person to talk about the deceased and the circumstances of the death or other loss.
- Encourage the free expression of feelings about the loss (including feelings of sadness, guilt or anger).
- Offer reassurance that recovery will take time. Some reduction in burdens (eg work) may be necessary.
- Explain that intense grieving will fade slowly over several months, but that reminders of the loss may continue to provoke feelings of loss and sadness.
- Take into account the cultural context of the loss.[27]

Medication

Avoid medication if possible. If the grief reaction becomes abnormal (see **Differential diagnosis** above), see **Depression — F32#**, page 47, for advice on the use of antidepressants. Disturbed sleep is to be expected. If severe insomnia occurs, the short-term use of hypnotic drugs may be helpful, but their use should be limited to 2 weeks (see *BNF*, Section 4.1.1). Avoid the use of anxiolytics.

Referral

Recommend the chaplain and voluntary organisations, eg CRUSE, for support through the normal grieving process. Probation officers may provide practical advice and support for women whose children have been taken into care.

Referral to the secondary mental-health services is advised:
- if the patient is severely depressed or showing psychotic features (see the relevant disorder) and

- non-urgently, if the symptoms have not resolved by 1 year despite bereavement counselling.

Consider an in-house counsellor, if available, or non-statutory bereavement counsellors[13] in all other cases where symptoms persist.

Refer bereaved people who have learning disabilities to the specialist disability team or a specialist learning disability counsellor.

Resources for patients and primary support groups

After Adoption Helpline: 08456 010168 (Monday, Wednesday and Thursday, 10 am–12 pm, 2 pm–4 pm; Tuesday, 10 am–12 pm, 2 pm–7 pm; 0161 839 4932 (office); E-mail: aadoption@aol.com (office)
12–14 Chapel Street, Manchester M3 7NN
(For people whose children have been adopted or may be adopted, those who have lost a child to adoption and are now caring for another child, and those who have been adopted themselves in the North West, Yorkshire and Wales. Provides information, advice, support, individual and group counselling by person, telephone and letter; also books and tapes, and training for professionals. Experience of providing counselling to a prison under contract)

Compassionate Friends Helpline: 0117 953 9639 (Monday–Sunday, 9:30 am–10:30 pm)
(Befriending and support for bereaved parents, grandparents and siblings)

Cruse Bereavement Care Helpline: 08701 67 1677
(One-to-one bereavement counselling; self-referral preferred)

Family Rights Group: 0800 731 1696 (freephone adviceline: Monday–Friday, 1.30–3.30 pm); 0800 783 0697 (freephone adviceline in Turkish: Tuesday, 10 am–12 pm); 020 7923 2628 (office)
The Print House, 18 Ashwin Street, London E8 3DL. E-mail: office@frg.u-net.com
(Callers speak in confidence to a social worker or solicitor who offers advice and written information free of charge. Offers advice, advocacy and publications to families whose children are involved with social services. Advice sheets, some in Turkish, Somali, Punjabi, Urdu and Bengali, include ones on reuniting children with their families, assistance for young people leaving care, child protection and many more. *Adoption: Guide for Birth Families.* £2.50 plus postage and packing)

Foundation for the Study of Infant Deaths (FSID): 020 7233 2090 (24-hour helpline)

Papyrus: 01706 214449
Rosendale GH, Union Road, Rawtenstall, Rosendale BB4 6NE
(Refers to support groups for parents of young people who have committed suicide)

Still Birth and Neonatal Death Society (SANDS): 020 7436 5881
(Monday–Wednesday, Friday, 10 am–3 pm)
(Information, emotional and physical support to parents who have lost a baby)

Talk Adoption: 0808 808 1234 (national helpline: Monday–Friday, 3 pm–9 pm); (confidential e-mail: helpline@talkadoption.org.uk)
(For young people under 25 who have children who have been or may be adopted or have been adopted themselves)

Bipolar disorder — F31

Presenting complaints

Patients may have a period of depression, mania or excitement, with the pattern described below. Referral may be made by others due to lack of insight, complaining of aggression, frequent adjudications, self-harm or food refusal.

Diagnostic features

Periods of mania with:

- increased energy and activity
  — elevated mood or irritability
  — rapid speech
  — loss of inhibitions
  — decreased need for sleep and
  — increased importance of self.
- Patient may be easily distracted.
- Patient may also have periods of depression with:
  — low or sad mood or
  — loss of interest or pleasure.
- The following associated symptoms are frequently present:
  — disturbed sleep
  — poor concentration
  — guilt or low self-worth
  — disturbed appetite
  — fatigue or loss of energy or
  — suicidal thoughts or acts.

Either type of episode may predominate. Episodes may alternate frequently or may be separated by periods of normal mood. In severe cases, patients may have hallucinations (hearing voices or seeing visions) or delusions (strange or illogical beliefs) during periods of mania or depression.

Differential diagnosis

- **Alcohol misuse — F10** or **Drug-use disorder — F11** (pages 18 and 55) can cause similar symptoms.
- Antisocial personality disorder: it can be difficult to assess mood if the patient's premorbid personality is not known. If possible, obtain information from their relatives, staff or former general practitioner.

Essential information for the patient and primary support group

- Unexplained changes in mood and behaviour can be symptoms of an illness.
- Effective treatments are available. Long-term treatment can prevent future episodes.
- If left untreated, manic episodes may become disruptive or dangerous. Manic episodes often lead to legal problems, loss of a job or financial problems (in the

community) and problems with debt, adjudications or high-risk sexual behaviour (in prison). When the first, milder symptoms of mania or hypomania occur, referral is often indicated and the patient should be encouraged to see the doctor straight away.

- Inform patients who are on lithium of the signs of lithium toxicity (see **Medication** below).

Advice and support to the patient and primary support group

- If it is decided that it is safe for the patient to live on ordinary location, seek patient permission to involve the residential manager and other relevant staff (eg workshop manager, teacher, chaplain) in implementing a management plan, including the location, activities, signs of lithium toxicity and planned response to relapse or mood swings. Inform staff that bipolar disorder carries the highest suicide risk of all mental disorders.
- During depression, assess the risk of suicide. (Has the patient frequently thought of death or dying? Does the patient have a specific suicide plan? Has he/she made serious suicide attempts in the past? Can the patient be sure not to act on suicidal ideas?) Close supervision by staff may be needed. Ask about the risk of harm to others (see **Depression — F32#** and **Assessing and managing people at risk of suicide**, pages 47 and 204).
- During manic periods:
  — avoid confrontation unless necessary to prevent harmful or dangerous acts
  — advise staff that aggression may be a sign of the illness and to avoid automatic use of disciplinary action
  — assess the risk of violence (see 'Assessing risk of violence' in **Aggression**, page 282)
  — advise caution about impulsive or dangerous behaviour
  — close observation by staff is often needed
  — if agitation or disruptive behaviour are severe, transfer to a prison healthcare centre or NHS hospital may be required.
- During depressed periods, consult the management guidelines for depression (see **Depression — F32#**, page 47).
- Describe the illness and the possible future treatments to the patient.
- Encourage staff to refer the patient when signs of depression arise, even if the patient is reluctant.
- Work with the patient and staff to identify early warning symptoms of mood swings to avoid a major relapse.
- For patients able to identify early symptoms of a forthcoming 'high', advise:
  — ceasing the consumption of tea, coffee and other caffeine-based stimulants
  — avoiding stimulating or stressful situations
  — planning for a good night's sleep
  — taking relaxing exercise during the day, eg gym or relaxation exercise in the cell
  — avoid taking major decisions or
  — if relevant, taking steps to limit capacity to spend money.[28]

Medication

- If the patient displays agitation, excitement or disruptive behaviour, antipsychotic medication may be needed initially[29] (see *BNF*, Section 4.2) (eg haloperidol, 1.5–4 mg up to three times per day). The doses should be the lowest possible for the relief of symptoms,[30] although some patients may require higher doses. If antipsychotic medication causes acute dystonic reactions (eg muscle spasms) or marked extrapyramidal symptoms (eg stiffness or tremors), anti-Parkinsonian medication (see *BNF*, Section 4.9), eg procyclidine, 5 mg orally up to three times per day, may be helpful. Routine use is not necessary.

- Benzodiazepines may also be used in the short-term in conjunction with antipsychotic medication to control acute agitation **and disturbance**[31] (see *BNF*, Section 4.1.2). Examples include diazepam (5–10 mg up to four times per day) or lorazepam (1–2 mg up to four times per day). If required, diazepam can be given rectally, or lorazepam IM (although it must be kept refrigerated).

- Lithium can help relieve mania[32] and depression,[33] and can prevent episodes from recurring.[34] One usually commences or stops taking lithium only with specialist advice. Some general practitioners are confident about restarting lithium treatment after a relapse. Alternative mood-stabilising medications include carbamazepine and sodium valproate. If used in the acute phase, lithium takes several days to show effects. If lithium is prescribed:
  — there should be a clear agreement between the referring general practitioner and the specialist about who is monitoring the lithium treatment. Lithium monitoring is ideally carried out using an agreed protocol. If carried out in primary care, monitoring should be done by a suitably trained person
  — the levels of lithium in the blood should be measured frequently when adjusting the dose, and every 3 months in stable patients 10–14 hours post-dose (desired blood level is 0.4–0.8 mmol l^{-1}).[N35] **If blood levels are > 1.5 or there is diarrhoea and vomiting, stop the lithium immediately.** If there are other signs of lithium toxicity (eg tremors, diarrhoea, vomiting, nausea, confusion), stop the lithium and check the blood level. Renal and thyroid function should be checked every 2–3 months when adjusting the dose, and every 6 months to 1 year in stable patients.[36]
    — **Never stop lithium abruptly** (except in the presence of toxicity) — relapse rates are twice as high under these conditions.[37] Lithium should be continued for at least 6 months after symptoms resolve (longer-term use is usually necessary to prevent recurrences).
    — If the patient is on ordinary location, ensure that a residential manager and, if the patient goes to the gym frequently, the physical education staff are aware of the signs of lithium toxicity. The leaflet on lithium toxicity on the disk may be helpful 💾.

- Antidepressant medication is often needed during phases of depression but can precipitate mania when used alone (see **Depression — F32#**, page 47). Bupropion may be less likely than other antidepressants to induce mania.[38] Doses should be as low as possible and used for the shortest time necessary. If the patient becomes hypomanic, stop the antidepressant.

Referral

Referral to the in-house or secondary mental-health services is advised:

- as an emergency if the patient is very vulnerable, eg if there is significant risk of suicide or disruptive behaviour or
- urgently if significant depression or mania continues despite treatment.

Non-urgent referral is recommended:

- for all new patients for assessment, care planning and allocation of key-worker under the Care Programme Approach

- before starting lithium
- to discuss relapse prevention and
- for women on lithium planning a pregnancy.

Where a patient is diagnosed with bipolar disorder for the first time, inform his/her solicitor, with patient permission, as the illness may have relevance to the offence.

If release is planned, work cooperatively with both probation or throughcare-planning officers to ensure that appointments with a general practitioner and specialist mental healthcare are arranged, and that housing, money for food, clothes and heating are arranged.

See **Managing the interface with the NHS and other agencies** (page 149) for more information on referral and throughcare.

Resources for patients and primary support groups

Manic Depression Fellowship: 020 7793 2600
(Advice, support, local self-help groups and publications list for people with manic depressive illness)

Manic Depression Fellowship (Scotland): 0141 400 1867

Resource leaflets:
Lithium Toxicity

Inside Out: A Guide to Self-Management of Manic Depression. Available from: Manic Depression Fellowship, Castle Works, 21 St George's Road, London SE1 6ES

Mary Ellen Copeland. *Living Without Depression and Manic Depression: A Workbook for Maintaining Mood Stability.* USA: New Harbinger. £11.95 Oakland 2001

Chronic fatigue, fatigue syndrome and neurasthenia — F48.0

Presenting complaints

Patients may report:

- a lack of energy
- aches and pains
- feeling tired easily or
- an inability to complete tasks.

Diagnostic features

- Mental and physical fatigue, made worse by physical and mental activity.
- Tiredness after minimal effort, with rest bringing little relief.
- Lack of energy.

Other common, often fluctuating, symptoms include:

- dizziness
- headache
- disturbed sleep
- inability to relax
- irritability
- aches and pains, eg muscle pain, chest pain, sore throat
- decreased libido and
- poor memory and concentration.

The disorder may be preceded by infection, trauma or another physical illness.

Fatigue syndrome is considered to be severe and chronic when substantial physical and mental fatigue lasts more than 6 months, significantly impairs daily activities and where there are no significant findings on physical examination or laboratory investigation. It is associated with other somatic symptoms.[39]

Differential diagnosis

- **Many medical disorders can cause fatigue.** A full history and physical examination are necessary, which can be reassuring for the doctor and therapeutic for the patient. Basic investigations include a full blood count, erythrocyte sedimentation rate (ESR) or CRP, thyroid function tests, urea and electrolytes, liver function tests, blood sugar and C-reactive protein. A medical disorder should be suspected where there is:
  — any abnormal physical finding, eg weight loss
  — any abnormal laboratory finding
  — unusual features of the history, eg recent foreign travel, or the patient is very young or very old or
  — symptoms occurring only after exertion and unaccompanied by any features of mental fatigue.

- **Depression — F32#** (page 47) if a low or sad mood is prominent.
- **Chronic mixed anxiety and depression — F41.2** (page 33).
- **Panic disorder — F41.1** (page 67) if anxiety attacks are prominent.
- **Unexplained somatic complaints — F45** (page 94) if unexplained physical symptoms are prominent.

Depression and anxiety may be somatised. Social, relationship or other life problems may cause or exacerbate distress.

- **Postviral fatigue syndrome and benign myalgic encephalomyelitis** (classified under G93.3 'Neurological disorders') are diagnosed where there is excessive fatigue following a viral disease and the symptoms do not fulfil the criteria for F48.0. 'Fatigue syndromes', both chronic and not, both with and without an established physical precursor, may be classified under F48.0 'Neurasthenia'. In practice, there is extensive overlap in symptoms (up to 96%). The choice of coding reflects different recording practices and uncertainty about the aetiology of these syndromes. Although classification is controversial, treatment is similar whatever choice is made about coding.

Essential information for the patient and primary support group

- Periods of fatigue or exhaustion are common and are usually temporary and self-limiting.
- Treatment for mild-to-moderate fatigue syndrome is possible and usually has good results, although the outcome for fatigue syndrome that is severe and chronic is more variable.[40]

Advice and support to the patient and primary support group

- Explore what the patient thinks his/her symptoms mean. Offer appropriate explanations and reassurance (eg symptoms are genuinely disabling and not 'all in the mind' but that symptoms following exertion do not mean physical damage and long-term disability).
- Advise a gradual return to usual activities. This may take time.
- The patient can build endurance with a programme of gradually increasing physical activity. Start with a manageable level and increase a little each week.
- Emphasise pleasant or enjoyable activities. Encourage the patient to resume activities that have helped in the past.
- Discuss sleep patterns. Encourage a regular sleep routine and avoid day time sleep (see **Sleep problems [insomnia] — F51**, page 91).
- Avoid excessive rest and/or sudden changes in activity.
- Severe chronic fatigue is less common than uncomplicated chronic fatigue. In severe chronic fatigue, a behavioural approach, including cognitive-behavioural therapy and/or a cautious graded programme of exercise and assessment of and assistance with activities of daily living, can be helpful.[41,42] Ideally, this would take place in a primary-care setting using clinical psychologists, nurse practitioners, practice counsellors, physiotherapists, occupational therapists or other suitably trained practitioners.

Medication

- To date, no pharmacological treatment for chronic fatigue has been established.[43]

- Depression and anxiety are common in severe chronic fatigue and may respond to pharmacological treatment. In treating depression, selective serotonin re-uptake inhibitors (SSRIs) (see *BNF*, Section 4.3.3) may be neutral or activating, and tricyclic antidepressants (TCAs) (see *BNF*, Section 4.3.1) at full dosage may be sedating.

- In the absence of depression, consider low dose tricyclic antidepressants (eg amitriptyline, 50–100 mg day^{-1}, or imipramine, 20 mg day^{-1}) (see *BNF*, Section 4.3.1), which may be effective for pain and poor sleep.[44,45]

Referral

See **General referral criteria** (page 152).

- Consider referral to a physician if the general practitioner is uncertain about diagnosis (see **Differential diagnosis** above).

- Referral to the secondary mental-health services or a liaison psychiatrist, if available, should be considered if there are:
  — comorbid mental disorders, eg eating disorder or bipolar disorder
  — a significant risk of suicide (see **Assessing and managing people at risk of suicide**, page 204) or
  — no improvement despite the above measures.

Resources for patients and primary support groups

Institute of Psychiatry's website (URL: http://www.kcl.ac.uk/cfs) includes a full patient-management package for the more severe symptoms of chronic fatigue syndrome. It includes information about the disorder and suggestions to aid self-management. It is a useful resource for the practitioner who is working with the patient to overcome the condition

Trudie Chalder. *Coping with Chronic Fatigue.* 1995 Sheldon, London. Self-help manual shown to improve the outcome in primary-care patients with chronic fatigue

M Sharpe, F Campling. *Chronic Fatigue Syndrome: The Facts.* Oxford: Oxford University Press, 2000. Self-help advice for more severe symptoms

For a review of the evidence for the full range of treatments for CFS/ME, see Bagnall AM, Whiting T, Wright J, Sowden AJ. *The Effectiveness of Interventions Used in the Treatment/Management of CFS and/or Myalgic Encephalomyelitis in Adults and Children.* York: NHS Centre for Reviews and Dissemination, University of York, 2001. URL: http://www.york.ac.uk/inst/crd/cfsrep.pdf

Chronic mixed anxiety and depression — F41.2

Presenting complaints

The patient may present with one or more physical symptoms (eg various pains, poor sleep or fatigue) accompanied by a variety of anxiety and depressive symptoms that will have been present for more than 6 months. These patients may be well known to their doctors and have often been treated by a variety of psychotropic agents over the years.

Diagnostic features

- Low or sad mood.
- Loss of interest or pleasure.
- Prominent anxiety or worry.
- Multiple associated symptoms are usually present, eg:
  — disturbed sleep
  — disturbed appetite
  — tremor
  — suicidal thoughts or acts
  — fatigue or loss of energy
  — dry mouth
  — palpitations
  — loss of libido
  — poor concentration
  — tension and restlessness
  — dizziness
  — irritability.

Differential diagnosis

- If more severe symptoms of depression or anxiety are present, see **Depression — F32#** or **Generalised anxiety — 41.1** (pages 47 and 64).
- If somatic symptoms predominate, which do not appear to have an adequate physical explanation, see **Unexplained somatic complaints — F45** (page 94).
- If the patient has a history of manic episodes (eg excitement, elevated mood, rapid speech), see **Bipolar disorder — F31** (page 26).
- If the patient is or has recently been drinking heavily or using drugs, see **Alcohol misuse — F10** and **Drug-use disorders — F11#** (pages 18 and 55).

Unexplained somatic complaints, alcohol or drug disorders may also coexist with mixed anxiety and depression.

Essential information for the patient and primary support group

- Stress or worry have many physical and mental effects and may be responsible for many of their symptoms. Symptoms are likely to be at their worst at times of personal stress. Aim to help the patient to reduce his/her symptoms.

- These problems are not due to weakness or laziness: patients are trying to cope.
- Regular structured visits can be helpful — state their frequency and include arranged visits to other professionals (to assess the progress of any physical disorder and give any advice on handling life stresses).

Advice and support to the patient and primary support group

- If physical symptoms are present, discuss the link between physical symptoms and mental distress (see **Unexplained somatic complaints — F45**, page 94).
- If tension-related symptoms are prominent, advise on relaxation methods to relieve physical symptoms. The *Managing Anxiety* leaflet on the disk includes a relaxation exercise.
- Advise a reduction in caffeine intake,[46] if appropriate, and a balanced diet, including plenty of complex carbohydrates and vitamins.[47]
- Discuss ways to challenge negative thoughts or exaggerated worries:
  — Identify exaggerated worries or pessimistic thoughts (eg when a visitor does not arrive on time, the patient worries that they no longer want contact with them).
  — Discuss ways to question these exaggerated worries when they occur, eg 'I am starting to be caught up in worry again. My visitor is only a few minutes late. He will probably be here soon.'
- Structured problem-solving methods[48] can help patients to manage current life problems or stresses that contribute to anxiety symptoms. Support the patient to carry out the following steps:
  — Identifying events that trigger excessive worry. (For example, a young woman presents with worry, tension, nausea and insomnia. These symptoms began after she learned that her son had been behaving badly in school following her conviction).
  — Listing as many possible solutions as the patient can think of, eg discussing her concerns with a close friend or relative, applying for an extended family visit, writing to her son's general practitioner, contacting a voluntary organisation that helps families of prisoners.
  — Listing the advantages and disadvantages of each possible solution. (The patient should do this, perhaps between appointments).
  — Choosing his/her preferred approach.
  — Working out the steps necessary to achieve the plan.
  — Setting a date to review the plan. Identify and reinforce things that are working.
- Help the patient plan activities that are relaxing, distracting or confidence building. Exercise may be helpful.[49,50] If necessary, consider advocating for improved access to appropriate activities.
- Assess the risk of suicide. (Has the patient thought frequently about death or dying? Does the patient have a specific suicide plan? Has he/she made serious suicide attempts in the past? Can the patient be sure not to act on suicidal ideas?) See **Assessing and managing people at risk of suicide** (page 204).
- Encourage self-help books, tapes and/or leaflets if appropriate.[51] If the patient has reading difficulties, a member of the healthcare team or another member of staff may be able to discuss the contents of the leaflets *Managing Depression* and *Managing Anxiety* (which are on the disk) with him/her.

Medication

- Medication should be simplified: it should be reviewed periodically and the patient should only be prescribed a drug if it is definitely helping. Multiple psychotropics should be avoided.
- An antidepressant with sedative properties can be prescribed if marked symptoms of depression or anxiety are present, but warn of drowsiness[N52] (see BNF, Section 4.3) For the severity threshold for initiating antidepressants and for specific guidance on these drugs, see **Depression — F32#** (page 47).
- *Hypericum perforata* (known as St John's Wort and available from health food stores) is often taken for mild and moderate symptoms of depression.[53] It has mild monoamine oxidase inhibitory (MAOI) properties,[54] so it should not be combined with other antidepressants and caution may in theory be needed with diet.[N55] *Hypericum* is an active agent and interactions with prescribed drugs may occur. For further information, see the advice from the Committee for Safety of Medicines.[N56]

Referral

See **General referral criteria** (page 152).

Referral to in-house or secondary mental-health services is advised:

- if the suicide risk is significant (see **Assessing and managing people at risk of suicide,** page 204) or
- non-urgently for psychological treatments, as available.

Consider recommending voluntary/non-statutory/self-help organisations. Stress/anxiety management,[N57] problem-solving,[N58] cognitive therapy,[59] cognitive-behavioural therapy[N60] or counselling[13] may be helpful and may be provided in primary care or the voluntary sector, as well as in the secondary mental-health services.

Resources for patients and primary support groups

For more resources, see **Depression — F32#** and **Generalised anxiety — F41.1** (pages 47 and 64).

Listeners/buddies, chaplain, the Samaritans

CITA (Council for Involuntary Tranquilliser Addiction): 0151 949 0102
(Monday–Friday, 10 am–1 pm)
Cavendish House, Brighton Road, Waterloo, Liverpool
(Confidential advice and support)

Samaritans: 08457 90 90 90 (24-hour, 7 days per week helpline)
(Support by listening for those feeling lonely, despairing or suicidal)

Resource leaflets:
Managing Anxiety
Managing Depression

Helping You Cope: A Guide to Starting and Stopping Tranquillisers and Sleeping Tablets. Available from: Mental Health Foundation, UK Office, 20/21 Cornwall Terrace, London NW1 4QL. Tel: 020 7535 7400; Fax: 020 7535 7474; E-mail: mhf@mhf.org.uk; URL: http://www.mentalhealth.org.uk

Chronic psychotic disorders — F20#

Includes schizophrenia, schizotypal disorder, persistent delusional disorders, induced delusional disorder and other non-organic psychotic disorders

Presenting complaints

Patients may present with:
- difficulties with thinking or concentration
- reports of hearing voices
- strange beliefs, eg having supernatural powers or being persecuted
- extraordinary physical complaints, eg having animals or unusual objects inside one's body
- poor hygiene
- problems in managing life in prison, work, education or relationships
- self-harm
- food refusal (may have delusions that food is being poisoned) or
- problems or questions related to antipsychotic medication.

Staff or a solicitor may seek help because of apathy, withdrawal, poor hygiene or strange behaviour.

Diagnostic features

- Chronic problems with the following features:
  — social withdrawal
  — low motivation, interest or self-neglect or
  — disordered thinking (exhibited by strange or disjointed speech).
- Periodic episodes of:
  — agitation or restlessness
  — bizarre behaviour
  — hallucinations (false or imagined perceptions, eg hearing voices) or
  — delusions (firm beliefs that are often false, eg the patient is related to royalty, receiving messages from the television, being followed or persecuted).

Differential diagnosis

- **Depression — F32#** (page 47) if a low or sad mood, pessimism and/or feelings of guilt.
- **Bipolar disorder — F31** (page 26) if symptoms of mania excitement, elevated mood or exaggerated self-worth are prominent.
- **Alcohol misuse — F10** or **Drug-use disorders — F11#** (pages 18 and 55). Chronic intoxication or withdrawal from alcohol or other substances (stimulants, hallucinogens) can cause psychotic symptoms.

Patients with chronic psychosis may also abuse drugs and/or alcohol.

Essential information for the patient and primary support group

- Agitation and strange behaviour can be symptoms of a mental illness.
- Symptoms may come and go over time.

- Medication is a central component of treatment. It will both reduce current difficulties and prevent relapse.
- Safe, stable living conditions (eg freedom from bullying, occupation) are a prerequisite for effective rehabilitation.
- Voluntary organisations can provide valuable support to the patient and support group.

Advice and support to the patient and primary support group

- Seek the patient's permission to discuss a treatment plan with staff involved in the care of the patient and obtain their support for it. A multidisciplinary care plan might consider options for location, occupation, ways of minimising unnecessary stress, an early response to signs of relapse and the monitoring of medication. Combination locations may be appropriate, eg sheltered work during the day, healthcare or Vulnerable Prisoners Unit (VPU) at night. Jointly establish appropriate expectations for the individual, to avoid inappropriate relegation to 'basic' status. The information leaflet on the disk for staff about psychotic disorder may be helpful 💾.
- Explain that medication will help prevent relapse, and inform the patient of the side-effects. Be vigilant to ensure that the patient is not persuaded/bullied into giving the medication to someone else. (They have currency, as antipsychotics may have a sedative and anti-Parkinsonian drugs a mood-elevating effect)
- Encourage the patient to function at the highest reasonable level in work and other daily activities.
- Minimise stress and stimulation:
  - Do not argue with psychotic thinking.
  - Avoid confrontation or criticism.[3] Staff should respond gently and with reassurance to slow responses to orders (eg slowness in going into a cell). Use of control and restraint should be a last resort.
  - During periods when the symptoms are more severe, rest and withdrawal from stress may be helpful.
- Keep the patient's physical health, including health promotion, obesity and smoking, under review.[61] Weight gain related to medication can be extreme. Heavy smokers may use tobacco to counteract the sedative effects of their antipsychotic medication. If this happens, consider a less sedating antipsychotic. If you suspect co-occurring substance misuse, check for possible physical problems (eg anaemia, chest problems) and nutritional deficiencies.
- If the illness has a relapsing course, work with the patient and staff to try to identify early warning signs of relapse.
- Encourage the patient to build relationships with key members of the healthcare team, eg by seeing the same doctor or nurse at each appointment. Use the relationship to discuss the advantages of medication and to review the effectiveness of the care plan.
- For advice on the management of agitated or excited states, see **Acute psychotic disorders — F23** (page 11).
- If care is shared with the in-house or NHS mental-health services, agree with them who is to do what.
- Especially if the patient becomes depressed, consider options for support, education and reassurance about their psychotic illness, including possible relapse and their future life chances. Mental-health staff may be able to provide individual counselling, goal planning and monitoring of early warning signs of relapse.

If the patient is also using substances:

- Express concern for the patient's well-being and avoid moral disapproval (eg 'I'm really not happy about you taking drugs as it makes your schizophrenia worse'). Focus on building a relationship with the patient, not on pushing an unmotivated patient towards abstinence.

- Discuss the benefits and costs of drug use (including the implications of continuing any form of illicit drug use while in prison) from the patient's perspective. Assess the patient's commitment to change. Thought disorder, suspiciousness and depression may make it difficult for the patient to make such a commitment.

- Educate the patient about the effect of alcohol and other drugs on the body and on schizophrenia (eg 'Drugs such as cannabis, LSD, stimulants and ecstasy all exacerbate the mood you are in when you take it, and so can make you more paranoid, anxious or depressed'). Feedback the results of tests, eg urine tests, changes in weight or other physical examinations.

- Consider options for dealing with prison-related problems that may be increasing the substance use (eg boredom, bullying, low-level depression). Consider:
  — encouraging the patient to spend more time out of the cell and in enjoyable activities, eg attend education, gym, work
  — liaising, with patient permission, with wing officers about reducing stress on the unit (eg noise, bullying, teasing) or increasing activities
  — encouraging the patient to talk to any trusted friend or staff member (eg personal officer, teacher, listener, chaplain) if day-to-day problems arise rather than turning to drugs.

For more information, see **Comorbidity** (page 191).

Medication

- Antipsychotic medication may reduce psychotic symptoms (see *BNF*, Section 4.2.1). Examples include haloperidol (1.5–4 mg up to three times day^{-1}), or an atypical antipsychotic[N6] (eg olanzapine, 5–10 mg day^{-1}, or risperidone, 4–6 mg day^{-1}).

- The dose should be the lowest possible for relief of symptoms. The drugs have different side-effect profiles. Indications for atypical drugs include uncontrolled acute extrapyramidal effects, uncontrolled hyperprolactinaemia and predominant, unresponsive, negative symptoms (eg withdrawal and low motivation). For more information on the different types of antipsychotic drugs and their side-effect profiles, see *Maudsley Prescribing Guidelines*.[10]

- Inform the patient that continued medication will reduce the risk of relapse. In general, antipsychotic medication should be continued for at least 6 months following a first episode of illness, and longer after a subsequent episode.[N9]

- Monitor compliance and the call up for review if more than two doses are missed.

- If, after team support, the patient is reluctant or erratic in taking medication, injectable long-acting antipsychotic medication may ensure the continuity of treatment and reduce the risk of relapse.[N62] It should be reviewed at 4–6-monthly intervals. Doctors and nurses who give depot injections in primary care need training to do so.[63] If available, specific counselling about medication also is helpful.[N64] Advise the nurse administering the medication to seek out the patient should he/she fail to attend an appointment.

- Discuss the potential side-effects with the patient. Common motor side-effects include:

— Acute dystonias or spasms that can be managed with anti-Parkinsonian drugs (see *BNF*, Section 4.9) (eg procyclidine, 5 mg three times per day, or orphenadrine, 50 mg three times per day).

— Parkinsonian symptoms (eg tremor and akinesia), which can be managed with oral anti-Parkinsonian drugs (see *BNF*, Section 4.9) (eg procyclidine, 5 mg up to three times per day, or orphenadrine, 50 mg three times per day). Withdrawal of anti-Parkinsonian drugs should be attempted after 2–3 months without symptoms as these drugs are liable to misuse and may impair memory.

— Akathisia (severe motor restlessness) may be managed with dosage reduction, or β-blockers (eg propranolol, 30–80 mg day^{-1}) (see *BNF*, Section 2.4). Switching to a low-potency antipsychotic (eg olanzapine or quetiapine) may help.

— Other possible side-effects include weight gain, galactorrhoea and photosensitivity. Patients suffering from drug-induced photosensitivity are eligible for sunscreen on prescription.

Referral

Referral to the secondary mental-health services is advised:

- urgently, if there are signs of relapse, unless there is an established previous response to treatment
- non-urgently:
  — to clarify diagnosis and ensure the most appropriate treatment
  — if there is non-compliance with treatment, problematic side-effects or breakdown of the living arrangements, eg problems on ordinary location or with occupation
  — for all new patients with a diagnosis of psychosis to obtain information about and review any existing care plan
  — for all patients who also abuse substances to review their medication to ensure that unwanted side-effects (eg sedation) are not increasing drug use.

Patients with a range of mental-health, occupational, social and financial needs are normally managed by specialist services. Referral for a key-worker under the Care Programme approach should always be considered.

The community mental-health services may be able to provide compliance therapy,[N64] family interventions,[N65] cognitive-behaviour therapy[66] and rehabilitative facilities.

Refer patients who are misusing substances and express some motivation to reduce for substance abuse counselling.[25] Liaise with the substance-misuse service to ensure the continued prescription of antipsychotic medication. Stress to the patient that relapses are to be expected, are not signs of failure and will not mean a loss of your support and respect (see **Comorbidity**, page 191).

If release is planned, work cooperatively with both probation or throughcare-planning officers to ensure that appointments with a general practitioner and specialist mental healthcare are arranged and that housing, money for food, clothes and heating are arranged.

If release is not planned, inform the local mental-health services that the patient may present to A&E in the area and advise them to look out for him/her.

For more detail on throughcare, see **Managing the interface with the NHS and other agencies** (page 149).

Resources for patients and primary support groups

Hearing Voices Network: 0161 834 5768
(Self-help groups to allow people to explore their voice hearing experiences)

MIND Infoline: 08457 660 163 (outside London); 020 8522 1728 (Greater London)

National Schizophrenia Fellowship: 020 8974 6814 (adviceline: Monday–Friday, 10:30 am–3 pm); 020 7330 9106 (office)

National Schizophrenia Fellowship (Northern Ireland): 02890 402 323

National Schizophrenia Fellowship (Scotland): 0131 557 8969

SANELine: 08457 678000 (12 pm–2 am, 7 nights)

Education and workshops may provide opportunities for creative expression
Education or Psychology Departments may provide basic social skills training

Resource leaflets:
Coping with the Side-effects of Medication
Working with a Prisoner with Severe Mental Illness
Early Warning Signs Form

Healthy Living with Schizophrenia. London: Health Education Authority 1998. Available from: Marsdon Book Services. Tel: 01235 465565

R Coleman, M Smith. *Working With Voices.* Handsell, 1997 Newton le Willows. Workbook to help voice hearers manage their voices

Delirium — F05

Presenting complaints

- Staff may request help because the patient is confused or agitated.
- Patients may appear uncooperative or fearful.
- Delirium may occur in patients hospitalised for physical conditions.

Diagnostic features

Acute onset, usually over hours or days, of:
- confusion (patient appears disoriented and struggles to understand surroundings) and
- clouded thinking or awareness.

Often accompanied by:
- poor memory
- agitation
- emotional upset
- loss of orientation
- wandering attention
- hearing voices
- withdrawal from others
- visions or illusions
- suspiciousness
- disturbed sleep (reversal of sleep pattern) and
- autonomic features, eg sweating, tachycardia.

Symptoms often develop rapidly and may change from hour to hour.
  Delirium may occur in patients with previously normal mental function or in those with dementia. Milder stresses (eg medication and mild infections) may cause delirium in older patients or in those with dementia.

Differential diagnosis

Identify and correct the possible underlying physical causes of the delirium, such as:
- alcohol intoxication or withdrawal
- drug intoxication, overdose or withdrawal (including prescribed drugs)
- infection
- metabolic changes, eg liver disease, dehydration, hypoglycaemia
- head trauma
- hypoxia or
- epilepsy.

If symptoms persist, delusions and disordered thinking predominate, and no physical cause is identified (see **Acute psychotic disorders — F23**, page 11).

Essential information for the patient and primary support group

Strange behaviour or speech and confusion can be symptoms of a medical illness.

Advice and support to the patient and primary support group[67]

- Take measures to prevent the patient from harming him/herself or others, eg remove unsafe objects, restrain if necessary but use the minimum amount of restraint required and take extra care to ensure no physical harm to the patient (see 'Restraint' in **Aggression**, page 282).
- Supportive contact with familiar people can reduce confusion.
- Provide frequent reminders of time and place to reduce confusion.
- A transfer to hospital may be required because of agitation or because of the physical illness that is causing delirium. There is an appreciable mortality rate with delirium. Patients may need to be admitted to a medical ward in order to diagnose and treat the underlying disorder. In an emergency, where there is risk to life and safety, a medically ill patient may be taken to a general hospital for treatment under common law. In such a case, a medical doctor may make this decision without involvement of a psychiatrist (see **Emergency treatment under common law**, page 168).

Medication[68]

- Avoid the use of sedative or hypnotic medications (eg benzodiazepines) except for the treatment of alcohol or sedative withdrawal.
- Antipsychotic medication in low doses (see *BNF*, Section 4.2.1) may sometimes be needed to control agitation, psychotic symptoms or aggression. Beware of drug side-effects (drugs with anticholinergic action and anti-Parkinsonian medication can exacerbate or cause delirium) and drug interactions.

Referral

Referral to the secondary mental-health services is rarely indicated. Referral to a physician is nearly always indicated if:

- the cause is unclear
- the cause is clear and treatable but treatment cannot safely be provided within the establishment or
- drug or alcohol withdrawal, overdose or another underlying condition necessitating in-patient medical care is suspected.

Dementia — F00#

Presenting complaints

- Patients may complain of forgetfulness, a decline in mental functioning or of feeling depressed, but they may be unaware of memory loss. Patients and staff may sometimes deny, or be unaware of, the severity of memory loss and other deterioration in function.
- Staff or the patient's solicitor may ask for help initially because of failing memory, disorientation and change in personality or behaviour. In the later stages of the illness, they may seek help because of behavioural disturbance, wandering or incontinence or an episode of dangerous behaviour.
- Dementia may also be diagnosed during consultations for other problems, as staff may believe deterioration in memory and function is a natural part of ageing.
- Changes in behaviour and functioning (eg poor personal hygiene or social interaction) in an older patient should raise the possibility of a diagnosis of dementia.

Diagnostic features

- Decline in memory for recent events, thinking, judgement, orientation and language.
- Patients may have become apparently apathetic or uninterested, but may also appear alert and appropriate despite a deterioration in memory and other cognitive function.
- Decline in everyday function, eg dressing, washing.
- Changes in personality or emotional control — patients may become easily upset, tearful or irritable, as well as apathetic.
- Common with advancing age (5% over 65 years, 20% over 80 years),[69] very rare in youth or middle age.

Progression is classically stepwise in vascular dementia, gradual in Alzheimer's and fluctuating in Lewy body dementia (fluctuating cognition, visual hallucinations and Parkinsonism), but the clinical picture is often not clear-cut.

Owing to the problems inherent in taking a history from people with dementia, it is very important that information about the level of current functioning and possible decline in functioning should also be obtained from an informant (eg relative who visits frequently or residential staff).

Tests of memory and thinking include:

- the ability to repeat the names of three common objects (eg apple, table, penny) immediately and recall them after 3 minutes
- the ability to identify accurately the day of the week, the month and the year and
- the ability to give their name and full postal address.

A very short screening test is set out in the resource section on the disk 💾.

Differential diagnosis

Examine and investigate for treatable causes of dementia. The common causes of cognitive worsening in the elderly are:

- urinary tract, chest, skin or ear infection
- onset or exacerbation of cardiac failure
- prescribed drugs, especially psychiatric and anti-Parkinsonian drugs, and alcohol and
- cerebrovascular ischaemia or hypoxia.

Less common causes include:
- severe depression
- severe anaemia in the very old
- vitamin B_{12} or folate deficiency
- hypothyroidism and hyperparathyroidism
- slow-growing cerebral tumour
- renal failure and
- communicating hydrocephalus.

Sudden increases in confusion, wandering attention or agitation will usually indicate a physical illness (eg acute infectious illness) or toxicity from medication (see **Delirium — F05**, page 41).

Depression may cause memory and concentration problems similar to those of dementia, especially in older patients. If low or sad mood is prominent, or if the impairment is patchy and has developed rapidly, see **Depression — F32#** (page 47).

Helpful tests include: MSU, full blood count (FBC), B_{12}, folate, LFTs, TFTs, U&E, Ca^{2+} and glucose.

Essential information for the patient and primary support group

- Dementia is frequent in old age but is not inevitable.
- Memory loss and confusion may cause behaviour problems (eg agitation, suspiciousness, emotional outbursts, apathy and an inability to take part in normal social interaction).
- Memory loss usually proceeds slowly, but the course and long-term prognosis varies with the disease causing dementia. Discuss the diagnosis, the likely progress and prognosis with the patient and, with patient permission, with his/her primary support group.
- Physical illness or other stress can increase confusion.
- Advise staff that the patient will have great difficulty in learning new information. Avoid placing the patient in unfamiliar places or situations
- The supply of information on dementia for staff involved in care of the patient is essential.

Advice and support to the patient and primary support group

- Seek patient permission to discuss a treatment plan with staff involved in the care of the patient and obtain their support for it. Regularly assess the risk (balancing safety and independence), especially at times of crisis. As appropriate, discuss arrangements for support in the establishment.
- Consider contacting the patient's solicitor, with patient permission, to discuss the possible application for release on grounds of ill-health.
- Regularly review the patient's ability to perform daily tasks safely as well as their behavioural problems and general physical condition.

- If memory loss is mild, consider the use of memory aids or reminders.
- Encourage the patient to make full use of their remaining abilities.
- Encourage maintenance of the patient's physical health and fitness through good diet and exercise, plus swift treatment of intercurrent physical illness.
- Discuss the planning of legal and financial affairs. An information sheet is available from the Alzheimer's Society (see **Resources Directory** page 316). A probation officer may be able to provide further information.

Medication

- Try non-pharmacological methods of dealing with difficult behaviour first. For example, staff may be able to deal with repetitive questioning if they are given the information that this is because the dementia is affecting the patient's memory.
- Antipsychotic medication in very low doses (see *BNF*, Section 4.2.1) may sometimes be needed to manage some behavioural problems (eg aggression or restlessness). Behavioural problems change with the course of the dementia; therefore, withdraw the medication every few months on a trial basis to see if it is still needed and discontinue if it is not. Beware of drug side-effects (eg Parkinsonian symptoms, anticholinergic effects) and drug interactions (avoid combining with tricyclic antidepressants (TCA), alcohol, anticonvulsants or L-dopa preparations). Antipsychotics should be avoided in Lewy body dementia.[70]
- Avoid using sedative or hypnotic medications (eg benzodiazepines) if possible. If other treatments have failed and severe management problems remain, use very cautiously and for no more than 2 weeks; they may increase confusion.
- Aspirin in low doses may be prescribed for vascular dementia to attempt to slow deterioration.
- In Alzheimer's disease, consider referring the patient to secondary care for an assessment and the initiation of anticholinesterase drugs[71] depending on locally agreed policies.

Referral

- Refer to a specialist to confirm diagnosis in complicated or atypical cases.
- Call a case conference with the relevant staff (eg probation officer, residential staff, occupational therapist, if available) to arrange the practicalities of managing the patient in the establishment.
- Refer to a physician if there is complex medical comorbidity or a sudden worsening of dementia.
- Refer to the psychiatric services if there are intractable behavioural problems or if a depressive or psychotic episode occurs.

If release is planned, work cooperatively with both probation or throughcare-planning officers to ensure that appointments with a general practitioner, specialist mental healthcare and socialcare are arranged, and that housing, money for food, clothes and heating are arranged.

For more detail on throughcare, see **Managing the interface with the NHS and other agencies** (page 149). See PSI 21/2001 for details of the Prison Service requirements about the provision of coordinated health- and socialcare to older people in prison.

Resources for patients and primary support groups

Alzheimer's Society and CJD Support Network: 0845 300336 (helpline); 020 7306 0606 (office)
(Support and advice to people with dementia of all kinds, ie not just Alzheimer's, and their family and friends)

Age Concern England: 0800 009966 (freephone helpline: Monday–Sunday, 7 am–7 pm); 020 8765 7200 (office)
(Information and advice relating to older people)

Age Concern Northern Ireland: 02890 245729

Age Concern Cymru: 02920 399562

Age Concern Scotland: 0131 220 3345

Help the Aged: 020 7253 0253

Counsel and Care: 020 7485 1550 (Monday–Friday, 10:30 am–12 pm, 2 pm–4 pm)
(Advice and information on issues including residential care, for older people and their carers)

Benefits Enquiry Line: 0800 882200 (freephone)
(For people with disabilities)

Carers' National Association: 020 7490 8818; 0808 808 7777 (carersline: 10 am–12 pm, 2:30 pm–4 pm)

H Cayton, N Graham, J Warner, *Alzheimer's At Your Fingertips*. Class, 1997 London. £11.95. A good book for patients and carers that answers commonly asked questions about all types of dementia

Depression — F32#

Presenting complaints

The patient may present initially with one or more physical symptoms, such as pain or 'tiredness all the time'. Further enquiry will reveal a low mood or severe and persistent loss of interest.

Irritability or increased aggression is sometimes the presenting problem.

A wide range of presenting complaints may accompany or conceal depression. These include anxiety or insomnia, worries about social problems such as financial or marital difficulties, increased drug or alcohol use, or (in a new mother) constant worries about her baby or fear of harming the baby.

Some groups are at higher risk (eg those who have recently given birth, those given a life sentence or a longer sentence than they expected, and those with physical disorders, eg Parkinson's disease or multiple sclerosis).

Diagnostic features

- Low or sad mood.
- Loss of interest and pleasure for most of the day for at least 2 weeks.

Plus at least four of the following:
- disturbed sleep
- disturbed appetite; food refusal
- increased irritability and aggression
- guilt or low self-worth
- pessimism or hopelessness about the future
- fatigue or loss of energy
- agitation (eg pacing) or slowing of movement or speech
- diurnal mood variation
- poor concentration
- suicidal thoughts or acts
- loss of self-confidence
- decreased libido.

Symptoms of anxiety or nervousness are also frequently present.

The more severe the depression, usually the greater number of symptoms and (most importantly) the greater the degree of interference with normal social or occupational functioning. Biological symptoms are more common in more severe depression.

Differential diagnosis

- **Adjustment reaction — F43.2** (page 15). Where symptoms are caused by recent stress (eg being given a prison sentence or bullying; loss of confidence may be caused by the individual's position in the prison hierarchy). Depression is diagnosed when symptoms are severe and continue for more than 1 month, irrespective of whether or not they are linked to life stresses.

- **Alcohol misuse — F10** or **Drug-use disorder — F11#** (pages 18 and 55) if heavy alcohol or drug use is present. Substance misuse may cause or increase depressive symptoms. It may also mask underlying depression. Depressive symptoms improve in 80% of patients after detoxification. Depression is diagnosed if major symptoms persist or worsen after alcohol, stimulant or opiate withdrawal (see **Comorbidity**, page 191).
- **Acute psychotic disorder — F23** (page 11) if hallucinations, eg hearing voices, or delusions, eg strange or unusual beliefs, are present.
- **Bipolar disorder — F31** (page 26) if the patient has a history of manic episodes, eg excitement, rapid speech and elevated mood.
- **Chronic mixed anxiety and depression — F41.2** (page 33).

Some medications may produce symptoms of depression (eg β-blockers, other antihypertensives, H$_2$-blockers, oral contraceptives and corticosteroids).

Unexplained somatic complaints, anxiety, alcohol or drug disorders may coexist with depression.

Essential information for the patient and primary support group

- Feelings of helplessness, hopelessness, anxiety and emotional swings are all symptoms of the illness. They do not mean that you are going mad. Depression is a common illness and effective treatments are available.
- It is normal to be sad when separated from family and friends. Depression is diagnosed when symptoms are severe and go on for a long time. Then people often need help to reduce the symptoms so that they can tackle their problems and get on with life.
- Some people use drugs and alcohol as a way of escaping from painful feelings and these may come back when the drugs are stopped. If you are still depressed a few weeks after being drug free, it usually means that there is a problem with depression. This could be an opportunity to try and deal with some of the problems that contributed to your depression and to your substance use.
- Depression is not weakness or laziness.
- Depression can affect people's ability to cope.
- Recommend information leaflets or audiotapes to reinforce the information.[51] If the patient has reading difficulties, a member of the healthcare team or another member of staff may be able to discuss the contents of the leaflet *Managing Depression* (it is on the disk 💾) with him/her.

Advice and support for the patient and primary support group

- Assess the risk of suicide. Ask questions about thoughts, plans and intent (eg Has the patient often thought of death or dying? Does the patient have a specific suicide plan? Has he/she made suicide attempts in the past? Can the patient be sure not to act on suicidal ideas? Involve the mental-health team. There should be close supervision, move to healthcare centre or use of care suite may be needed (see **Assessing and managing people at risk of suicide**, page 204).
- Ask about risk of harm to others (see 'Assessing risk of violence' in **Aggression**, page 282).
- Identify the current life problems or social stresses, including precipitating factors, and what help he/she needs in resolving them. Wing officers may be

helpful, especially where problems involve the wing hierarchy. Focus on small, specific steps patients might take towards reducing or improving management of these problems (for agencies providing help for particular problems, see **Resource directory**, page 316). Advise the patient to avoid major decisions or life changes while he/she is depressed.

- Plan short-term activities that give the patient enjoyment or build confidence. Exercise may be helpful.[72]
- If appropriate, advise a reduction in caffeine intake[46] and drug use.
- Support the development of good sleep patterns and encourage a balanced diet.[47]
- Encourage the patient to resist pessimism and self-criticism, not to act on pessimistic ideas (eg ending a marriage) and not to concentrate on negative or guilty thoughts.
- Identify someone the patient can confide in. Encourage him/her to seek practical and emotional help from others. Inform the patient about the role and availability of the prison healthcare team and any other support available. Consider supporting him/her to obtain additional telephone calls to family and friends outside or extended family visits.
- If physical symptoms are present, discuss the link between physical symptoms and mood (see **Unexplained somatic symptoms — F45**, page 94).
- Involve the patient in discussing the advantages and disadvantages of the available treatments. Inform the patient that medication usually works more quickly than psychotherapies.[N74,N75] Where patients choose not to take medication, explore their reasons and dispel any misconceptions, but if they remain of the same mind, respect their decision and arrange another appointment to monitor progress.
- After improvement, plan with the patient the action to be taken if signs of relapse occur.

Liaison and advice to residential and other staff

Ask the patient's permission to discuss the following with the other staff caring for him/her. Inform him/her that you will only do this with their permission, except where there is a significant risk of suicide or harm to others.

- Discuss the outcome of the assessment of risk and discuss ways of managing the risk including the level of monitoring required. Discuss the location, including the shared room or care suite. Discuss the options for staff support outlined on the leaflet on the disk 💾.
- Advise staff not to make judgements about whether giving up on life is to be expected in the face of the patient's life situation.
- Inform staff of the likely impact of the illness on the individual's functioning, eg irritability and aggression can cause an increase in arguments with other inmates or with visitors.
- Promote contact with family and friends, eg extended family visits, telephone calls.
- Consider advocating for access to an appropriate activity, eg art materials, suitable work placement.
- If the patient's illness means that he/she can no longer manage his/her previous routine, eg work placement, discuss the options for replacement activities, eg art, exercise, easier work.

Medication

- There is no evidence that people with only few or very mild depressive symptoms respond to antidepressants.[76] Moderate-to-severe episodes will need treatment with antidepressants. Consider medication at the first visit.
- Antidepressants are effective even when depression is linked to the presence of life stresses or physical illness. Treatment is indicated by the severity and duration of symptoms.
- Discuss the aims of the treatment and the side-effects; explore the patient's perceptions of treatment.

Choice of medication

At present, there is no evidence to suggest that any antidepressant is more effective than others.[77,78] However, their side-effect profiles differ and, therefore, some drugs will be more acceptable to particular patients than others (see *BNF*, Section 4.3).

- If the patient has responded well to a particular drug in the past, use that drug again.
- If the patient is older or physically ill, use medication with fewer anticholinergic and cardiovascular side-effects.
- If the patient is suicidal, avoid tricyclic antidepressants (TCAs) or consider supervised ingestion.
- If the patient is anxious or unable to sleep, use a drug with more sedative effects, but warn of drowsiness and problems with machinery.
- If the patient is about to be released and is unwilling to give up alcohol, choose one of the SSRI antidepressants which do not interact with alcohol (eg fluoxetine, paroxetine and citalopram). (See *BNF* Section 4.3.3)
- *Hypericum perforata* (known as St John's Wort and available from health food stores) is often taken for mild and moderate symptoms of depression, both acute and chronic.[53] It has mild monoamine oxidase-inhibiting (MAOI) properties[54] so it should not be combined with other antidepressants and caution may be needed with diet.[N55] *Hypericum* is an active agent and interactions with prescribed drugs may occur (for further information, see the advice from the Committee for Safety of Medicines[N56]).

If antidepressants are prescribed, explain to the patient that:

- the medication must be taken every day
- the drug is not addictive
- improvement will build up over 2–3 weeks after starting the medication
- mild side-effects may occur, eg dry mouth, blurred vision, sedation with TCAs and agitation and stomach upset with selective serotonin re-uptake inhibitors (SSRIs), but they usually fade in 7–10 days and
- stress that the patient should consult the doctor before stopping medication. All antidepressants should be withdrawn slowly, preferably over 4 weeks in weekly decrements.

Continue full-dose antidepressant medication for at least 4–6 months after the condition improves to prevent relapse.[79,80] Review regularly during this time. Consider, jointly with the patient, the need for further continuation beyond 4–6 months. If the patient has had several episodes of major depression, consider carefully long-term prophylactic treatment.[N81] Obtain a second opinion at this point, if available.

If using TCA medication, build up over 7–10 days to the effective dose, eg dothiepin: start at 50–75 mg and build to 150 mg nocte; or imipramine: start at 25–50 mg each night and build to 100–150 mg.[N82]

Withdraw antidepressant medication slowly and monitor for withdrawal reactions to ensure that remission is stable. Gradual reduction of SSRIs can be achieved by using syrup in reducing doses or taking a tablet on alternate days.

Referral

The following structured therapies, delivered by properly trained practitioners, have been shown to be effective for some people with depression.[N83]

- Cognitive-behavioural therapy (CBT).
- Behaviour therapy.
- Interpersonal therapy.
- Structured problem solving.

Patients with chronic, relapsing depression may benefit more from CBT or a combination of CBT and antidepressants than from medication alone.[84,85] Counselling may be helpful, especially in milder cases and if focused on specific psychosocial problems which are related to the depression, eg relationships, bereavement.[N13]

Referral to the secondary mental-health services is advised:

- as an emergency, if there is a significant risk of suicide or danger to others, psychotic symptoms, severe agitation or retardation with impaired food/fluid intake and
- as a non-emergency, if:
  — significant depression persists despite treatment in primary care (antidepressant therapy has failed if the patient remains symptomatic after a full course of treatment at an adequate dosage. If there is no clear improvement with the first drug, it should be changed to another class of drug) or
  — there is a history of severe depression, especially bipolar disorder.

If drug or alcohol misuse is also a problem, see the guidelines for these disorders.

Involve non-healthcare support (eg chaplain, counsellor, listener/buddy, voluntary support group) in all other cases where symptoms persist, where the patient has a poor or non-existent support network, or where social or relationship problems are contributing to the depression.[86]

Severely depressed adolescents are difficult to assess and manage, and referral is recommended (see **Emotional disorders in young people**, page 126).

For more details on referral, see **Managing the interface with the NHS and other agencies** (page 149).

Resources for patients and primary support groups

Association for Post Natal Illness: 020 7386 0868

Depression Alliance: 020 7633 0557 (answerphone)

SAD (Seasonal Affective Disorder) Association: 01903 814942

Samaritans: 08457 909090 (24-hour, 7 days per week helpline)

UK Register of Counsellors: 08704 435232
(Provides a list of BACP-accredited counsellors)

Resource leaflets:
Problem-solving
Coping with Depression

Dorothy Rowe. *Depression: Way Out of Your Prison*. An explanatory book

Erika Harvey. *The Element Guide to Postnatal Depression: Your Questions Answered*. Shaftesbury: Element, 1999

Dissociative (conversion) disorder — F44

Presenting complaints

Patients exhibit unusual or dramatic physical symptoms such as seizures, amnesia, trance, loss of sensation, visual disturbances, paralysis, aphonia, identity confusion and 'possession' states. The patient is not aware of their role in their symptoms — they are not malingering.

Diagnostic features

Physical symptoms are:
- unusual in presentation and are
- not consistent with known disease.

Onset is often sudden and related to psychological stress or difficult personal circumstances.

In acute cases, symptoms may:
- be dramatic and unusual
- change from time to time or
- be related to attention from others.

In more chronic cases, patients may appear unduly calm in view of the seriousness of the complaint.

Differential diagnosis

Carefully consider the physical conditions that may cause symptoms. A full history and physical (including neurological) examination are essential. The early symptoms of neurological disorders (eg multiple sclerosis) may resemble conversion symptoms.
- If other unexplained physical symptoms are present, see **Unexplained somatic complaints — F45** (page 94).
- **Depression — F32#** (page 47). Atypical depression may present in this way.

Essential information for the patient and primary support group

- Physical or neurological symptoms often have no clear physical cause. Symptoms can be brought about by stress.
- Symptoms usually resolve rapidly (from hours to a few weeks), leaving no permanent damage.

Advice and support to the patient and primary support group

- Encourage the patient to acknowledge recent stresses or difficulties (though it is not necessary for the patient to link the stresses to current symptoms).
- Give positive reinforcement for improvement. Try not to reinforce symptoms
- Advise the patient to take a brief rest and relief from stress, then to return to usual activities.
- Advise against prolonged rest or withdrawal from activities.

Medication

Avoid anxiolytics or sedatives.

In more chronic cases with depressive symptoms, antidepressant medication may be helpful.

Referral

See general referral criteria (page 152).

Non-urgent referral to the secondary mental-health services is advised if confident of the diagnosis:

- if symptoms persist
- if symptoms are recurrent or severe or
- if the patient is prepared to discuss a psychological contribution to symptoms.

If you are unsure of the diagnosis, consider referral to a physician before referral to the secondary mental-health services.

If release is planned, work cooperatively with both probation or throughcare-planning officers to ensure that appointments with a general practitioner and specialist mental healthcare are arranged along with other needs such as housing.

For more detail on throughcare, see **Managing the interface with the NHS and other agencies** (page 149).

Resource for patients and primary support groups

UK Register of Counsellors: 08704 435232
(Supplies names and addresses of BAC-accredited counsellors).

Drug-use disorders — F11#

Presenting complaints

Patients may present in a state of withdrawal or (more rarely) of intoxication or with physical complications of drug use, eg abscesses or thromboses. They may also present with the legal or social consequences of their drug use, eg prosecution or debt. Occasionally, covert drug use may manifest itself as bizarre, unexplained behaviour.

Patients may have: depressed mood, nervousness or insomnia.

Patients may present with a direct request for prescriptions for narcotics or other drugs, a request for help to withdraw, or for help with stabilising their drug use.

Signs of drug withdrawal include the following.

- Opioids: nausea, sweating, aching, stomach cramps, gooseflesh, dilated pupils
- Sedatives: anxiety, tremors, perceptual distortions, fits
- Stimulants: depression, moodiness, hunger, excessive sleep.

Staff may request help before the patient (eg because the patient is irritable or has a positive result to a drug test). Whatever their motivation for seeking help, the aim of treatment is to assist the patient in remaining healthy until, if motivated to do so and with appropriate help and support, he/she can achieve a drug-free life.

Diagnostic features

- Drug use has caused physical harm (eg injuries while intoxicated), psychological harm (eg symptoms of mental disorder due to drug use) or has led to harmful social consequences (eg criminality, loss of job, severe family problems)
- Habitual and/or harmful or chaotic drug use
- Difficulty controlling drug use
- Strong desire to use drugs
- Tolerance (can use large amounts of drugs without appearing intoxicated)
- Withdrawal (eg anxiety, tremors or other withdrawal symptoms after stopping use).

Diagnosis will be aided by the following.

- History: including a reason for presentation, past and current (ie in the past 4 weeks) drug use, a history of injecting and the risk of HIV and hepatitis, past medical and psychiatric history, social (and especially child care) responsibilities, forensic history and past contact with treatment services
- Examination: motivation, physical (needle tracks or complications, eg thrombosis or viral illness), mental state
- Investigations: haemoglobin, LFTs, urine drug screen, hepatitis B and C, HIV.

Differential diagnosis

- **Alcohol misuse — F10** (page 18) can coexist. Polydrug use is common
- Symptoms of anxiety or depression may also occur with heavy drug use. If these continue after a period of abstinence (eg about 4 weeks), see **Depression — F32#** and **Generalised anxiety — F41.1** (pages 47 and 64)

- **Psychotic disorders — F23, F20#** (page 11 and 36)
- Acute organic syndromes.

Essential information for the patient and primary support group

- Drug misuse is a chronic, relapsing condition. Controlling or stopping use often requires several attempts. It is particularly hard when the patient also has another mental disorder. Relapse is common
- Abstinence should be seen as a long-term goal. Harm reduction (especially reducing intravenous drug use) may be a more realistic goal in the short- to medium-term
- Stopping or reducing drug use will bring psychological, social and physical benefits
- Using some drugs during pregnancy risks harming the baby[N87]
- For intravenous drug users, there is a risk of transmitting HIV infection, hepatitis or other infections carried by body fluids. Discuss the appropriate precautions, eg use condoms and do not share needles, syringes, spoons, water or any other injecting equipment
- Where the patient also has a psychotic disorder, advise that substance abuse makes acute symptoms of psychosis (eg hallucinations) worse, even when antipsychotic medication is taken.

Advice and support to the patient and primary support group

Advice should be given according to the patient's motivation and willingness to change.[88] For some patients with chronic, relapsing opioid dependence, the treatment of choice is maintenance on long-acting opioids (usually methadone).[89]
For all patients, do the following.

- Discuss the benefits and costs of drug use (including the links between drug use and offending) from the patient's perspective
- Feedback information about the health risks, including the results of investigations
- Emphasise the personal responsibility for change
- Give clear advice to change
- Assess and manage the physical health problems (eg deep vein thrombosis [DVT], abscesses, infections, hepatitis, HIV, anaemia, chest problems) and nutritional deficiencies
- Consider the options for problem-solving or targeted counselling to deal with life problems related to drug use.

For patients not willing to stop or change their drug use immediately, do the following.

- Do not reject or blame
- Advise on harm-reduction strategies (eg if the patient is injecting, advise on the risks of needle sharing, not injecting alone, not mixing alcohol, benzodiazepines and opiates) (see the patient leaflet *Harm Reduction* on the disk 💾)
- Clearly point out medical, psychological, social and offending problems caused by drugs
- Make a future appointment to reassess health (eg well-woman checks, immunisation) and discuss drug use.

If reducing drug use is a reasonable goal (or if a patient is unwilling to quit):
- Negotiate a clear goal for decreased use
- Discuss strategies to avoid or cope with high-risk situations (eg release, social situations, stressful events)
- Plan for self-monitoring procedures upon release (eg a diary of drug use) and for safer drug-use behaviours (eg time restrictions, slowing down rate of use)
- Consider options for counselling and/or rehabilitation.

If maintenance on substitute drugs is a reasonable goal (or if a patient is unwilling to quit):
- Negotiate a clear goal for less harmful behaviour. Help the patient develop a hierarchy of aims, eg stopping illicit use and maintenance on prescribed, substitute drugs, reduction of substitute drugs
- Discuss strategies to avoid or cope with high-risk situations, eg release, social situations or stressful events
- Consider withdrawal symptoms and how to avoid or reduce them
- Consider options for counselling or rehabilitation, or both.

For patients willing to stop immediately:
- Consider withdrawal symptoms and how to manage them
- Discuss strategies to avoid or cope with high-risk situations, eg release, social situations or stressful events
- Make specific plans to avoid drug use, eg how to respond to friends who still use drugs
- Identify family or friends who will support stopping drug use
- Consider options for counselling or rehabilitation, or both.

For patients who do not succeed or who relapse or transfer to a different drug while in prison:
- Identify and give credit for any success
- Discuss situations that led to the relapse
- Return to the earlier steps.

Self-help organisations such as Narcotics Anonymous are often helpful.

Medication

To withdraw a patient from benzodiazepines, convert to a long-acting drug such as diazepam and reduce gradually over 2–6 months (see *BNF*, Section 4.1). For more information, see 'Guidelines for the prevention and treatment of benzodiazepine dependence'.[90]
   Withdrawal from stimulants or cocaine is distressing and may require medical supervision. The risk of suicide and self-harm during and following withdrawal from stimulants and cocaine is particularly high. For more information, see **Comorbidity** (page 191).
   Both long-term maintenance of a patient on substitute opiates (usually methadone) and withdrawal from opiates should be done as part of a shared-care scheme.[91] A multidisciplinary approach is essential and should include drug counselling/therapy[N92] and possible future rehabilitation needs.[93] The doctor signing the prescription is wholly responsible for prescribing; this cannot be delegated. For more information, see *Drug Misuse and Dependence: Guidelines on Clinical Management.*[94]

- Careful assessment, including urine analysis and, where possible, dose assessment, is essential before prescribing any substitute medication, including methadone. Addicts often try to obtain a higher-than-needed dose. Dosages will depend on the results of the assessment
- For long-term maintenance or stabilisation before gradual withdrawal, the dose should be titrated up to that needed both to block withdrawal symptoms and the craving for opiates[N95]
- For gradual withdrawal after a period of stabilisation, the drug can be slowly tapered (eg by 5 mg per fortnight)
- Daily dispensing and supervised ingestion are recommended
- In the UK at present, methadone mixture BNF 1 mg ml^{-1} is the most often-used substitute medication for opioid addiction[96] (see *BNF*, Section 4.10). Other, newer drugs are, or may become, available (eg Buprenorphine[97]). Specialist advice should be obtained before prescribing these
- Withdrawal from opiates for patients whose drug use is already well controlled can be managed with Lofexidine[98] (see *BNF*, Section 4.10).

Referral

Consider referral:

- To a Detoxification Unit if the patient is dependent upon drugs
- Involve the in-house or secondary mental-health services in addition if the patient has an associated severe psychiatric disorder, or if the symptoms of mental illness persist after detoxification and abstinence. Ideally, treatment should be provided by clinicians skilled in treating both substance misuse and mental disorder[25]
- To counselling, assessment, referral, advice and throughcare services (CARATS) workers for counselling targeted at problems associated with/triggering drug use and relapse prevention work
- To in-house rehabilitation programmes and therapeutic communities.

Before release:

- If possible, arrange in good time for on-going rehabilitation support in the community. Help with life problems, employment and social relationships is an important component of treatment[99]
- Where the patient has both a mental illness and a drug misuse problem and expresses some motivation to reduce use, if either the psychiatric or substance misuse problem appears to predominate, refer them initially to that service. Make the rationale clear in the letter/fax. If both types of disorder are of equal significance, then negotiate with both agencies about the preferred initial referral route. It may be that the individual will require support and input by both agencies. Some can provide services jointly. Ideally, a modified form of motivational interviewing that takes account of the additional problems of a patient with a severe mental illness will be used. Liaise with the service to ensure continued prescription of psychotropic medication, if appropriate
- Stress to the patient that relapses are to be expected, are not signs of failure and will not mean a loss of your support and respect.

See **Comorbidity** (page 191).

Resources for patients and primary support groups

ADFAM National: 020 7928 8900 (helpline)
(For families and the friends of drug users)

CITA (Council for Involuntary Tranquilliser Addiction): 0151 949 0102
(Monday–Friday, 10 am–1 pm)
Cavendish House, Brighton Road, Waterloo, Liverpool
(Confidential advice and support)

Heroin Adviceline: 020 7729 9904
(Advice, support and information to drug users and their friends and families on all aspects of drug use and drug-related legal problems)

Narcotics Anonymous: 020 7730 0009

National Drugs Helpline: 0800 776600 (24-hour freephone)
(Confidential advice, including information on local services)

Release Out of Hours: 020 7603 8654 (helpline: Monday–Friday, 6 pm–10 pm; Saturday and Sunday, 8 am–12 midnight)

Resource leaflets:
Harm Minimization Advice
Drug Use Diary

Eating disorders — F50

Presenting complaints

The patient may indulge in binge-eating and extreme weight-control measures such as self-induced vomiting, excessive use of diet pills and laxative abuse. This may be recognised first on reception into prison when low weight is recorded, or it may become more apparent after a period in prison when abnormal eating behaviours have been observed.

Both anorexia and bulimia may present as physical disorders, eg amenorrhoea, seizures and cardiac arrhythmias that require monitoring or treatment.

Diagnostic features

Common features are:

- unreasonable fear of being fat or gaining weight
- extensive efforts to control weight, eg strict dieting, vomiting, use of purgatives, excessive exercise
- denial that weight or eating habits are a problem
- low mood, anxiety/irritability
- obsessional symptoms
- relationship difficulties
- increasing withdrawal and
- school and work problems.

Patients with anorexia nervosa typically show:

- severe dieting despite very low weight: body mass index (BMI) < 17.5 kg m^{-2} (BMI = weight [kg]/height [m^2])
- a distorted body image, ie an unreasonable belief that one is overweight and
- amenorrhoea.

Patients with bulimia typically show:

- binge-eating, ie eating large amounts of food in a few hours and
- purging: attempts to eliminate food by self-induced vomiting or via diuretic or laxative use.

A patient may show both anorexic and bulimic patterns at different times. Binge-eating may be very difficult in a prison setting and the inability to use this coping mechanism may result in increased anxiety and the use of alternative maladaptive coping strategies, eg deliberate self-harm, aggression.

The medical consequences of severe weight loss include amenorrhoea, dental problems, muscle weakness, renal stones, constipation and liver dysfunction. Medical complications of purging include dental problems, salivary-gland swelling, kidney stones, cardiac arrhythmias and seizures.

Eating disorders are rarer in men than in women. There is an association between eating disorders and childhood abuse.

Differential diagnosis

- **Depression — F32#** (page 47) may occur along with bulimia or anorexia.
- Physical illness may cause weight loss.
- There may be coexisting problems such as drugs and alcohol misuse or self-harm.

Essential information for the patient and primary support group

- Purging and severe starvation may cause serious physical harm. Anorexia nervosa can be life-threatening.
- Purging and severe dieting are ineffective ways of achieving lasting weight control.
- Self-help groups, leaflets and books may be helpful in explaining the diagnosis clearly and involving the patient in treatment.

Advice and support to the patient and primary support group

The prison doctor can undertake some simple steps to treat eating disorders, ideally with the help of the counsellors, healthcare staff and/or a dietitian.

In anorexia nervosa:

- Expect denial and ambivalence. Elicit the patient's concerns about the negative effects of anorexia nervosa on aspects of their life. Ask the patient about the benefits that anorexia has for them, eg the feeling of being in control, feeling safe, being able to get care and attention from family. Do not try to force the patient to change if he/she is not ready.
- Educate the patient about food and weight.
- Weigh the patient regularly and chart their weight. Set manageable goals in agreement with the patient (eg aim for a 0.5 kg increase per week; this requires a calorie intake of about 2500 kcal day^{-1}). A supportive member of staff who the patient trusts may be able to help the patient achieve this. Consultation with a dietitian may be helpful to establish the normal calorie and nutrient intake and the regular patterns of eating.
- A return to normal eating habits may be a distant goal.
- Provide counselling, if available, about traumatic life events and difficulties (past and present) that seem significant in the onset or maintenance of the disorder (see **Counselling and other psychological therapies** below).

In bulimia nervosa:

- Use a collaborative approach.
- A food diary can be a useful therapeutic tool in discussions with the patient.
- Educate the patient about the need to eat regularly throughout the day (three meals plus two snacks) to reduce urges to binge.
- Set mutually agreed, gradual goals to increase number of meals eaten, the variety of foods allowed, and to reduce vomiting and laxatives.
- Help the patient identify the psychological and physiological triggers for binge-eating and make clear plans to cope more effectively with these trigger events, eg plan an alternative behaviour.
- Discuss the patient's biased beliefs about weight, shape and eating (eg carbohydrates are fattening) and encourage a review of their rigid views about body image, eg patients believe no one will like them unless they are very thin. Do not simply state that the patient's view is wrong.

Provide counselling, if available, about the difficulties underlying or maintaining the disorder, eg childhood abuse, relationship difficulties or concurrent problems with substance abuse (see **Counselling and other psychological therapies** below).

Additional advice to staff (with patient permission)

- Support will be required around eating to reduce anxiety at those times — critical comments or exhortations to eat will not help.
- Encouraging reasonable levels of activity and exercise to promote a healthy lifestyle is important and can help in re-establishing eating habits and appetite.
- Help to develop alternative coping strategies. Attendance at education and/or work will be helpful.
- Explanations about the disorder and the treatment approaches for personal officers will help them be supportive of the patient day to day.

Medication

- In bulimia nervosa, antidepressants (eg fluoxetine, 60 mg) are effective in reducing bingeing and vomiting in a proportion of cases.[N100] However, compliance with medication may be poor (see *BNF*, Section 4.3).
- No pharmacological treatment for anorexia has been established to date.[N101] Psychiatric conditions (eg depression) may co-occur and may respond to pharmacological treatment.
- Order blood tests for urea and electrolytes.

Referral

Refer for urgent assessment (if possible, to the secondary mental-health services with expertise in eating disorders) if:

- BMI < 13.5 kg m^{-2}, especially if there has been rapid weight loss
- potassium < 2.5 mmol l^{-1}
- there is severe bone marrow dysfunction with loss of platelets
- there is evidence of proximal myopathy
- there are significant gastrointestinal symptoms from repeated vomiting, eg blood in vomitus
- there is significant risk of suicide or
- there are other complicating factors, eg substance or alcohol abuse.

Refer to specialist mental-health services for assessment if there is a lack of progress despite the above measures.

Counselling and other psychological therapies

If available, consider family therapy for appropriate patients, including anorexic patients (under 18 years),[102] individual psychotherapy for anorexic patients over 18, and cognitive-behavioural therapy[103] for those with bulimia. If detention in prison has revealed an eating disorder for the first time, liaison with community providers for access to therapeutic interventions on release is important.

Consider non-statutory/voluntary services/self-help groups.

Where the patient is on remand or on a short sentence, and especially if the traumatic life events include severe childhood abuse, appropriate types of help will encourage the patient to focus on the present and help him/her deal with current problems for which solutions may be possible.

Resources for patients and primary support groups

Eating Disorders Association: 01603 621 414 (helpline: 9 am–6.30 pm)
(Self-help support groups for sufferers, and their relatives and friends. Assists in putting people in touch with sources of help in their own area)

Centre for Eating Disorders (Scotland): 0131 668 3051
(Information, private psychotherapy, self-help manuals, information packs and a helpline)

Anorexia Bulimia Careline (Northern Ireland): 02890 614440

Overeaters Anonymous: 01454 857158 (recorded message)
(Self-help groups for those suffering from eating disorders or overeating)

Resource leaflet:
Food and Behaviour Diary

U Schmidt, J Treasure, 1993, *Getting Better Bit(e) by Bit(e) Survival Guide for Sufferers of Bulimia Nervosa and Binge Eating Disorders.* Lawrence Erlbaum, 1993 Hove. (Self-help manual of proven efficacy for sufferers of bulimia and binge-eating disorders)[104]

J Treasure. *Anorexia Nervosa: A Survival Guide for Families, Friends and Sufferers.* London: Psychology Press, 1997

Both the above books are available from the Institute of Psychiatry: URL: http://www.iop.kcl.ac.uk/IoP/Departments/PsychMed/EDU/GuidedSelfCare .stm; or the distributors Taylor & Francis. Tel: 01264 343071

CG Fairburn. *Overcoming Binge Eating.* New York: Guilford, 1995. Advice tested in controlled research

Generalised anxiety — F41.1

Presenting complaints

The patient may present initially with tension-related physical symptoms (eg headache or a pounding heart) or with insomnia. Enquiry will reveal prominent anxiety.

Diagnostic features

Multiple symptoms of anxiety or tension include:

- physical arousal, eg dizziness, sweating, a fast or pounding heart, a dry mouth, stomach pains or chest pains
- mental tension, eg worry, feeling tense or nervous, poor concentration, fear that something dangerous will happen and the patient will not be able to cope and
- physical tension, eg restlessness, headaches, tremors or an inability to relax.

Symptoms may last for months and recur regularly. Often they are triggered by stressful events in those prone to worry.

Differential diagnosis

- **Alcohol misuse — F10** or **Drug-use disorders — F11#** (pages 18 and 55) if heavy alcohol or drug use is present. Anxiety is a common symptom during detoxification/withdrawal. It may also underlie substance misuse and become prominent after withdrawal. Substances may be used to self-medicate for anxiety. If symptoms of anxiety remain or increase following detox, suspect an underlying anxiety disorder and/or benzodiazepine dependence (see **Comorbidity**, page 191).
- **Depression — F32#** (page 47) if a low or sad mood is prominent.
- **Chronic mixed anxiety and depression — F41.2** (page 33).
- **Panic disorder — F41.0** (page 67) if discrete attacks of unprovoked anxiety are present.
- **Phobic disorders — F40** (page 79) if fear and avoidance of specific situations are present.
- Certain physical conditions (eg thyrotoxicosis) or medications (eg methylxanthines, β-agonists) may cause anxiety symptoms.
- Anxiety can be a symptom of post-traumatic stress disorder. **Post-traumatic stress disorder — F43.1** (page 82).

Essential information for the patient and primary support group

- Stress and worry have both physical and mental effects.
- Where drugs or alcohol have previously been used to deal with underlying anxiety, prison presents an opportunity to learn alternative ways of dealing with it.
- Learning skills to reduce the effects of stress (not sedative medication) is the most effective relief.[105]

Advice and support to the patient and primary support group

- Encourage the patient to use relaxation methods daily to reduce the physical symptoms of tension. The *Managing Anxiety* leaflet on the disk includes a relaxation exercise 💾. If the patient has reading difficulties, a member of the healthcare team or other member of staff may be able to go over the contents of the leaflet with the patient.
- Advise a reduction in caffeine consumption, if appropriate.[46]
- Try to avoid using cigarettes, other drugs or alcohol to cope with anxiety.
- Help the patient plan activities that are relaxing, pleasurable or confidence building. Exercise may be helpful.[49,50] If necessary, consider advocating for improved access to appropriate activities.
- Identify and challenge exaggerated worries to help the patient reduce anxiety symptoms:
  — Identify exaggerated worries or pessimistic thoughts, eg when a visitor does not arrive on time, the patient worries that they no longer want contact with them.
  — Discuss ways to question these exaggerated worries when they occur, eg 'I am starting to be caught up in worry again. My visitor is only a few minutes late. He will probably be here soon.
- Structured problem-solving methods[48] can help patients to manage current life problems or stresses that contribute to anxiety symptoms. Support the patient to carry out the following steps:
  — Identifying events that trigger excessive worry. (For example, a young woman presents with worry, tension, nausea and insomnia. These symptoms began after she learned that her son was behaving badly in school following her conviction).
  — Listing as many possible solutions as the patient can think of (eg discussing her concerns with a close friend or relative, applying for an extended family visit, writing to her son's general practitioner, contacting a voluntary organisation that helps families of prisoners).
  — Listing the advantages and disadvantages of each possible solution. (The patient should do this, perhaps between appointments).
  — Choosing his/her preferred approach.
  — Working out the steps necessary to achieve the plan.
  — Setting a date to review the plan. Identify and reinforce things that are working).
- Identify possible resources for problem solving, relaxation, yoga (eg counsellor, voluntary agency teaching meditation/relaxation; see **Resources Directory** page 316).

Medication

Medication is a secondary treatment in the management of generalised anxiety.[105,106] It may be used, however, if significant anxiety symptoms persist despite the measures suggested above.

Anti-anxiety medication[N107] (see *BNF*, Section 4.1.2) can only be used for ≤ 2 weeks. Avoid short-acting benzodiazepines; consider diazepam. Longer-term use may lead to dependence and is likely to result in the return of symptoms when discontinued.

Antidepressant drugs,[108] eg imipramine, clomipramine, paroxetine or venlafaxine, may be helpful, especially if the symptoms of depression are present. They do not lead to dependence or rebound symptoms, but can lead to withdrawal symptoms and so should be tapered gradually (see *BNF*, Section 4.3).

β-Blockers may help control physical symptoms such as tremor.[109]

Referral

See **General referral criteria** (page 149).

Non-urgent referral to the secondary mental-health services is advised if the patient's symptoms are sufficiently severe or enduring to interfere with his/her social or occupational functioning.

If available, consider cognitive-behavioural therapy or anxiety management.[N110] Self-care classes and 'assisted bibliotherapy' can also be effective in the primary care of milder anxiety.[111,112]

Resources for patients and primary support groups

No Panic Helpline: 01952 590545 (10 am–10 pm); 0800 7831531 (freephone infoline)
(Helpline, information booklets and local self-help groups for people with anxiety, phobias obsessions, panic)

Prison Phoenix Trust: 01865 512521/512522
Prison Phoenix Trust, PO Box 328, Oxford OX2 7HF. Fax: 01865 516011
(Teaches and encourages the use of techniques such as meditation and yoga among prisoners, through correspondence and a network of teachers)

Stresswatch Scotland 01563 574144 (helpline); 01563 570886 (office)
(Advice, information, materials on panic, anxiety, stress phobias. Thirty-five local groups)

Triumph Over Phobia (TOP) UK: 01225 330353
(Structured self-help groups. Produces self-help materials)

Resource leaflets:
Coping with Anxiety

Mind Publications produces booklets on *Understanding Anxiety* and other relevant topics. Available from: Mind England and Wales. Tel: 020 8519 2122; Northern Ireland Tel: 02890 237937; Scotland: Tel: 0141 568 7000

Alice Neville. *Who's Afraid…? Coping With Fear, Anxiety and Panic Attacks.* Arrow, 1991

Panic disorder — F41.0

Presenting complaints

Patients may present with one or more physical symptoms (eg chest pain, dizziness or shortness of breath) or unexplained episodes of intense fear. Further enquiry shows the full pattern described below.

Diagnostic features

The patient experiences unexplained attacks of anxiety or fear, which begin suddenly, develop rapidly and may last only a few minutes.

The panics often occur with physical sensations such as palpitations, chest pain, sensations of choking, churning stomach, dizziness, feelings of unreality or fear of personal disaster (losing control or going mad, sudden death or having a heart attack).

A panic often leads to fear of another panic attack and avoidance of places where panics have occurred.

Differential diagnosis

Many medical conditions may cause symptoms similar to panic, eg arrhythmia, cerebral ischaemia, coronary disease, asthma or thyrotoxicosis. It is not uncommon for individuals with these conditions additionally to suffer from panic. History and physical examination should exclude many of these and should reassure the patient. However, avoid unnecessary medical tests or therapies.

- Drugs may induce the symptoms of panic.
- **Phobic disorders** — F40 (page 79) if panics tend to occur in specific situations.
- **Depression** — F32# (page 47) if a low or sad mood is also present.

Essential information for the patient and primary support group

- Panic is common and can be treated.
- Anxiety often produces frightening physical symptoms. Chest pain, dizziness or shortness of breath are not necessarily signs of a physical illness; they will pass when anxiety is controlled. Explain how the body's arousal reaction provides the physical basis for their symptoms and how anxiety about a physical symptom can create a vicious cycle. A diagram may be helpful.
- Panic anxiety also causes frightening thoughts (eg fear of dying, a feeling that one is going mad or will lose control) and vice versa. These also pass when anxiety is controlled.
- Mental and physical anxiety reinforce each other. Concentrating on physical symptoms will increase fear.
- A person who withdraws from or avoids situations where panics have occurred will only strengthen his/her anxiety.

Advice and support to the patient and primary support group[N106]

- Advise the patient to identify the early warning signs of an impending panic attack and take the following steps at the first sign of a panic:

— Stay where you are until the panic passes, which may take up to 1 hour. Do **not** leave the situation. Start slow, relaxed breathing, counting up to four on each breath in and each breath out. Breathing too deeply (hyperventilation) can cause some of the physical symptoms of panic. Controlled breathing will reduce the physical symptoms. Do something to focus your thinking on something visible, tangible and non-threatening, eg look at a picture on the wall.

— If hyperventilation is severe, sit down and breathe into a paper bag so that the increased carbon dioxide will slow down your breathing (unless the patient has asthma or cardiovascular disease).

— Concentrate on controlling anxiety and not on the physical symptoms

— Tell yourself that this is a panic attack and that the frightening thoughts and sensations will eventually pass. Note the time passing on your watch. It may feel like a long time but it will usually only be a few minutes.

• Identify exaggerated fears that occur during panic, eg patient's fears that he/she is having a heart attack.

• Discuss ways to challenge these fears during panic, eg the patient reminds him/herself: 'I am not having a heart attack. This is a panic, and it will pass in a few minutes'.

• If possible, identify someone (a member of the healthcare team or other staff member) who the patient trusts who may support him/her in taking the above actions.

• Monitor and, if necessary, reduce caffeine intake.

• Try to avoid using cigarettes or other drugs to cope with anxiety.

• Self-help groups, books, tapes or leaflets may help the patient manage panic symptoms and overcome fears.[113] If the patient has reading difficulties, a member of the healthcare team or another member of staff may be able to discuss the contents of the leaflet *Managing Anxiety* on the disk with him/her 💾.

Medication

Many patients will benefit from the above measures and will not need medication, unless their mood is low.

• If attacks are frequent and severe or if the patient is significantly depressed, antidepressants, including tricyclics (TCAs) and selective serotonin re-uptake inhibitors (SSRIs), may be helpful.[N114] Paroxetine and citalopram are currently licensed for panic (see *BNF*, Section 4.3). There can be a slight worsening of symptoms initially, so advise the patient to plan reduced activities for the week following the first prescription.

• Encourage patients to face fears without the use of benzodiazepines. However, where the feared situation is rare, occasional short-term use of anti-anxiety medication may be helpful.[N115] Regular use may lead to dependence and is likely to result in a return of symptoms when discontinued.

Referral

See **General referral criteria** (page 149).

Non-urgent referral to the secondary mental-health services or a counsellor with appropriate special training is advised for assessment for cognitive-behavioural psychotherapy for patients who do not improve or those whose lifestyle is severely compromised. (This can be particularly effective for patients with panic disorder.[116,117]) Cognitive-behavioural therapy (CBT), which has been developed in specialist settings, also appears to be effective in primary care.[118]

Panic commonly causes physical symptoms; avoid unnecessary medical referral for physical symptoms if you are certain of the diagnosis.

Consider self-help/voluntary/non-statutory services.

Resources for patients and primary support groups

No Panic Helpline: 01952 590545 (10 am–10 pm); 0800 7831531 (freephone infoline)
(Helpline, information booklets and local self-help groups for people with anxiety, phobias, obsessions and panic)

Stresswatch Scotland: 01563 574144 (helpline); 01563 570886 (office)
(Advice, information, materials on panic, anxiety, stress phobias. Thirty-five local groups)

Triumph Over Phobia (TOP) UK: 01225 330353
(Structured self-help groups. Produces self-help material)

Resource leaflets:
Managing Anxiety

Mind Publications produces booklets on *How To Cope With Panic Attacks* and other relevant topics. Available from: Mind England and Wales: Tel: 020 8519 2122; Northern Ireland: Tel: 02890 237973; Scotland: 0141 568 7000

Isaac Marks. *Living with Fear*. New York: McGraw Hill 1978. Self-help manual

Alice Neville. *Who's Afraid…? Coping With Fear, Anxiety and Panic Attacks*. Arrow, 1991

Personality (behavioural) disorders — F60–69

Introduction

Many people in prison have a personality disorder. Some have suffered extremes of abuse and neglect as children leading to very disturbed behaviours and ways of relating to others. People with personality disorders are very difficult to manage. However, treatable mental disorders occur frequently in people with personality disorders. The aims of this guideline are to help primary-care staff to do the following.

- Form and maintain a therapeutic relationship with these patients:
  - to treat comorbid mental and physical disorders
  - to recognise and reinforce the patient's capacity to change their immediate situation at times of crisis and
  - to offer support and thus contribute to avoiding further deterioration.
- Identify those patients who may benefit from further assessment and treatment for their behavioural problems by specialists.
- Participate in the multidisciplinary management of very difficult patients.

Presenting complaints

Most patients present with complaints of another disorder rather than the personality problem itself. They may present with anxiety, depression, eating problems or deliberate self-harm, or they may repeatedly seek psychotropic medication. People with personality disorder may experience high levels of distress. Staff or other inmates may express concern about the patient's behaviour, eg overly hostile and/or frequent attempts at self-harm. The patient's personality problem often interferes with treatment for another mental disorder.

Diagnostic features

The features of personality disorder are displayed in a patient's behaviour and relationships, and may also affect the organisation around them.

Behaviour

The patient displays a long-term, stable pattern of experience and behaviour that started in early life, deviates markedly from cultural norms and leads to distress and impairment. The patient behaves in this way most or all the time, in some or all of a range of settings (eg work, home, when out with friends, in prison) without learning from the negative responses of others towards them. There are many different kinds of personality disorders and in prison people most often have features of more than one type. The types of personality disorders most commonly found in prison are the following.

Antisocial or dissocial personality disorder

Most individuals in prison are inclined towards an antisocial lifestyle. Sometimes this rises to the level of a disorder. The features of the disorder include the following.

- A disregard for and a violation of the rights of others, eg violence, theft, cruelty to animals.
- Deceitfulness.
- Reckless disregard for safety.
- Consistent irresponsibility and a disregard for rules and regulations.
- Inability to maintain relationships for any length of time.
- Low tolerance for frustration, leading to aggression or violence.
- Lack of remorse; a tendency to blame others or rationalise their own behaviour.
- Tendency not to learn from experience, particularly from punishment.
- Often superficially cooperative and charming.

Emotionally unstable disorder (also known as 'borderline personality disorder')

Individuals may be emotionally unstable and, in some, this may rise to the level of a disorder. The features of the disorder include the following.

- Unstable and intense interpersonal relationships, eg extremes of idealising and denigrating the other person, sometimes friendly, sometimes intensely angry, fearful of abandonment.
- Highly reactive, sudden mood swings, eg intense, inappropriate anger, transient, stress-related paranoid thoughts.
- Chronic feeling of emptiness, clinging dependency and terror of being left alone.
- Marked impulsiveness that is potentially self-damaging, eg reckless driving, sexual promiscuity, excessive spending sprees, binge-eating.
- Poor ability to plan ahead and to solve problems.

Paranoid personality disorder

Many individuals in prison display paranoid characteristics and, in some, this may rise to the level of a disorder. The features of the disorder include the following.

- Distrust and suspiciousness, eg unjustified suspicions that others are exploiting or harming him/her, reluctance to confide in others, bears grudges, will not accept rational explanation.
- Being tense, anxious, irritable or angry.
- Preoccupation with justice and rules.

Individual relationships

The individual's problems and feelings of fear, humiliation, anger and need are played out in their relationships. For example, they may:

- bully and attempt to dominate those around them, eg via non-verbal intimidation, critical questioning, threats of complaints or violence
- use charm, flattery, friendly support to obtain special privileges or develop a 'special relationship' that goes beyond the boundaries of a professional relationship
- become very dependent upon you or other staff
- be resistant to authority or
- be critical of you or others who are working with them.

The genuine distress the patient feels may be experienced by the other person as manipulation.

Organisational relationships

The intense feelings and disturbed behaviours and relationships commonly affect both staff teams and the relationships between departments. For example, the patient may idealise and denigrate different members of staff causing the favoured staff member to doubt the good will or professional ability of the denigrated one. This may cause division and conflict within the healthcare staff team and the healthcare staff and other staff, eg discipline officers, probation officers, chaplain, psychologist.

Differential diagnosis

Personality disorder commonly coexists with mental disorder. A history from a relative or close friend may be useful to distinguish the two. Personality disorder is a disorder of relating to others and those symptoms become visible in relationships with others. The symptoms of mental illness are visible when the patient is alone. In mental illness, the patient's behaviour becomes different from what is normal for that patient. In personality disorder, the behaviour is normal for that patient but is different from the norm in his/her culture.

If behaviour, eg 'out of character' aggression, has developed for the first time in adulthood, is of recent onset or is temporary, consider the following.

- **Depression** and **Anxiety disorders** (pages 47 and 33). Aggression and/or irritability may be a sign of depression.
- **Acute or chronic psychosis** (pages 11 and 36).
- **Post-traumatic stress disorder** (page 82).
- **Adjustment disorder** (page 15).
- Abuse of stimulants or hallucinogenic drugs (see **Drug misuse**, page 55).
- Medical condition causing personality change, eg brain injury, dementia.

Also, consider the patient's cultural, social and family background. Check that the person's behaviour is constant across a number of different settings. For example, ask: 'Do even little things get you very angry?' 'Was this true at home as well as here in prison?' Check the available records such as the inmate medical record (IMR) and probation records. If criminal behaviour is undertaken for gain and other features are absent, consider 'no mental or behavioural disorder'.

Diagnosis of personality disorder is difficult as many of the diagnostic features are present (though in a lesser degree) in all people. A formal diagnosis of personality disorder should only be made by a specialist and where there is reason to believe that such a diagnosis will lead to the patient being offered improved management, eg assessment for medication or transfer to a therapeutic prison.

Comorbidity

A person may have a personality disorder **and** a mental disorder. Mental disorder (eg psychosis, anxiety, depression) may emerge in times of stress. For example, a personality-disordered prisoner spending time in segregation may experience psychotic symptoms.

- **Self-harm** (eg cutting, drug overdoses) is common in borderline and antisocial types, especially where there are real or perceived relationship problems, rejections or losses.

- **Depression and substance abuse** are common and increase the risk of suicide.
- Someone with personality disorder may experience **psychotic episodes** when under particular stress.
- Most people in prison with personality disorder show features of more than one type of personality disorder.

Information for the patient and primary support group

With patient permission, the following information may be given to others.

- Change is possible but it is very difficult and requires insight (ie the ability to see that the patient plays some part in causing or maintaining his/her own distress; that it is not all the fault of others) and substantial motivation. Where that motivation is present, long-term specialist treatment is required.
- Depression, anxiety, transient psychotic illness and substance abuse can be treated.
- Problem-solving skills can help the patient cope with particular problems, but they will not change the overall personality.
- Treatment of any sort (including for associated conditions) requires the patient's active involvement. The relationship with the professional(s) concerned is crucial.

Advice and support to the patient

All patients

- Show respect for the patient and afford them dignity, but do not expect to like them.
- Consider your own safety at all times (see **Managing aggression**, page 282).
- Assess the risk of danger to yourself, others and the patient (depression and self-harming behaviour are common).
- Be very clear about your role and its boundaries. For example:
  — the timing and duration of appointments
  — do not buy or bring things in for patients
  — do not discuss your own personal details with them and
  — do not develop a 'special relationship' that is secret from your colleagues.
- Be honest, though sympathetic, in communications. Keep promises; conversely, do not make promises you cannot keep.
- Communicate with others in your team and, as much as is possible within confidentiality, with staff in other departments who are involved with the patient. Tell them about the approach you are taking. Ensure a consistent approach.
- Treat comorbid conditions.
- Focus on immediate, everyday problems. The aim is not to cure the personality disorder but to help the patient deal with everyday life.
- Liaise, with the patient's permission, with other staff who may be able to help address any immediate, practical problem. For example, wing staff about bullying, probation about resettlement following release. Be aware of the potential for division and conflict between staff (see **Organisational relationships** above). If problems occur, try seeing the patient together with the other staff concerned.
- Support and reinforce any legal actions or interests that develop self-esteem, eg work, creativity, education, exercise. Help them to develop any existing strengths, but aim low. Modest success can build into larger gains later; failures can undo good work.

Very difficult patients

It is **essential** that very difficult patients are managed in a multidisciplinary way. Consider convening a case conference involving healthcare, mental-health staff, work supervisor, residential (wing) manager, probation officer, psychologist and chaplain as appropriate. Agree a management plan and inform the patient of that plan in the presence of all participants. Sharing responsibility can reduce stress/burnout and risk of dependence on a patient worker (see **Managing prisoners with complex presentations and very difficult behaviours**, page 202).

Antisocial behaviours

- Aim to maintain an open and trusting atmosphere.
- Identify clearly the reason the patient is seeking help. Ask the patient, 'Why did you come to the Centre?' 'What do you think are your difficulties?'
- Start from the standpoint that there is a legitimate problem underlying most requests, eg 'I may not be able to help you with medication at this centre. I could perhaps help you if you were prepared to tell me why you think you need this medication. But otherwise there is nothing I can do for you'.
- Do not accept all information at face value. Seek further evidence to support the patient's statements. For example, if the patient says he/she is depressed, seek out symptoms normally associated with depression using open questions such as 'What other problems have you been experiencing?' 'What have you been doing with your time?' rather than closed questions such as 'And have you lost interest in the things you normally enjoy?' Allow the person adequate personal space — do not crowd them.
- Do not take the patient's comments personally.
- Allow the patient a chance to talk freely about his/her concerns.
- Set limits and clear guidelines about expected behaviour, eg verbal abuse will not be tolerated.
- It is safest to treat all patients in this way, as you may not know in advance which are difficult.

Emotionally unstable (borderline) behaviours

- Set clear limits. Have a very clear management plan: how frequently you will see the patient, what expectations they have and what you can realistically offer them.
- Try to avoid expressing anger or irritation with the patient — remain outwardly calm and objective. Aim to be firm yet caring and do not argue with the patient.
- It may be counter-productive to tell patients that you believe them to have a personality disorder. It may be better to use terms such as 'exceptionally sensitive', ie they react with more pain, fear and anger to the ups and downs of life than do most people, and so tend to experience many crises in their lives. You can then attempt to agree a plan with the patient, and with other staff, to help them deal a bit better with their crises and other day-to-day problems when they arise.
- Make an agreement about contact between scheduled appointments, eg allow only scheduled appointments, or define what constitutes an 'emergency' which will mean that an unscheduled appointment is allowed.

- Establish a team approach. Establish a clear protocol for how all members of the team will respond to this patient if on duty during a crisis. Crisis contacts should be brief, focused and goal-oriented. If possible, give the patient some responsibility for resolving the crisis. The crisis care plan should involve other staff who are involved in responding to incidents of self-harm, eg chaplain, personal officer, suicide prevention team.
- While formal contracts, sometimes signed by all relevant parties, can sometimes help, they require meticulous attention to detail, require regular updating in the light of progress or deterioration and should not be introduced when the professionals concerned are angry.

Paranoid behaviours

- Assess dangerousness, especially if the patient is aggressive as well as paranoid. Be aware of hidden weapons as paranoid patients may hide weapons to protect themselves.
- Avoid over friendly or inquisitive behaviour — be professional.
- Listen to the patient's concerns.
- Accept but do not confirm the patient's beliefs.
- Plan clear and mutual goals, eg 'How can we work this out together?'
- Explain **everything**, all treatments, medications, etc.
- Empathise with the patient's anxiety, eg 'I realise it can be upsetting to talk about yourself to someone you don't know well. If you have questions, please ask'.
- Share information with the patient, eg allow him/her to read letters you have written about him/her. Write letters bearing in mind that the patient may see a copy at some stage.
- Keep careful notes, documenting interactions where appropriate. Paranoid patients may be litigious.

Advice and liaison with wing and other staff

- If hostility or paranoia is focused on a particular inmate, member of staff, or type of inmate such as a particular ethnic group, make staff aware. Steps should be taken to protect staff and inmates who may be involved in the patient's paranoid thinking. For example, a paranoid inmate should not share a cell.
- Recommend that these patients have an experienced officer as personal officer. There should not be only one unskilled person working alone.
- Ensure the manager of the wing/unit where the patient is located has a copy of the information sheet on *Personality Disorders*, which is on the disk 💾.
- The prison regime is an important part of management. Discuss work, education, exercise and opportunities to be creative.
- Staff working with this group of individuals, whether on wings or in the healthcare centre, need supervision and support to prevent breaches of role boundaries, eg developing a special relationship that is secret from colleagues.
- For very challenging patients, identify a core, multidisciplinary group (wing manager, psychologist and others as appropriate) to develop and monitor a management plan.

Medication

Offer treatment for associated illness.

- See **Depression** and **Anxiety** (pages 47 and 33) for advice on medication for these conditions. If the patient is **abusing substances**, interactions with prescribed medication are possible and the efficacy of antidepressants is lessened. Benzodiazepines should be avoided because of possible interactions with illegal substances.
- People with a personality disorder may suffer episodes of **psychosis** when under stress. For information about medication, see page 70.

There are no drugs for the treatment of personality disorder. Medication may be tried for certain behavioural problems, though evidence of effectiveness is weak. Careful assessment of the benefit versus side-effects must be made. Decisions about patient consent and capacity are also particularly difficult. Therefore, a careful clinical evaluation by a specialist is required before medication for the long-term treatment of behaviours associated with personality disorder is started.[119] If there is a poor relationship between the clinician and patient, there is a danger of medication being used by the clinician purely for control or by the patient to self-harm, or to sell to others. Drugs that a specialist may prescribe include:

- **Sedative antipsychotics**: may be helpful if paranoid or dissocial behaviours are prominent and the patient is highly aroused.
- **Antipsychotic drugs**: may help patients who harm themselves impulsively and those who display symptoms suggestive of (but falling short of) frank psychotic illness.[120]
- **Serotonin re-uptake inhibitor (SSRI) antidepressants**: have been reported as useful in reducing aggression in some patients with dissocial and borderline personality disorder.[121]
- **Carbamazepine treatment**: has been shown to help reduce aggressive behaviour, especially in patients with a history of head injury, genuine amnesia for assaults, the *déjà vu* phenomenon, olfactory hallucinations and abnormalities shown by electroencephalography or brain imaging.[122] Careful monitoring is required.

Dealing with cutting or self-harm in the context of personality disorder

Admission to psychiatric hospital or prison healthcare centre should be for treatment of comorbid disorders or indicated by suicide risk. Admission should be part of a carefully prepared crisis plan, agreed in advance by all parties. In-patient contracts, drawn up and signed by the patient and staff, may be helpful but must not make support contingent on ceasing of the self-harming behaviour immediately and should not be drawn up when clinicians are angry (for further advice, see **Assessment and management following an act of self-harm**, page 211). Not everyone who cuts, burns or otherwise mutilates themselves displays the full pattern of behaviour of a personality disorder.

Specialist consultation or referral

Refer urgently to mental-health services if:

- paranoia is marked, excessive, there is a past history of extreme violence and the patient is threatening violence (forensic services are to be preferred, if available) and
- psychotic illness is evident.

Refer for assessment to mental-health services if you are unsure if the diagnosis is personality disorder, mental illness or both.

Although the evidence base for the following treatments is poor, these psychological interventions may be useful for patients motivated to undertake them.

- **Anger management**:
  - If the patient shows problems controlling and expressing anger, if they have no, or only very mild, paranoid features, and they can discuss their own behaviour, anger management may be useful in reducing maladaptive behaviour at least in the short-term.[123]
  - If problems in controlling anger or aggression have led to the crime the patient has committed and the patient has at least 1 year of their sentence still to serve, the patient may be eligible for one of the relevant Prison Service offending behaviour courses.

  For more details, see **Offending behaviour programmes** (page 117).
- **Structured problem-solving** may be useful for associated problems that trigger self-harming behaviour, though it has not been tested specifically in personality-disordered patients.[120]
- **Assertiveness training, anxiety management, social skills training or cognitive-behaviour therapy** may help if the patient is chronically over-anxious, dependent and fearful.[124]
- **Dialectical behaviour therapy** has been shown to reduce the frequency of deliberate self-harm in people with emotionally unstable (borderline) personality disorder. This therapy is complicated and time-intensive to administer.[125]
- **Psychotherapy** for personality-disordered patients needs to be long- not short-term.[119]

Consider referral to HMP Grendon Underwood if the patient has:

- a curiosity and a wish to tell their story
- psychological mindedness
- motivation
- ability to see that other people might have another point of view
- more than 2 years left in current sentence
- no appeal against their sentence, current or pending
- objective evidence of being free of substance misuse for 6 months
- no psychoactive medication for 3 months or while at Grendon or
- satisfactory reports from the wing officer, probation officer, chaplain, psychologist and medical officer.

Other prison treatment centres (TCs) include HMP Wormwood Scrubs (Max Glitt Unit), HMP Dovegate TC and the lifers' TC at HMP Gartree.

Prerelease plans

Ensure patients are assessed in good time for both the risk and treatment facilities that may help them if they are willing to engage in treatment. This is particularly important for emotionally unstable patients who react badly to real or imagined abandonment.

For details of prerelease planning appropriate for all patients, see **Managing the interface with the NHS and other agencies** (page 149).

Facilities that provide services for people with a personality disorder include the following.

- **Henderson Hospital**: a centrally funded outreach service based in Birmingham and Crewe that treats people with enduring emotional, relationship and behavioural problems, including impulsive, violent and self-harming behaviour and other associated problems. Patients are expected to be free of medication and not currently detained under the Mental Health Act 1983. South East and London NHS Regions, contact: Dr Alex Esterhuyzen, Henderson Hospital, 2 Homeland Drive, Sutton SM2 5LT. Tel: 020 8661 1611. West Midlands and South West NHS Regions, contact: Dr Ian Birtle, Main House, c/o South Birmingham Mental Health NHS Trust Therapeutic Community Service, 22 Summer Road, Acocks Green, Birmingham B27 7UT. Tel: 0121 678 3244; Northern and North West NHS Regions, contact: Dr Keith Hyde, Webb House, c/o Mental Health Services of Salford, Victoria Avenue, Crewe CW2 7SQ. Tel: 01270 580 770. For patients from outside these areas or those from Scotland, Wales and Northern Ireland, contact the NHS Mental Health Trust nearest the patient's home address.
- **Cassell Hospital**: treats women with less severe personality disorders. 1 Ham Common, Richmond TW10 7JF. Tel: 020 8940 8181.
- **Francis Dixon Lodge**: provides group-orientated self-help programmes for those with personality and emotional difficulties. Gipsy Lane, Leicester LE5 0TD. Tel: 0116 2256800.

Resources for patients and primary support groups

Listener or buddy scheme. Where the patient is considered dangerous, steps should be taken to protect listeners, eg personal alarms

Alcoholics Anonymous: 08457 697555 (24-hour helpline)
(Gives telephone support numbers and self-help groups across the UK for men and women trying to achieve and maintain sobriety)

Borderline website: URL: http://www. BPDCentral.com
(Mainly for families of people with borderline personality disorder)

Gamblers Anonymous: 020 7384 3040
PO Box 88, London SW10 0EU
(Provides advice and support to patients with addiction/habit disorders)

Narcotics Anonymous: 020 7730 0009 (helpline); 020 7251 4007 (office)
202 City Road, London EC1V 2PH
(Provides advice and support to patients with drug disorders)

Samaritans: 08457 90 90 90

Understanding Personality Disorders. Available from: MIND Publications, 15–19 Broadway, London E15 4BQ. Tel: 020 8 519 2122. Leaflet with straightforward explanations. It is useful for family members, staff and others

Phobic disorders — F40

Includes claustrophobia, agoraphobia and social phobia

Presenting complaints

Patients may avoid or restrict activities because of fear. They may have difficulty travelling in the prison transport van, taking part in association or eating in front of others. Some common phobias (eg agoraphobia, social phobia) may not manifest in closed prison conditions, but may become evident when the patient transfers to more open conditions.

Patients sometimes present with physical symptoms, eg palpitations, shortness of breath or 'asthma'. Questioning will reveal specific fears.

Diagnostic features

The patient experiences an unreasonably strong fear of people, specific places or events. Patients often avoid these situations altogether.

Commonly feared situations include:

- eating in public
- open spaces
- being confined in an enclosed space
- crowds or public places
- travelling in buses, cars, trains or planes or
- social events.

Patients may avoid being alone because of fear.

Differential diagnosis

- **Panic disorder — F41.0** (page 67) if anxiety attacks are prominent and not brought on by anything in particular.
- **Depression — F32#** (page 47) if a low or sad mood is prominent.

Panic disorder and depression may coexist with phobias.

Many of the guidelines below also may be helpful for specific (simple) phobias, eg fear of water or of heights.

Essential information for the patient and primary support group

- Phobias can be treated successfully.
- Avoiding feared situations allows the fear to grow stronger.
- Following certain steps can help someone overcome fear.

Advice and support to the patient and primary support group[105]

- Assess the patient's understanding of the problem and their readiness to change.
- Encourage the patient to practise **controlled breathing methods** to reduce physical symptoms of fear (see advice on **Panic disorders — F41.0**, page 67).
- Ask the patient to make a list of all situations that he/she fears and avoids although other people do not.

- Discuss ways to challenge these exaggerated fears (eg patient reminds him/herself, 'I am feeling anxious because there is a large crowd. The feeling will pass in a few minutes').
- Help the patient to plan a series of progressively more challenging steps whereby they confront and get used to feared situations:
  — Identify a small, first step toward the feared situation, eg if they are afraid of eating in public, eat the meal in the cell, take a cup of coffee into the dining area, sit down but do not drink it.
  — Practise this each day until it is no longer frightening.
  — If entering the feared situation still causes anxiety, carry out slow and relaxed breathing, saying the panic will pass within 30–60 minutes (see advice on **Panic disorder — F41.0**, page 67).
  — Do not leave the feared situation until the fear subsides. Do not move on to the next step until the current situation is mastered.
  — Move on to a slightly more difficult step and repeat the procedure, eg eat a meal in the cell but sit with a friend in the dining area and drink a cup of coffee.
  — Take no anti-anxiety medicine for at least 4 hours before practising these steps.
- Ask a friend or member of the healthcare staff to help plan exercises to overcome the fear. Self-help groups can assist in confronting feared situations.
- Keep a diary of the confrontation experiences described above to allow step-by-step management.
- Avoid using benzodiazepines to cope with feared situations.

Medication

With the use of these behavioural methods, many patients will not need medication.[N105]

- If depression is also present, antidepressant medication may be indicated. Paroxetine may be helpful in social phobia[N126] (see *BNF*, Section 4.3.3).
- Encourage patients to face fears without the use of benzodiazepines. Where the feared situation is rare, however, occasional short-term use of anti-anxiety medication may be helpful.[N115] Regular use may lead to dependence and is likely to result in a return of symptoms when it is discontinued.
- For management of performance anxiety, eg fear of public speaking, β-blockers may reduce the physical symptoms.[109]

Referral

See **General referral criteria** (page 152).
Non-urgent referral to the secondary mental-health services is advised:

- if disabling fears persist and
- to prevent problems with long-term sickness and disability.

If available, cognitive-behavioural psychotherapy and exposure[127] may be effective for patients who do not improve with simple measures outlined above.

Recommend self-help/non-statutory/voluntary services, eg Triumph Over Phobia, in all other cases where symptoms persist.

Resources for patients and primary support groups

Stresswatch Scotland: 01563 574144 (helpline); 01563 570886 (office)
(Advice, information, materials on panic, anxiety, stress phobias. Thirty-five local groups)

Triumph Over Phobia (TOP) UK: 01225 330353
(Structured self-help groups for those suffering from phobias or obsessive-compulsive disorder. Produces self-help materials)

Resource leaflet:
Managing Anxiety

Isaac Marks. *Living With Fear*. New York: McGraw Hill. Self-help manual

Post-traumatic stress disorder — F43.1

Presenting complaints

The patient may present initially with:

- irritability
- memory and/or concentration problems
- associated difficulties in interpersonal relationships
- impaired occupational functioning
- low mood
- loss of interest and
- physical problems.

Presentation may be delayed for several months following the trauma.

Diagnostic features

- History of a stressful event or situation (either short or long lasting) of an exceptionally threatening or catastrophic nature, which is likely to cause pervasive distress to almost anyone. The trigger event may have resulted in death or injury and/or the patient may have experienced intense horror, fear or helplessness.
- Intrusive symptoms: memories, flashbacks, nightmares.
- Avoidance symptoms: avoidance of thoughts, activities, situations and cues reminiscent of the trauma, with a sense of 'numbness', emotional blunting, detachment from other people, unresponsiveness to surroundings or anhedonia.
- Symptoms of autonomic arousal, eg hypervigilance, increased startle reaction, insomnia, irritability, excessive anger and impaired concentration and/or memory.
- Symptoms of anxiety and/or depression.
- Drug and/or alcohol abuse are commonly associated with this condition.
- Significant functional impairment.

Where the traumatic event is related to the index offence, the patient may be reluctant to talk about it, especially before the trial, thus complicating a diagnosis.

Differential diagnosis

- **Depression — F32#** (page 47) if preoccupation with, and ruminations about, a past traumatic event have emerged during a depressive episode.
- **Phobic anxiety disorders — F40** (page 79) if the patient avoids specific situations or activities after a traumatic event, but has no re-experiencing symptoms.
- Obsessive-compulsive disorder if recurrent, intrusive thoughts or images occur in the absence of an event of exceptionally threatening or catastrophic nature.

Essential information for the patient and primary support group

- Traumatic or life-threatening events often have psychological effects. For the majority, symptoms will subside with minimal intervention. The information leaflet *Reactions to Traumatic Stress: What to Expect* on the disk may be helpful in reinforcing information 💾. If the patient has reading difficulties, a member of the healthcare team or another member of staff may be able to discuss its contents with him/her.

- For those who continue to experience symptoms, effective treatments are available.
- Post-traumatic stress disorder (PTSD) is not a weakness and does not mean the patient has gone 'mad'. The patient needs support and understanding and must not be told to 'snap out of it'.

Advice and support to the patient and primary support group

- Educate the patient and, with patient permission, staff about PTSD, thus helping them understand the patient's changes in attitude and behaviour.
- Avoiding discussion about the event that triggered the condition is usually unhelpful, but be aware of cultural differences in the ways of coping with past difficulties. Encourage the patient to talk about the event when they are ready and in their own way. This may include not talking about more extreme experiences. The recognition that certain experiences are 'there' but 'unutterable' can be positive.[1]
- Explain the role of avoidance of cues associated with the trauma in reinforcing and maintaining fears and distress. Encourage the patient to face avoided activities and situations gradually. It may be possible to involve staff in supporting the patient in this, eg in initially accompanying the patient into an area where they were assaulted and are now avoiding.
- Explain that suppression of painful memories and thoughts may reinforce them and make them more persistent. Encourage the patient, if possible, simply to allow the thoughts to pass through his/her head and not to suppress them actively.
- Where the patient has become scared of going to sleep because of repeated nightmares, it may be helpful for them to talk with someone they trust about the dream, or to write it down, describing it in detail, perhaps several times, and to remind themselves 'It's a dream. It cannot hurt me'.
- Ask about suicide risk, particularly if marked depression is present (see **Assessing and managing people at risk of suicide**, page 204).
- Encourage the patient to use any existing, available sources of support or solace, eg chaplain and other religious leaders, traditional healers, friends, listeners/buddies, the Samaritans.
- Try to avoid using cigarettes or other drugs to cope with anxiety.

Medication

- Consider antidepressant for concurrent depressive illness (see **Depression — F32#**, page 47).
- Antidepressant medication, including tricyclics (TCAs) and selective serotonin re-uptake inhibitors (SSRIs), may be useful for the treatment of intrusion and avoidance symptoms[N128] (see *BNF*, Section 4.3). Drug treatments for this condition generally need to be used in higher doses and for longer periods than those used for treating depression. There may be a latent period of 8 weeks or more before the effects are seen.
- Startle and hyperarousal symptoms may be helped by β-blockers[N128] (see *BNF*, Section 2.4).

Referral

See **General referral criteria** (page 149).

Referral to the secondary mental-health services is advised if the patient is still having severe intrusive experiences and avoidance symptoms, and there is a marked functional disability despite the above measures. If available, consider behaviour therapy (exposure) or cognitive techniques.[N129,N130] The specialist assessment should include cultural factors. Where possible, advise patients of agencies able to provide appropriate therapy after release.

See **Immigration detainees** and **People who have been sexually assaulted** (pages 326 and 260) for more information about the needs of these groups.

Resources for patients and primary support groups

CombatStress: 01372 841600
(Formerly known as the Ex-Services Mental Welfare Association, it supports men and women discharged from the armed services and Merchant Navy who suffer from mental-health problems, including PTSD. Has a regional network of welfare officers who visit people at home or in hospital. Some practical and financial help)

Medical Foundation for the Care of Victims of Torture: 020 7813 7777
(Provides survivors of torture with medical treatment, social assistance and psychotherapeutic support)

Refugee Support Centre: 020 7820 3606
(Provides counselling to refugees, asylum seekers; plus training and information to health- and socialcare professionals on psychosocial needs of refugees)

Trauma Aftercare Trust (TACT): 0800 1696814 (24-hour freephone helpline); 01242 890306
(Provides information about counselling and treatment)

Victim Support Supportline: 0845 3030900 (Monday–Friday, 9 am–9 pm; Saturday and Sunday, 9 am–7 pm; Bank Holidays, 9 am–5 pm); 020 7735 9166
(Emotional and practical support for victims of crime)

---

[1] Professor Papadopoulos, Tavistock Clinic Refugee Centre, personal communication, quoted in CVS Consultants and Migrant and Refugee Community Forum. *A Shattered World: The Mental-Health Needs of Refugees and Newly Arrived Communities.* London: CVS Consultants, 1999.

Sexual disorders — F52

Sexual disorders — female

Presenting complaints

Patients may be reluctant to discuss sexual matters. They may instead complain of physical symptoms, depressed mood or relationship problems. There may have been sexual abuse — in childhood or later.

Patients may ask for advice about problems with partners outside, or inside, the prison. They may be confused about their sexual orientation. They may ask for help in adjusting to sexual lifestyle changes that relate only to their time in prison. Occasionally, a request for help with gender reassignment may be made.

Special problems may occur in cultural minorities.

Patients may present sexual problems during a routine cervical-smear test.

Diagnostic features

Common sexual disorders presenting in women are:
- a lack or loss of sexual desire, arousal or enjoyment
- vaginismus or spasmodic contraction of vaginal muscles on attempted penetration
- dyspareunia (pain in the vagina or pelvic region during intercourse) or
- anorgasmia (an inability to achieve orgasm or climax).

Differential diagnosis

- If a low or sad mood is prominent, see **Depression — F32#** (page 47). Depression may cause low desire, or may result from sexual and relationship problems.
- Relationship problems: where there is persistent discord in the relationship, relationship counselling should precede or accompany specific treatment of the sexual dysfunction.
- Gynaecological disorders, eg vaginal infections, pelvic infections (salpingitis) and other pelvic lesions (eg tumours or cysts), although vaginismus rarely has a physical cause. Gynaecological complaints and disorders are common in women in prison. It is important to take them seriously and consider investigation and referral to specialist physical help as appropriate.
- Adjustment to sexual lifestyle changes in the prison situation, eg temporary lesbianism or bisexuality. Consider giving sexual health information and counselling. Consider the possibility that the patient is being exploited or bullied.
- Alcohol intoxication and chronic abuse of illicit drugs (eg opioids, cocaine, amphetamines, sedatives, anxiolytics) may decrease sexual interest and cause arousal problems.
- Side-effects of medication, eg selective serotonin re-uptake inhibitor (SSRI) antidepressants, oral contraceptives, β-blockers.
- Physical illnesses may contribute, eg multiple sclerosis, diabetes, spinal injury
- Lack of desire may be related to confusion about sexual orientation, especially in young people.

- Rarely, sexual problems may relate to the patient's feeling that she is really a man and that she wishes to become a man physically. This is very difficult to manage in prison as the usual community management (living as a man and/or treatment with male hormones for at least 1 year before any irreversible surgical steps are taken) is especially difficult. Be aware of the danger of bullying and of serious self-mutilation. Obtain expert advice, including from the prison Health Policy Unit, and refer to a forensic psychiatrist, who may in turn refer to a gender identity clinic. Consider relocation within the prison to reduce the risk of bullying.

Lack or loss of sexual desire

Essential information for the patient and partner

The level of sexual desire varies widely between individuals. Loss of or low sexual desire has many causes, including relationship problems, earlier traumas, fear of pregnancy, postnatal problems, and physical and psychiatric illnesses and stress. The problem can be temporary or persistent.

Advice and support to the patient and partner

Discuss the patient's beliefs about sexual relations. Check whether the patient and/or the partner have unreasonably high expectations. Ask the patient about traumatic sexual experiences and negative attitudes to sex. Accept that this may take more than one appointment. Give advice about treatment approaches that may be appropriate in the community. Inform the patient that doctors often see partners together as well as individually. Suggest planning sexual activity for specific days. Suggest ways of building self-esteem (eg exercise, education), and advise time and space to herself.

Vaginismus

Essential information for the patient and partner

Vaginismus is an involuntary spasm of the pubococcygeal muscles accompanied by intense fear of penetration and anticipation of pain. It is usually caused by psychosocial factors (eg previous negative sexual experiences). It can be overcome with specific psychosexual therapy.

Advice and support to the patient and partner

Exercises are recommended for the patient, and, later, for the partner, with graded dilators or finger dilation, accompanied by Kegel exercises, relaxation exercises, treatment for anxiety and couple counselling. Treatment often requires intensive therapy, but it has a promising outcome.

Dyspareunia

Essential information for the patient and partner

There are many physical causes, both of deep and superficial dyspareunia. In some cases, however, anxiety, poor lubrication and muscle tension are the main factors. Even where there has been a physical cause and it has resolved, anticipation of pain may frequently maintain the dyspareunia.

Advice and support to the patient and partner

Check if the patient experiences desire/arousal/lubrication. Relaxation, prolonged foreplay and careful penetration may overcome psychogenic problems. Referral to a gynaecologist or GUM clinic is advisable if simple measures are unsuccessful.

Anorgasmia

Essential information for the patient and partner

Many women cannot experience orgasm during intercourse but can often achieve it by clitoral stimulation.

Advice and support to the patient and partner

Discuss the couple's beliefs and attitudes. Encourage self-pleasuring, manually or by using a vibrator. The couple should be helped to communicate openly and reduce any unrealistic expectations. Books, leaflets or educational videos may be useful (see **Resources** below).

Referral

After release, patients can refer themselves to:
- Relate
- Brook Advisory Centres
- family planning clinics and
- genitourinary medicine clinics

Consider referral to a psychosexual specialist if the patient and doctor cannot enter into a programme of treatment or if primary-care treatment has failed.

Sexual disorders — male

Presenting complaints

Patients may be reluctant to discuss sexual matters. They may complain instead of physical symptoms, depressed mood or relationship problems.

Patients may ask for advice about problems with partners outside, or inside, the prison. They may be confused about their sexual orientation. They may ask for help in adjusting to sexual lifestyle changes that relate only to their time in prison. Occasionally, a request for help with gender reassignment may be made.

Special problems may occur in different cultures. Sexual problems are often somatised, expectations may be high, and psychological explanations and therapies may not be readily accepted.

Diagnostic features

Common sexual disorders presenting in men are:
- erectile dysfunction or impotence
- premature ejaculation
- retarded ejaculation or orgasmic dysfunction (intravaginal ejaculation is greatly delayed or absent but ejaculation can often occur normally during masturbation) or
- a lack or loss of sexual desire.

Differential diagnosis

- **Depression** — **F32#** (page 47).
- Problems in relationships with partners often contribute to sexual disorder, especially those of desire. Where there is persistent discord in the relationship, relationship counselling should precede or accompany specific treatment of the sexual dysfunction.
- Adjustment to sexual lifestyle changes in the prison situation, eg temporary homosexuality or bisexuality. Consider giving sexual health information, counselling about harm minimisation and access to condoms. Consider the possibility that the patient is being exploited or bullied (see **Victims of sexual assault**, page 260).
- Alcohol intoxication and chronic abuse of illicit drugs (eg opioids, cocaine, amphetamines, sedatives, anxiolytics) may decrease sexual interest and cause arousal problems.
- Rarely sexual problems may relate to the patient's feeling that he is really a woman and that he wishes to become a woman physically. This is very difficult to manage in prison as the usual community management (living as a woman and/or treatment with female hormones for at least 1 year before any irreversible surgical steps are taken) is especially difficult. Be aware of the danger of serious self-mutilation and of bullying. Obtain expert advice, including from the prison Health Policy Unit, and refer to a forensic psychiatrist, who may in turn refer to a gender identity clinic. Consider relocation within the prison to reduce the risk of bullying.
- Specific organic pathology is a rare cause of orgasmic dysfunction or premature ejaculation.
- Physical factors that may contribute to erectile dysfunction include alcohol abuse and chronic abuse of illicit drugs (eg opioids, cocaine, amphetamines, sedatives, anxiolytics), diabetes, hypertension, smoking, medication (eg antidepressants, antipsychotics, diuretics and β-blockers), multiple sclerosis and spinal injury.
- Patients may have unreasonable expectations of their own performance.
- Lack of desire may be related to confusion about sexual orientation, especially in young people.

Erectile dysfunction (failure of genital response, impotence)

Essential information for the patient and partner

Erectile dysfunction is often a temporary response to stress or loss of confidence and it responds to psychosexual treatment especially if morning erections occur. It may also be caused by physical factors (neurological, vascular), by medication or may be secondary to the ageing process.

Advice and support to the patient and partner

Advise the patient and their partner to refrain from attempting intercourse for 2–3 weeks. Encourage them to practise pleasurable physical contact without intercourse during that time, commencing with non-genital touching and moving through mutual genital stimulation to a gradual return to full intercourse at the end of that period. Progression along this continuum should be guided by the return of consistent, reliable erections. A book containing self-help exercises (see **Resources** below) may be helpful. Inform the patient and his partner of the possibilities of physical treatment by penile rings, vacuum devices, intracavernosal injections and medication.

Medication

- Oral: sildenafil 50–100 mg taken on an empty stomach 40–60 minutes before intercourse enhances erections in 80% of patients, whether the cause is psychogenic or neurological.[131] Beware of danger of interaction with cardiac nitrates (see *BNF*, Section 7.4.5).
- Intra-urethral: MUSE (prostaglandin E₁) 125–1000 µg inserted 10 minutes before intercourse produces erections in 40–50% of patients[132] (see *BNF*, Section 7.4.5).
- Intracavernosal: prostaglandin E₁ 5–20 µg injected 10 minutes before intercourse produces erections in 80–90% of patients,[133] but long-term acceptability is low.

These medications are less effective in predominantly vasculogenic cases.

See the current NHS Executive guidelines for prescription of the above, either privately or on the NHS.

Premature ejaculation

Essential information for the patient and partner

Control of ejaculation is possible and can enhance sexual pleasure for both partners.

Advice and support to the patient and partner

Reassure the patient that ejaculation can be delayed by learning new approaches, eg the squeeze or stop–start technique. This and other exercises are set out in self-help books (see **Resources** below). In some cases, delay can also be achieved with clomipramine or selective serotonin re-uptake inhibitor (SSRI) medication, but relapse is very common on cessation. Local anaesthetic sprays, if used cautiously, can delay ejaculation.

Orgasmic dysfunction or retarded ejaculation

Essential information for the patient and partner

This is a more difficult condition to treat; however, if ejaculation can be brought about in some way (eg through masturbation) the prognosis is better. Individual psychotherapy may be required.

Advice and support to the patient and partner

Recommend exercises such as penile stimulation with body oil or masturbation close to the point of orgasm, followed by penetration.

Lack or loss of sexual desire

Essential information for the patient and partner

The level of sexual desire varies widely between individuals. Lack or loss of sexual desire has many causes, including physical and psychiatric illnesses, stress and relationship problems and, rarely, hormonal deficiencies. It may merely represent different expectations.

Advice and support to the patient and partner

Encourage relaxation, stress reduction, open communication, appropriate assertiveness and cooperation between partners. Educational leaflets, books or videos may be helpful.

Referral

When released, patients can refer themselves to:
• Relate
• family planning clinics and
• genitourinary medicine clinics.

Consider referral if the patient and doctor cannot enter into a programme of treatment or if primary-care treatment has failed:
• To a urologist for erectile dysfunction if it is unresponsive to medication and counselling.
• To a psychosexual specialist if the problem is predominantly psychogenic.

Resources for patients and primary support groups

Beaumont Society Infoline: 01582 412220 (24 hours, 7 days per week)
27 Old Gloucester Street, London WC1N 3XX
(National self-help organisation for transvestites, transsexuals, and their partners and families. Advice and information on issues of cross-dressing and gender dysphoria; social functions)

Brook Advisory Centres: 020 7617 8000 (24-hour helpline)
(Free counselling and confidential advice on contraception and sexual matters especially for young people [those under 25])

Out-Side In: 01689 835566
PO Box 119, High Street, Orpington BR6 9ZZ
(Befriending pen-pal service for gay and lesbian prisoners)

Relate: 01788 573241
(Relationship counselling for couples or individuals over 16. Sex therapy for couples. Clients pay on a sliding scale)

Books for women:
Heiman J, LoPiccolo J. *Becoming Orgasmic: A Sexual Growth Program for Women.* Englewood Cliffs: Prentice-Hall, 1988. Self-help exercises for anorgasmia

Brown P, Faulder C. *Treat Yourself to Sex.* Harmondsworth: Penguin, 1977

Goodwin AJ, Agronin Marc E, MD. *A Woman's Guide to Overcoming Sexual Fear and Pain.* Oakland: New Harbinger, 1997

Books for men:
How to Cope with Doubts About Your Sexual Identity and *Gender Dysphoria.* Available for £1.00 each from: Mind Publications, 15–19 Broadway, London E15 4BQ. Tel: 020 8519 2122

Zilbergeld, B. *Men and Sex.* London: Fontana, 1980. Self-help exercises for erectile dysfunction and premature ejaculation

Yaffe M, Fenwick E. *Sexual Happiness.* London: Dorling Kindersley, 1986

Sleep problems (insomnia) — F51

Presenting complaints

Patients are distressed by persistent insomnia and are sometimes disabled by the daytime effects of poor sleep.

Diagnostic features

- Difficulty falling asleep.
- Restless or unrefreshing sleep.
- Frequent or prolonged periods of being awake.

Differential diagnosis

- Short-term sleep problems may result from stressful life events such as coming into prison for the first time, bullying, acute physical illnesses or changes in their schedule.
- Persistent sleep problems may indicate another cause, for example:
  — **Depression — F32#** (page 47) if a low or sad mood and loss of interest in activities are prominent.
  — **Generalised anxiety — F41.1** (page 64) if daytime anxiety is prominent.
  — **Post-traumatic stress disorder — F43.1** (page 82) if the patient fears going to sleep because of repeated nightmares.
- Sleep problems can be a presenting complaint of alcohol misuse or substance abuse (see **Alcohol misuse — F10** or **Substance abuse — F11#**, pages 18 and 55). A patient may also seek benzodiazepines because he/she is still dependent upon them. Enquire about their current substance use and the presence of other withdrawal symptoms. Withdrawal from benzodiazepines needs sometimes to be very gradual (months not weeks)
- Profound sleep deprivation is a part of the experience of major drug withdrawal. Sleep problems may persist for some weeks thereafter. Treatment may be indicated during the very early stages of withdrawal.
- Consider medical conditions that may cause insomnia, eg heart failure, pulmonary disease, pain conditions.
- Consider medications that may cause insomnia, eg steroids, theophylline, decongestants, some antidepressant drugs.
- Consider life style causes: the patient may spend most of the day asleep in his/her cell.
- If the patient snores loudly while asleep, consider sleep apnoea. It may be helpful, with patient consent, to take a history from the cellmate. Patients with sleep apnoea often complain of daytime sleepiness but are unaware of night-time awakenings.
- The patient may be seeking drugs to sell or may be being pressured by others to obtain drugs on their behalf. Wing staff may have useful information where this is suspected.

Essential information for the patient and primary support group

- Temporary sleep problems are common at times of stress or physical illness.
- Sleep requirements vary widely and usually decrease with age.
- Improvement of sleeping habits (not sedative medication) is the best treatment.[134]
- Worry about not being able to sleep can worsen insomnia.
- Stimulants (including coffee and tea, especially if taken in the evening) can cause or worsen insomnia.

Advice and support to the patient and primary support group

- Encourage the patient to maintain a regular sleep routine by:
  — relaxing in the evening
  — keeping to regular hours for going to bed and getting up in the morning, trying not to vary the schedule or 'sleep in' on the weekend
  — getting up at the regular time even if the previous night's sleep was poor and
  — avoiding daytime naps since they can disturb the next night's sleep.
- Daytime exercise can help the patient to sleep regularly, but evening exercise may contribute to insomnia. Consider promoting daytime exercise through custody/sentence planning.
- Simple measures may help, eg a milk drink or use of ear plugs or eye shades.
- Recommend relaxation exercises to help the patient to fall asleep.
- Advise the patient to avoid caffeine in the evenings.
- If the patient cannot fall asleep within 30 minutes, advise him/her to get up and try again later when feeling sleepy.
- Self-help leaflets and books may be useful. The *Getting a Good Night's Sleep* leaflet on the disk includes a relaxation exercise ▉. If the patient has reading difficulties, a member of the healthcare team or another member of staff may be able to go through the contents of the leaflet with the patient.
- Sleep diaries are often useful in the assessment and monitoring of progress.

Medication

- Treat the underlying psychiatric or physical conditions.
- Make changes to medication, as appropriate.
- Consider strictly short-term use of a hypnotic in the very early stages of withdrawal from drugs if sleep deprivation is profound. Explain the risk of developing dependence on these medications to the patient.
- Hypnotic medication may be used intermittently.[135] The risk of dependence increases significantly after 14 days of use. Avoid hypnotic medication in cases of chronic insomnia (where insomnia is experienced for most nights over at least 3 weeks).
- Consider the timing and method of administering the medication. Sedatives given at 4 or 5 pm by supervised ingestion will be less effective than sedatives taken later in the evening.
- Valerian may have a weak effect on sleep but without a hangover effect the next day.[136]

Referral

See **General referral criteria** (page 152).

If available, consider referral to the in-house therapeutic day centre for relaxation sessions.

Referral to the secondary mental-health services is rarely helpful.

Refer to a sleep laboratory, if available, if more complex sleep disorders (eg narcolepsy, night terrors, somnambulism) are suspected.

Where symptoms are severe and long lasting and the above measures are unsuccessful, consider referral to a clinical psychologist or specially trained counsellor, if available, for therapies such as sleep hygiene training.[N137,138]

Resources for patients and primary support groups

British Snoring and Sleep Apnoea Association: 01249 701010
1 Duncroft Close, Reigate RH2 9DE. E-mail:
snoreshop@britishsnoring.demon.co.uk; URL:
http://www.britishsnoring.demon.co.uk

Insomnia Helpline: 020 8994 9874 (helpline: Monday–Friday, 6 pm–8 pm)

Narcolepsy Association UK (UKAN): 020 7721 8904
Craven House, 1st Floor, 121 Kingsway, London WC2B 6PA. E-mail:
info@narcolepsy.org.uk

Resource leaflet:
Getting a Good Night's Sleep

Unexplained somatic complaints — F45

Presenting complaints

- Any physical symptom may be present.
- Symptoms may vary widely across cultures.
- Complaints may be single or multiple and may change over time.

Diagnostic features

Medically unexplained physical symptoms (a full history and physical examination are necessary to determine this):

- Frequent medical visits in spite of negative investigations.
- Symptoms of depression and anxiety are common.

Some patients may be primarily concerned with obtaining relief from physical symptoms. Others may be worried about having a physical illness and be unable to believe that no physical condition is present (hypochondriasis).

Differential diagnosis

- **Drug-use disorders — F11#** (page 55), eg seeking narcotics for relief of pain.
- If low or sad mood is prominent, see **Depression — F32#** (page 47). People with depression are often unaware of everyday physical aches and pains.
- **Generalised anxiety disorder — F41.1** (page 64), if anxiety symptoms are prominent.
- **Panic disorder — F41.0** (page 67) misinterpretation of the somatic signs associated with panic.
- **Chronic mixed anxiety and depression — F41.2** (page 33).
- **Acute psychotic disorders — F23** (page 11) if strange beliefs about symptoms are present, eg belief that organs are decaying.
- An organic cause may eventually be discovered for the physical symptoms. Psychological problems can coexist with physical problems.

Depression, anxiety, alcohol or drug disorders may coexist with unexplained somatic complaints.

Essential information for the patient and primary support group

- Stress often produces or exacerbates physical symptoms.
- When people are forced to remain inactive for long periods, it is natural for them to focus on bodily sensations. The sensations may become exaggerated in the process.
- The focus should be on managing the symptoms, not on discovering their cause.
- Cure may not always be possible; the goal should be to live the best life possible even if the symptoms continue.

Advice and support to the patient and primary support group[139]

- Acknowledge that the patient's physical symptoms are real to them.

- Ask about the patient's beliefs (what is causing the symptoms?) and fears (what does he/she fear may happen?).
- Ask how the patient spends his/her day. How long do they spend in the cell? Encourage exercise and enjoyable activities. The patient need not wait until all symptoms are gone before undertaking activities. If necessary, advocate for increased access to appropriate activities. If the patient is under cellular confinement, advocate for access to art materials and, if literate, to reading materials.
- Be explicit early on about considering psychological issues. The exclusion of illness and exploration of emotional aspects can happen in parallel. Investigations should have a clear indication. It may be helpful to say to the patient, 'I think this result is going to be normal'.
- Offer appropriate reassurance, eg not all headaches indicate a brain tumour. Advise patients not to focus on medical worries.
- Discuss the emotional stresses present when the symptoms arose.
- Explain the links between stress and physical symptoms and how a vicious cycle can develop, eg 'Stress can cause a tightening of the muscles in the gut. This can lead to the development of abdominal pain or worsening of existing pain. The pain aggravates the tightening of the gut muscles'. A diagram may be helpful.
- Relaxation methods can help relieve symptoms related to tension, eg headache, neck or back pain.
- Treat associated depression, anxiety or substance misuse problems.
- For patients with more chronic complaints, time-limited appointments that are regularly scheduled can prevent more frequent, urgent visits.[140]
- Structured problem-solving methods may help patients to manage current life problems or stresses that contribute to symptoms.[48]
- Help the patient to:
  — identify the problem
  — list as many possible solutions as the patient can think of
  — list the advantages and disadvantages of each possible solution (the patient should do this, perhaps between appointments)
  — support the patient in choosing his/her preferred approach
  — help the patient to work out the steps necessary to achieve the plan and
  — set a date to review the plan. Identify and reinforce things that are working.

Medication

Avoid unnecessary diagnostic testing or prescription of new medication for each new symptom. Rationalise polypharmacy.

Where depression is also present, an antidepressant may be indicated (see **Depression — F32#**, page 47)

Low doses of tricyclic antidepressant (TCA) medication (eg amitriptyline, 50–100 mg day^{-1}, or imipramine, 20 mg day^{-1}) may be helpful in some cases, eg where there is headache or atypical chest pain.[141,142]

Referral

- Patients are best managed in primary healthcare settings. Consistency of approach within the practice is essential. Seeing the same person is helpful. Consider referral to a partner or other medical officer for a second opinion. Documenting discussions with colleagues can reduce stress by sharing responsibility within the primary-care team.

- Non-urgent referral to the secondary mental-health services is advised on grounds of functional disability, especially an inability to work, and for the duration of symptoms.
- Cognitive-behaviour therapy, if available, may help some patients, though the willingness of patients to participate is sometimes poor.[N143]
- Refer to a liaison psychiatrist, if available, for those who persist in their belief that they have a physical cause for their symptoms, despite good evidence to the contrary.
- Avoid multiple referrals to medical specialists. Documented discussions with appropriate medical specialists may be helpful from time to time as, in some cases, underlying physical illness eventually emerges.

Resources for patients and primary support groups

Listeners, buddies, chaplains and personal officers may offer emotional support and/or help with practical problems

Resource leaflets:
Coping with Depression
Getting a Good Night's Sleep
Managing Anxiety. Contains instructions for a relaxation exercise

References

References are graded A–C, I–V, as discussed in the Introduction and in the key on page 15.

1 Birchwood M. Early intervention in schizophrenia: theoretical background and clinical strategies. *Br J Clin Psychol* 1992; 31: 257–278. (BIV)

For more information about the early detection of psychosis, see the Early Psychosis Prevention and Intervention Centre (EPPIC). *The Early Psychosis Training Pack*. Cheshire: Gardiner-Caldwell Communications, 1997. Tel: 0393 422800.

2 World Health Organization. *Schizophrenia: An International Follow-up Study*. Chichester: Wiley, 1979. (AIV)

Large outcome study with a 2-year follow-up that showed that only 10–15% of patients did not recover from their illness in that 2 years. Another, shorter-term follow-up study showed 83% of first-episode psychotic patients treated with antipsychotic medication remitting by 1 year post-inpatient admission. Lieberman J, Jody D, Geisler S *et al*. Time course and biologic correlates of treatment response in first episode schizophrenia. *Arch Gen Psychiatry* 1993; 50: 369–376.

3 Kavanagh DJ. Recent developments in expressed emotion and schizophrenia. *Br J Psychiatry* 1992; 160: 601–620. (AIII)

Family support and education, which promotes a more supportive family environment, can reduce relapse rates substantially.

4 Driver and Vehicle Licensing Agency. *At a Glance Guide to Medical Aspects of Fitness to Drive*. Swansea: DVLA, 1998.

Further information is available from: Senior Medical Adviser, DVLA, Driver Medical Unit, Longview Road, Morriston, Swansea SA99 ITU.

5a Mental Health Commission. *Early Intervention in Psychosis: Guidance Note*. Wellington: Mental Health Commission, 1999.

b Falloon I, Coverdale J, Laidlaw T *et al*. Family management in the prevention of morbidity of schizophrenia: social outcome of a two-year longitudinal study. *Psychol Med* 1998; 17: 59–66.

Involvement of the family is vital. Education is important for engaging individuals and families in treatment and promoting recovery. Psychological therapies may be helpful.

6 Atypical antipsychotics appear to be better tolerated, with fewer extrapyramidal side-effects, than typical drugs at therapeutic doses. Even at low doses, extrapyramidal side-effects are commonly experienced with typical drugs. Whether atypicals improve the long-term outcome has yet to be established. Risperidone, amisulpride and possibly olanzapine have a dose-related effect. Selected references (BII):

a American Psychiatric Association. Practice guidelines: schizophrenia. *Am J Psychiatry* 1997; 154(Suppl 4): 1–49.

Reports that 60% of patients receiving acute treatment with typical antipsychotic medication develop significant extrapyramidal side-effects.

b Zimbroff D, Kane J, Tamminga CA. Controlled, dose–response study of sertindole and haloperidol in the treatment of schizophrenia. *Am J Psychiatry* 1997; 154: 782–791.

Haloperidol produced extrapyramidal symptoms at 4 mg day^{-1}.

c Mir S, Taylor D. Issues in schizophrenia. *Pharmaceut J* 1998; 261: 55–58.

Reviews evidence on the efficacy, safety and patient tolerability of atypical antipsychotics.

d Duggan L, Fenton M, Dardennes RM, El-Dosoky A, Indran S. Olanzapine for schizophrenia. Cochrane Library, Oxford 1999. Update software.

e Kennedy E, Song F, Hunter R, Gilbody S. Risperidone versus conventional antipsychotic medication for schizophrenia. Cochrane Library, Oxford 1998, issue 2.

7 People suffering a first episode of psychosis develop side-effects at lower doses of antipsychotic drugs than patients used to these drugs. For patients treated with high-potency typical antipsychotics who are used to the drugs, the mean dose at which extrapyramidal side-effects appear is below the average clinically effective dose. The average clinically effective dose for those suffering a first episode has not yet been established, but clinical practice indicates that it is significantly lower than for patients used to the drugs. Selected references (BIII):

a McEvoy JP, Hogarty GE, Steingard S. Optimal dose of neuroleptic in acute schizophrenia: a controlled study of the neuroleptic threshold and higher haloperidol dose. *Arch Gen Psychiatry* 1991; 48: 739–745.

First-episode patients developed extrapyramidal side-effects at mean doses of haloperidol of 2.1 ± 1.1 mg day^{-1}, whereas 'experienced' patients did so at a mean dose of 4.3 ± 2.4 mg day^{-1}.

b See reference 6a.

The optimal therapeutic dose for most patients appears to be in the range 6–12 mg day^{-1} haloperidol or equivalent. Evidence on the optimal dose for first-onset patients is not yet clear.

8 Bollini P, Pampallona S, Orza MJ. Antipsychotic drugs: is more worse? A meta-analysis of the published randomized control trials. *Psychol Med* 1994; 24: 307–316. (AI)

For most patients, higher than moderate doses bring increased side-effects but no additional therapeutic gains.

9 Al Dixon LB, Lehman AF, Levine J. Conventional antipsychotic medications for schizophrenia. *Schizophrenia Bull* 1995; 21: 567–577.

Presents overwhelming evidence that continuing maintenance therapy reduces the risk of relapse. It concludes that it is appropriate to taper or discontinue medication within 6 months to 1 year for first-episode patients who experience a full remission of symptoms.

10 Taylor D, McConnell D, Abel K, Kerwin R. *The Bethlem and Maudsley NHS Trust Prescribing Guidelines*. London: Martin Dunitz, 1999.

Available from: Martin Dunitz, 7–9 Pratt Street, London NW1 0AE. Tel: 020 7482 2202. £14.99 + £2.00 postage and packaging.

11 Consensus (BV). As people reacting to stresses such as unemployment or divorce are at a high risk of developing a mental disorder, studies on prevention in high-risk groups may be relevant. These support the offering of social support and problem-solving. NHS Centre for Reviews and Dissemination. Mental health promotion in high-risk groups. *Effect Health Care Bull* 1997; 3: 1–10.

12 Catalan J, Gath D, Edmonds G, Ennis J. The effects of not prescribing anxiolytics in general practice. *Br J Psychiatry* 1984; 144: 593–602.

Demonstrates that general practitioner advice and reassurance is as effective as administration of benzodiazepines. The mean time spent by the general practitioner for advice and reassurance was 12 minutes compared with 10.5 minutes for giving a prescription.

13a Department of Health. *Treatment Choice in Psychological Therapies and Counselling: Evidence Based Clinical Practice Guideline*. London, Department of Health, 2001.

Concludes that there is evidence of the benefit from counselling for mixed anxiety/depression in primary care but not for more severe disorders. The evidence is better for counselling used with specified client groups, eg postnatal mothers, bereaved groups.

b Rowland N, Bower P, Mellor Clark J et al. *The Effectiveness and Cost-Effectiveness of Counselling in Primary Care*. Cochrane Library, Oxford 2000.

14 Rosenberg H. Prediction of controlled drinking by alcoholics and problem drinkers. *Psychol Bull* 1993; 113: 129–139. (BII)

Qualitative review of the literature. The successful achievement of controlled drinking is associated with less severe dependence and a belief that controlled drinking is possible.

15 NHS Centre for Reviews and Dissemination. Brief interventions and alcohol use. *Effect Health Care Bull* 1993; 1: 1–12. (AI)

Brief interventions, including assessing drinking and related problems, motivational feedback and advice, are effective. They are most successful for less severely affected patients.

16 McCrady B, Irvine S. Self-help groups. In Hester R, Miller W, Wilmsford N (eds), *Handbook of Alcoholism Treatment Approaches*. New York: Pergamon, 1989. (AIV)

Discusses the characteristics of patients who are good candidates for Alcoholics Anonymous (AA). Several studies show AA to be an important support in remaining alcohol-free to patients who are willing to attend.

17 American Psychiatric Association. *Practice Guidelines: Substance Use Disorders*. Washington, DC: APA, 1996. (BIV)

Where patients have mild-to-moderate withdrawal symptoms, general support, reassurance and frequent monitoring are sufficient treatment for two-thirds of them without pharmacological treatment.

18 Duncan D, Taylor D. Chlormethiazole or chlordiazepoxide in alcohol detoxification. *Psychiatr Bull* 1996; 20: 599–601. (AIV)

Describes randomized, controlled trials that show chlordiazepoxide and chlormethiazole to be of equal efficacy, and uncontrolled studies showing that chlormethiazole has generally mild adverse effects, while those of chlordiazepoxide may be very serious.

19 Tallaksen C, Bohmer T, Bell H. Blood and serum thiamin and thiamin phosphate esters concentrations in patients with alcohol dependence syndrome before and after thiamin treatment. *Alcohol Clin Exp Res* 1992; 16: 320–325. (BIV)

20 Kranzler H, Burleson J, Del Boca F *et al*. Buspirone treatment of anxious alcoholics: a placebo-controlled trial. *Arch Gen Psychiatry* 1994; 51: 720–731. (BII)

21 Department of Health, Scottish Office, Welsh Office, DHSS Northern Ireland. *Drug Misuse and Dependence — Guidelines on Clinical Management*, 1999. Stationery Office, London

22 *Brief Interventions Guidelines*. London: Alcohol Concern, 1997.

Available from Alcohol Concern, Waterbridge House, 32–36 Loman Street, London SE1 0EE. Tel: 020 7928 7377.

23 Holder H, Longabaugh R, Miller W, Rubonis A. The cost effectiveness of treatment for alcoholism: a first approximation. *J Stud Alcohol* 1991; 52: 517–540. (AI)

Treatments aim to improve self-control and social skills, eg relationship skills, assertiveness and drink refusal.

24 Hunt G, Azrin N. A community reinforcement approach to alcoholism. *Behav Res Ther* 1973; 11: 91–104. (AI)

This approach uses behavioural principles and includes training in job-finding, support in developing alcohol-free social and recreational activities, and an alcohol-free social club.

25 Ideally a modified form of motivational interviewing that takes account of the additional problems of a patient with a severe mental illness will be used. Drake RE, McFadden C, Mueser K, McHugo GJ, Bond R. Review of integrated mental health and substance abuse treatments for patients with dual disorders. *Schiz Bull* 1998; 24: 589-608; Bellack AS, Diclemente CC. Treating substance abuse among patients with schizophrenia. *Psychiat Serv* 1999; 50: (1), 75–80.

26 Raphael B. Preventive intervention with the recently bereaved. *Arch Gen Psychiatry* 1977; 34: 1450–1454. (BIII)

Demonstrates that 'high-risk' bereaved people who receive counselling have fewer symptoms of lasting anxiety and tension than those who do not.

27 Murray Parkes C, Laungani P, Young B (eds), *Death and Bereavement Across Cultures*. London: Routledge, 1997. (AV)

28 Manic Depression Fellowship, *Inside Out: A Guide to Self-Management of Manic Depression*. London: MDF, 1995. (BV)

Available from: Manic Depression Fellowship, 8–10 High Street, Kingston-upon-Thames, London KT1 1EY. The advice in this book comes from the shared experience of people with manic depression who have tried these techniques.

29 Chou JC-Y. Recent advances in treatment of acute mania. *J Clin Psychopharm* 1991; 11: 3–21. (BII)

The author concludes that antipsychotics are effective in mania and they appear to have a more rapid effect than lithium.

30 Rifkin A, Doddi S, Karajgi B *et al*. Dosage of haloperidol for mania. *Br J Psych* 1994; 165: 113–116. (BII)

Concludes that doses of haloperidol > 10 mg day^{-1} in the management of mania confer no benefit.

31 American Psychiatric Association. *Practice Guidelines: Bipolar Disorder*. Washington, DC: APA, 1996. (AII)

Reviews four randomized control trials that show that benzodiazepines are effective in place of or in conjunction with a neuroleptic in sedating acutely agitated, manic patients.

32a Cookson J. Lithium: balancing risks and benefits. *Br J Psychiatry* 1997; 171: 113–119. (BIII)

b Dali I. Mania. *Lancet* 1997; 349: 1157–1160.

c Bowden C, Brugger A, Swann A *et al*. Efficacy of divolproex versus lithium and placebo in the treatment of mania. The Depakote Mania Study Group. *J Am Med Assoc* 1994; 271: 918–924.

33 Zornberg G, Pope H Jr. Treatment of depression in bipolar disorder: new directions for research. *J Clin Psychopharmacol* 1993; 13: 397–408. (BIII)

Review of nine controlled studies shows a high response rate to lithium for acute bipolar depression. A response may take 6–8 weeks to become evident, however.

34a Goodwin G. Lithium revisited: a re-examination of the placebo-controlled trials of lithium prophylaxis in manic-depressive disorder. *Br J Psychiatry* 1995; 167: 573–574. (BIII)

Trials show the prophylactic use of lithium to be effective, although most trials had methodological flaws.

b Berghofer A, Kossmann B, Muller-Oerlinghausen B. Course of illness and pattern of recurrence in patients with affective disorders during long-term lithium prophylaxis: a retrospective analysis over 15 years. *Acta Psychiatr Scand* 1996; 93: 349–354.

The prophylactic effect of lithium can be maintained over at least 10 years.

35 See reference 31.

The upper limits of the therapeutic range for lithium is 1.0 meq l^{-1}. However, although the efficacy of lithium at 0.6–0.8 meq l^{-1} has not been formally studied, this is the range commonly chosen by patients and their doctors as giving the best balance between effectiveness and side-effects.

36 Schou M. Effects of long-term lithium treatment on kidney function: an overview. *J Psychiatry Res* 1988; 22: 287–296.

Qualitative literature review.

37 Suppes T, Baldessanni RJ, Faedda GL. Risk of recurrence following discontinuation of lithium treatment in bipolar disorder. *Arch Gen Psych* 1991; 48: 1082–1088. (AIII)

38 Sachs G, Lafer B, Stoll A *et al*. A double-blind trial of bupropion versus desipramaine for bipolar depression. *J Clin Psychiatry* 1994; 55:391–393. (CII)

Preliminary evidence.

39 Reid S, Chalder T, Cleare A, Hotopf M, Wessely S. Chronic fatigue syndrome. In *Clinical Evidence*. London: *Br Med J* Publications, 1999: 397–405. (BV)

40 Joyce J, Hotopf M, Wessely S. The prognosis of chronic fatigue and chronic fatigue syndrome: a systematic review. *Quart J Med* 1997; 90: 223–233. (BIV)

41 Price JR, Couper J. Cognitive behaviour therapy for CFS. Cochrane Library, Oxford 1998, issue 4. (AI)

42 Fulcher KY, White PD. A randomised controlled trial of graded exercise therapy in patients with the chronic fatigue syndrome. *Br Med J* 1997; 314: 1647–1652. (AII)

43 See reference 39. (BIII)

44 Carette S, Bell MJ, Reynolds WJ *et al*. Comparison of amitriptyline, cyclobenzaprine, and placebo in the treatment of fibromyalgia. *Arthritis Rheum* 1994; 37: 32–40. (CII)

45 Hannonen P, Malminiemi K, Yli-Kerttula U *et al*. A randomised double-blind placebo controlled study of moclobemide and amitriptyline in the treatment of fibromyalgia in females without psychiatric disorder. *Br J Rheumatol* 1998; 37: 1279–1286. (CII)

46 Greden JF. Anxiety or caffeinism: a diagnosis dilemma. *Am J Psychiatry* 1974; 131: 1089–1092. (AV)

47 Wallin M, Rissanen A. Food and mood: relationship between food, serotonin and affective disorders. *Acta Psychiatr Scand* 1994; 377(Suppl): 36–40. (CV)

Quoted in *Guidelines for the Treatment and Management of Depression by Primary Health Care Professionals*. Wellington: National Health Committee of New Zealand, 1996.

48 Hawton K, Kirk J. Problem-solving. In Hawton K, Salkovskis PM, Kirk J, Clark DM (eds), *Cognitive Therapy for Psychiatric Problems: A Practical Guide*. Oxford: Oxford University Press, 1989. (AII)

49 Glenister D. Exercise and mental health: a review. *J Roy Soc Health* 1996; February: 7–13. (BIII)

50 McCann L, Holmes D. Influence of aerobic exercise on depression. *J Personal Social Psychol* 1984; 46: 1142–1147. (BIII)

Quoted in *Mental Health Promotion: A Quality Framework*. London: Health Education Authority, 1997.

51 Consensus, plus some, usually small, trials. For example, Donnan P, Hutchinson A, Paxton R *et al*. Self-help materials for anxiety: a randomised controlled trial in general practice. *Br J Gen Pract* 1990; 40: 498–501. (BV)

An audiotape and a booklet are given to patients with chronic anxiety. Intervention led to reduced scores for depression, as well as for anxiety.

52 The differences in outcome between the active drug and the placebo are less in primary-care depressions than among more severe cases. *Depression in Primary Care*. Clinical Practice Guideline Number 5. US Department of Health Human Services, Agency for Health Care Policy and Research, 1993; *Treatment of Major Depression*. AHCPR Publication 93-0551.

Fluoxetine does not produce better outcomes than tricyclic drugs in general primary-care depression; Simon G, VonKorff M, Heiligenstein J *et al*. Initial antidepressant choice in primary care: effectiveness and cost of fluoxetine versus tricyclic antidepressants. *J Am Med Assoc* 1996; 275: 1897–1902.

Paroxetine and citalopram are both licensed for panic as well as for depression, so they may be useful where panic symptoms are prominent. Both selective serotonin re-uptake inhibitors (SSRI) and tricyclic antidepressants (TCA) may initially worsen anxiety and panic symptoms, so they should be introduced at low doses and slowly increased.

53a Linde K, Mulrow CD. St John's Wort for depression. Cochrane Library, Oxford 1999; issue 1. (AI)

b Philip M, Kohnen R, Hiller K-O. Hypericum extract versus imipramine or placebo in patients with moderate depression: randomized, multi-centre study of treatment for 8 weeks. *Br Med J* 1999; 319: 1534–1539.

54 Thiede HM, Walper A. Inhibition of MAO and CoMT by *Hypericum* extracts and hypericin. *J Geriat Psychiatr Neurol* 1994; 7(Suppl 1): S54–S56.

55 Interactions with tyramine-containing foods (eg beans, some cheeses, yeast, Bovril, bananas, pickled herrings) are theoretically possible. However, there is to date an absence of spontaneous reports of these problems occurring.

56 Breckenbridge A. *Important Interactions between St John's Wort* (Hypericum perforata*) Preparations and Prescribed Medicines*. Committee for Safety of Medicines, 29 February 2000.

Letter advises that *Hypericum* reduces the therapeutic effect of indinavir, warfarin, cyclosporin, oral contraceptives, digoxin and theophylline, and may reduce the effect of other drugs — except topical medicines with limited systemic absorption and non-psychotropic medicines excreted renally. Adverse reactions may occur if combined with triptans (used to treat migraine) or selective serotonin re-uptake inhibitor (SSRI) antidepressants.

Information for professionals and the general public is available on the Medicines Control Agency website: URL: http://www.open.gov.uk/mca/mcahome.htm or Tel: 020 7273 0000 (health professionals) or NHS Direct: 0845 46 47 (public).

57 McLean J, Pietroni P. Self care — who does best? *Soc Sci Med* 1990; 30: 591–596. (BIII)

Describes a controlled trial of a general practice-based class teaching self-care skills, relaxation, stress management, medication, nutrition and exercise. Significant improvements were maintained after 1 year.

58 Catalan J, Gath DH, Anastasiades P *et al*. Evaluation of a brief psychological treatment for emotional disorders in primary care. *Psychol Med* 1991; 21: 1013–1018. (BII)

Describes a small, randomized controlled trial. Patients receiving problem-solving therapy did significantly better than those receiving routine care. Patients were selected on the basis of higher symptom scores, however. Another group of patients with lower symptom scores who were not treated showed equal improvement to the treated group.

59 Gloaguen V, Cottraux J, Cucherat M *et al*. A meta-analysis of the effects on cognitive therapy in depressed patients. *J Affect Disord* 1998; 49: 59–72. (AI)

Supports cognitive therapy in patients with mild-to-moderate depression.

60 Sheldon T, Freemantle N, House A *et al*. Examining the effectiveness of treatments for depression in general practice. *J Mental Health* 1993; 2: 141–156. (BI)

Review of four randomized controlled trials that concluded that there is some evidence of the effectiveness for cognitive therapy in depression in primary care, but that it is considerably weaker than cognitive therapy in a major depressive disorder in secondary care.

61 Brown S. Excess mortality of schizophrenia: a meta-analysis. *Br J Psychiatry* 1997; 171: 502–508. (AI)

Reports on life expectancy and excess mortality rate, including from physical illnesses, in patients with schizophrenia.

62 Adams CE, Eisenbruch M. Depot versus oral fluphenazine for those with schizophrenia. Cochrane Library, Oxford 1998, issue 2. (AI)

63 Kendrick T, Millar E, Burns T, Ross F. Practice nurse involvement in giving depot neuroleptic injections: development of a patient assessment and monitoring checklist. *Prim Care Psychiatry* 1998; 4: 149–154 (AIV)

Of the 25% of people with schizophrenia who have no specialist contact, many have a practice nurse as their only regular professional contact. The levels of knowledge of schizophrenia and its treatment of those nurses was often no better than that of lay people.

64 Kemp R, Kirov G, Everitt B, David A. A randomised controlled trial of compliance therapy: 18 month follow up. *Br J Psychiatry* 1998; 172: 413–419. (AII)

Patients who received specific counselling about their attitudes towards their illness and drug treatment were five times more likely to take medication without prompting than controls.

65 Mari JJ, Streiner D. Family intervention for people with schizophrenia. Cochrane Library, Oxford 1991, issue 1. (AI)

Families receiving this intervention, which promotes a more supportive family environment, may expect the family member with schizophrenia to relapse less and to be in hospital less.

66 Jones C, Cormac I, Mota J, Campbell C. Cognitive behaviour therapy for schizophrenia. Cochrane Library, Oxford, issue 4, 2001. (AI)

Four small trials show that cognitive-behaviour therapy is associated with substantially reduced risk of relapse.

67 Rabins PV. Psychosocial and management aspects of delirium. *Int Psychoger* 1991; 3: 319–324. (BV)

Reviews 21 papers. The evidence base is very thin.

68 Rummans TA, Evans JM, Krahn LE, Fleming KC. Delirium in elderly patients: evaluation and management. *Mayo Clinic Proc* 1995; 70: 989–998. (BV)

Reviews 55 papers. The evidence base is thin.

69 Eurodem Prevalence Research Group, Hofman PM, Rocca WA, Brayne C *et al.* The prevalence of dementia in Europe: a collaborative study of 1980–1999. *Int J Epidemiol* 1991; 20: 736–748.

70 Ballard C, Grace J, McKeith I *et al.* Neuroleptic sensitivity in dementia with Lewy bodies and Alzheimer's disease. *Lancet* 1998; 351: 1032–1033.

71a Stein K. *Donepezil in the Treatment of Mild to Moderate Dementia of the Alzheimer Type (SDAT)*. Report to the South and West Development and Evaluation Committee (DEC) No. 69, June. Bristol: NHS Executive, 1997.

b Rogers SL, Farlow MR, Doody RS *et al* and Donepezil Study Group. A twenty four week, double blind, placebo-controlled trial of donepezil in patients with Alzheimer's disease. *Neurology* 1998; 50: 136–145.

The limited number of studies available to date show that donepezil produces some improvement in a minority of patients with mild-to-moderate Alzheimer's disease (defined as those with a mini-Mental State Examination score between 10 and 26). There is no evidence to date that donepezil has any effect on the non-cognitive manifestations of Alzheimer's disease.

72 Martinsen E. Physical activity and major depressive disorder: clinical experience. *Acta Psychiatrica Scand* 1994; 377(Suppl): 23–27. (BIV)

Reviews 10 experimental studies that all indicate that aerobic exercise is more effective than no treatment for major depressive disorder.

73 Schuckit M. Alcohol and major depressive disorder: a clinical perspective. *Acta Psychiatrica Scand* 1994; 377: 28–32. (AIV)

74 Schulberg H, Katon W, Simon G, Rush AJ. Best clinical practice: guidelines for managing major depression in primary care. *J Clin Psychiatry* 1999; 60(Suppl 7): 19–24. (BII)

Concludes that recovery rates for an acute episode of major depression in primary care are similar for guideline-driven pharmacotherapy and depression-specific psychotherapies, such as interpersonal therapy and problem-solving treatments. Medication takes 4–6 weeks to show an effect and psychotherapies take 6–8 weeks.

75 Lave J, Frank R, Schulberg H, Kamlet M. Cost-effectiveness of treatments for major depression in primary care practice. *Arch Gen Psychiatry* 1998; 55: 645–651. (BII)

Describes a high-quality randomized controlled trial comparing the standardized treatment by nortriptyline, interpersonal psychotherapy and primary physician's usual care ($n > 90$ for each group) for major depression in primary care. Both standardized therapies were better than usual care, and more expensive. Those taking drugs did slightly better with respect to both quality of life and economic outcomes.

76 Paykel E, Hollyman J, Freeling P, Sedgwick P. Prediction of therapeutic benefit from amitriptyline in mild depression: a general practice, placebo-controlled trial. *J Affective Disord* 1988; 14: 83–95. (BIII)

Antidepressants do not show efficacy in mild acute depression. However, there is some evidence of efficacy in dysthemia (chronic, mild depressive syndrome that has been present for at least 2 years; Lima M, Moncrieff J. A comparison of drugs versus placebo for the treatment of dysthemia: a systematic review. Cochrane Database of Systematic Reviews, Depression, Anxiety and Neurosis Module. Cochrane Library, Oxford 1998, issue 2.

77 NHS Centre for Reviews and Dissemination, University of York. The treatment of depression in primary care. *Effect Health Care* 1993; March: 1–12. (AII)

78 See reference 74.

Another conclusion from this paper is that recent randomized controlled trials conducted in primary care show a 50–60% response rate to all classes of antidepressants in primary-care patients.

79 Prien R, Kupfer D. Continuation drug therapy for major depressive episodes: how long should it be maintained? *Am J Psychiatry* 1986; 143: 18–23. (BII)

Concludes that patients treated for a first episode of uncomplicated depression who respond well to an antidepressant should receive a full therapeutic dose for at least 16–20 weeks after achieving full remission.

80 Reimherr F, Amsterdam J, Quitkin F *et al.* Optimal length of continuation therapy in depression: a prospective assessment during long-term fluoxetine treatment. *Am J Psychiatry* 1998; 155: 1247–1253. (BIII)

81 Kupfer D, Frank E, Perel J *et al*. Five-year outcomes for maintenance therapy: possible mechanisms and treatments. *J Clin Psychiatry* 1998; 59: 279–288.

The study was carried out by psychiatric patients. There are no comparable clinical trials of maintenance treatments' efficacy in reducing recurrence of depression in primary care.

82 Donaghue J, Taylor D, David M. Sub-optimal use of antidepressants in the treatment of depression. *CNS Drugs* Vol 13(5), May 2000; 365–383. (BIII)

83a DeRubeis RJ, Crits-Cristoph P. Empirically supported individual and group psychological treatments for adult mental disorders. *J Consulting Clin Psychol* 1998; 66: 37–52. (BI)

Supports cognitive-behaviour therapy, behaviour therapy and structured problem-solving. The studies reviewed are based in secondary care.

b Schulberg HC, Bock MR, Madonia MJ *et al*. Treating major depression in primary care practice: eight month clinical outcomes. *Arch Gen Psychiatry* 1996; 53: 913–919. (BII)

Supports interpersonal therapy.

c Mynors-Wallis LM, Gath DH, Lloyd-Thomas AR, Tomlinson D. Randomised controlled trial comparing problem solving treatment with amitriptyline and placebo for major depression in primary care. *Br Med J* 1995; 310: 441–445. (AII)

Where the therapies have been compared with each other, none appears clearly superior to the others. More variance in outcomes may be due to the strength of the therapeutic relationship rather than to the treatment method used. Problem-solving is the easiest therapy to learn and can be provided by general practitioners and primary-care nurses. Brief cognitive-behaviour therapy is difficult to deliver, even using trained therapists (Scott C, Tacchi M, Jones R, Scott J. Abbreviated cognitive therapy for depression: a pilot study in primary care. *Behav Cogn Psychother* 1994; 22: 96–102), so the time taken is unlikely to be reduced to less than 8–10 hours (Scott J. Editorial: Psychological treatments for depression — an update. *Br J Psychiatry* 1995; 167: 289–292). Evidence for the effectiveness of therapies in depression in primary care tends to be weaker than in major depressive disorder in secondary care.

84 Thase M, Greenhouse J, Frank E *et al*. Treatment of major depression with psychotherapy or psychotherapy–pharmacotherapy combinations. *Arch Gen Psychiatry* 1997; 54: 1009–1015.

A Cochrane review on this topic is pending.

85 Evans M, Hollins S, De Rubeis R *et al*. Differential relapse following cognitive therapy and pharmacotherapy of depression. *Arch Gen Psychiatry* 1992; 49: 802–808.

86 Ostler KJ, Thompson C, Kinmonth ALK *et al*. Influence of socio-economic deprivation on the prevalence and outcome of depression in primary care: The Hampshire Depression Project. *Br J Psychiatry*. Vol 178, 2001, 12–17.

Shows strong link between high indices of deprivation and a poor prognosis for depression in primary care.

87 Kaltenbach K, Finnegan L. Children of maternal substance misusers. *Curr Opin Psychiatry* 1997; 10: 220–224.

Most harm caused is indirect, eg via ill-health of the mother, poor antenatal care or cigarette smoking. There is a smaller risk of direct harm caused by heroin — growth retardation — and cocaine and amphetamines.

88 Miller W, Rollnick S. *Motivational Interviewing: Preparing People to Change Addictive Behaviour*. New York: Guilford, 1991. (AV)

89 Gossop M, Stewart D, Marsden J. *NTORS at One Year: The National Treatment Outcome Research Study. Change in Substance Use, Health and Criminal Behaviour One Year After Intake*. London: Department of Health, 1998. (A1)

b Ward J, Mattick R, Hall W. *Maintenance Treatment and Other Opioid Replacement Therapies*. London: Harwood, 1997.

c Carnworth T, Gabbay M, Barnard J. A share of the action: General Practitioner involvement in drug misuse treatment in Greater Manchester Drugs, Education Prevention and Policy Vol 7(3), 2000, 235–250.

90 Lader M, Russel J. Guidelines for the prevention and treatment of benzodiazepine dependence: summary of a report from the Mental Health Foundation. *Addiction* 1993; 88: 1707–1708.

91 The Task Force to Review Services for Drug Misusers. *Report of an Independent Review of Drug Treatment Services in England*. London: Department of Health, 1995.

92 American Psychiatric Association. *Practice Guidelines: Substance Use Disorders*. Washington, DC: APA, 1996. (BII)

Reports a large randomized, controlled trial replicated in a controlled trial comparing drug counselling, drug counselling plus supportive psychotherapy, and drug counselling plus cognitive-behaviour therapy for methadone maintenance patients. Those with moderate-to-high depression or other psychiatric symptoms did better with either therapy in addition to drug counselling. For patients with low levels of psychiatric symptoms, all three treatments were equally effective.

93 Khantzian E. The primary care therapist and patient needs in substance abuse treatment. *Am J Drug Alcohol Abuse* 1988; 14: 159–167.

Reviews studies of relapse prevention through, for example, encouraging the improved social and other relationships and activities.

94 Department of Health, Scottish Office, Welsh Office and DHSS Northern Ireland. *Drug Misuse and Dependence: Guidelines on Clinical Management*, 1999 Stationery Office, London.

95 Although some patients may benefit from maintenance on low doses (eg 10–20 mg day^{-1}), in general, higher doses (> 60 mg day^{-1}, range 60–120, average 70–80) are associated with better outcome; Ball J, Ross A. *The Effectiveness of Methadone Maintenance Treatment*. New York: Springer, 1991 (a prospective cohort study). Doses for stabilization in withdrawal are also often > 60 mg day^{-1} and are determined by the patient's response based on objective signs of withdrawal. See reference 92.

96 Marsch LC. The efficacy of methadone maintenance interventions in reducing illicit opiate use, HIV risk behaviour and criminality: a meta-analysis. *Addiction* 1998; 93: 515–532. (A1)

97 Johnson R, Jaffe J, Fudala P. A controlled trial of beprenorphine treatment for opioid dependence. *J Am Med Assoc* 1992; 267: 2750–2755. (CIII)

Additional research is needed, particularly in a UK setting.

98 Bearn J, Gossop M, Strang J. Randomised double-blind comparison of lofexidine and methadone in the in-patient treatment of opiate withdrawal. *Drug Alcohol Depend* 1996; 43: 87–91. (BII)

Concludes that lofexidine is as efficacious as methadone.

99 McLellan AT, Arndt IO, Metzger DS. The effects of psychosocial services in substance abuse treatment. *J Am Med Assoc* 1993; 269: 1953–1959. (BII)

Patients who received employment help, psychiatric care and family therapy had better outcomes than those who received counselling, who in turn had better outcomes than those who received methadone only.

100 Imipramine, desipramine, trazodone and fluoxetine have all shown some efficacy. In the imipramine studies, most patients reduced their symptoms by at least half, and one-third became free of symptoms. Higher doses of fluoxetine are needed than those normally used for treating depression. Several trials of medication may be needed to establish the one most suitable for an individual patient. Fluoxetine is currently the only antidepressant licensed in the UK for bulimia nervosa. Selected references:

a Mitchell J, Raymond N, Specker S. A review of the controlled trials of pharmacotherapy and psychotherapy in the treatment of bulimia nervosa. *Int J Eating Disord* 1993; 15: 229–247. (BIII)

b American Psychiatric Association. *Practice Guidelines: Eating Disorders*. Washington, DC: APA, 1996. B(II)

101 Uncontrolled trials and one small controlled trial have suggested that fluoxetine may help some patients in the weight-maintenance phases, but many patients do not improve with this or any other currently available medication. However, for patients with persistent depression, the use of antidepressants should be considered. Consider medication with fewer cardiovascular side-effects. Selected references:

a See reference 101b. (AIII)

b Leach A. The psychopharmacotherapy of eating disorders. *Psychiatr Annals* 1995; 25: 628–633.

c Kaye W, Gendall K, Strober M. Serotonin neuronal function and selective serotonin re-uptake inhibitor treatment in anorexia and bulimia nervosa. *Biol Psychiatr* 1998; 44: 825–838. (CIII)

102 Russell GFM, Szmukler GI, Dare C, Eisler I. An evaluation of family therapy in anorexia nervosa and bulimia nervosa. *Arch Gen Psychiatr* 1987, 44: 1047–1056. (CIII)

Shows that patients with anorexia nervosa with onset at or before age 18, and with a duration less than 3 years, did better with family therapy than individual therapy. Moreover, older patients did better with individual therapy. However, a major UK review, while supporting these recommendations, states that there are currently no high-quality reviews of psychological treatments for anorexia nervosa (see reference 59).

103 Whitbread J, McGown A. The treatment of bulimia nervosa: what is effective? A meta-analysis. *Int J Clin Psychol* 1994; 21: 32–44. (BI)

A Cochrane review is currently in progress.

104 Treasure J, Schmidt U, Troop N *et al*. First step in managing bulimia nervosa: controlled trial of a therapeutic manual. *Br Med J* 1994; 308: 686–689. (BIII)

105 Shear K, Schulberg H. Anxiety disorders in primary care. *Bull Menninger Clinic* 1995; 59(2, Suppl A): 73–82. (BI)

Reviews studies of the provision of psycho-education and minimal interventions in primary care. Observations suggests that they show considerable promise as first-line interventions for anxiety disorders in primary care; however, more severely ill patients will require more sophisticated intervention.

106 See reference 12. (BII)

107a Gould RA, Otto MW, Pollack MH, Yap L. Cognitive behavioural and pharmacological treatment of generalised anxiety disorder: a preliminary meta-analysis. *Behaviour Ther* 1997; 28: 285–305. (BI)

Revealed the highest effect sizes for diazepam. Buspirone had a much lower effect size than either benzodiazepines or antidepressants, and its onset is slow (up to 4 weeks). However, problems with dependence and withdrawal are minimal compared with benzodiazepines.

b Lader MH, Bond AJ. Interaction of pharmacological and psychological treatments of anxiety. *Br J Psychiatry* 1998; 173(Suppl 34): 165–168.

Firm conclusions are not possible. Observations suggest using benzodiazepines for treating anxiety initially, as these produce rapid symptomatic improvement; then psychological treatments can take over.

108 Imipramine and paroxetine have both been shown to reduce anxiety symptoms in the short-term. Onset is slower than benzodiazepines but addiction is not a problem. Relapse rates following longer-term use are not known. Selected references (BII):

a Kahn R, Mcnair D, Lipman R *et al*. Imipramine and chlordiazepoxide in depressive and anxiety disorders II. Efficacy in anxious out-patients. *Arch Gen Psychiatry* 1986; 43: 79–85.

b Rocca P, Fonzo V, Scotta M *et al*. Paroxetine efficacy in the treatment of generalised anxiety disorder. *Acta Psychiatr Scand* 1997; 95: 444–450.

109 Tyrer P. Use of beta blocking drugs in psychiatry and neurology. *Drugs* 1980; 20: 300–308.

110 Gould RA, Otto MW, Pollack MH, Yap L. Cognitive behavioural and pharmacological treatment of generalised anxiety disorder: a preliminary meta-analysis. *Behaviour Ther* 1997; 28: 285–305. (BI)

Cognitive-behavioural therapy (CBT) and anxiety management were the most efficacious of psychological treatments. Medication and psychological therapies were equally efficacious in the short-term. Gains of CBT and anxiety management were maintained at 6 months.

111 Kupshik G, Fisher C. Assisted bibliotherapy: effective, efficient treatment for moderate anxiety problems. *Br J Gen Pract* 1999; 49: 47–48. (BIII)

Learning self-help skills through reading, supported by contact with a clinician, led to a significant improvement of symptoms. Greater numbers improved with a greater amount of clinician contact, especially patients with fewer educational achievements.

112 See reference 57. (BIII)

113 Swinson RP, Soulios C, Cox BJ, Kuch K. Brief treatment of emergency-room patients with panic attacks. *Am J Psychiatry* 1992; 149: 944–946. (BIII)

People presenting to A&E with panic provided with psycho-education and exposure instructions had a significantly better outcome than controls.

114 American Psychiatric Association. Practice guideline for the treatment of patients with panic disorder. *Am J Psychiatry* 1998; 155(Suppl): 1–26. (AII)

Concludes that tricyclic antidepressants (TCAs), selective serotonin re-uptake inhibitors (SSRIs), monoamine oxidase inhibitors (MAOIs) and benzodiazepines have roughly comparable efficacy in the short-term. Benzodiazepines are useful in the very short-term in situations where very rapid control of symptoms is critical. TCA side-effects may be problematic. Short-term use of medication commonly results in relapse, so longer-term use is recommended — 2–18 months — after which period the relapse rate is not known.

115 Benzodiazepines are effective in many cases in suppressing panic in the short-term. They are not an effective treatment for chronic panics or phobias as there is no evidence that gains made continue when drugs are withdrawn; there is some evidence that they do not. Where patients are undergoing exposure therapy, ie dealing with the fear by gradually facing it, there is some evidence that benzodiazepines may actually interfere with maintaining longer-term therapeutic gains. Selected references (BII):

a American Psychiatric Association. Practice guideline for the treatment of patients with panic disorder. *Am J Psychiatry* 1998; 155(Suppl): 1–26.

b Marks I, Swinson P, Basoglu M *et al*. Alprazolam and exposure alone and combined in panic disorder with agoraphobia. A controlled study in London and Toronto. *Br J Psychiatry* 1993; 162: 776–787.

116 See reference 13a.

Conclude that 85% of chronic patients stay well between the 1- and 2-year follow-up when treated using cognitive-behaviour therapy.

117 Marks I, Swinson RP. Alprazolam and exposure for panic disorder with agoraphobia; summary of London/Toronto results. *J Psychiatric Res* 1990; 24: 100–101. (AII)

Where agoraphobic fear and avoidance is present, with panic, exposure — a behavioural treatment — proved twice as effective as alprazolam.

118 Wade WA, Treat TA, Stuart GL. Transporting an empirically supported treatment for panic disorder to a service clinic setting; a benchmarking strategy. *J Consult Clin Psychol* 1998; 66: 231–239. (CIII)

119 Dolan B, Coid J. Psychopathic and antisocial personality disorders: treatment and research issues. London: Gaskell/Royal College of Psychiatrists, 1993, pp. 116–119.

120 Hawton K, Arensman E, Townsend E *et al*. Deliberate self harm: systematic review of efficacy of psychosocial and pharmacological treatments in preventing repetition. *Br Med J* 1998; 317: 441–447.

121 Coccaro EF, Kavoussi RJ. Fluoxetine and impulsive aggressive behaviour in personality-disordered subjects. *Arch Gen Psychiatry* 1997; 54: 1081–1088.

122 Greenberg WM. Sedative or antimanic effects of carbamazepine and treatment of behavioural dyscontrol. *Am J Psychiatry* 1986; 143: 1486–1487.

123 Stermac L. Anger control treatment for forensic patients. *J Interpersonal Violence* 1986; 1: 446–722.

124 Fleming G, Pretzer JL. Cognitive-behavioural approaches to personality disorders. In Hersen M, Eisler M, Miller PM (eds), *Progress in Behaviour Modification*, vol. 26. Beverly Hills: Sage, 1990, pp. 119–151; Appleby L, Joseph P. Management of personality disorder. *Int Rev Psychiatry* 1991; 3: 59–70.

125 Linehan MM, Heard HL, Armstrong He. Interpersonal outcome of cognitive-behavioural treatment for chronically suicidal borderline patients. *Am J Psychiatry* 1994; 151: 1771–1776.

126 Murray B, Stein M, Michael R *et al*. Paroxetine treatment of generalized social phobia (social anxiety disorder): a randomised controlled trial. *J Am Med Assoc* 1998; 280: 8. (CII)

Symptoms improved in short-term, ie 11-week trial. However, relapse rates are very high after discontinuation, and relapse rates after longer-term treatment are not known; Stein MB, Chartier MJ, Hazen Al *et al*. Paroxetine in the treatment of generalised social phobia: open-label treatment and double-blind, placebo-controlled discontinuation. *J Clin Psychopharmacol* 1996; 16: 218–222.

127 DeRubeis RJ, Crits-Cristoph P. Empirically supported individual and group psychological treatments for adult mental disorders. *J Consult Clin Psychol* 1998; 66: 37–52. (AII)

Exposure with cognitive therapy shows efficacy for social phobia; exposure with cognitive-behaviour therapy shows efficacy for agoraphobia. Efficacy of exposure behaviour therapy has proven twice that of alprazolam for agoraphobic fear and avoidance. See reference 118.

128 Fichtner C, Poddig B, deVito R. Post-traumatic stress disorder: pathophysiological aspects and pharmacological approaches to treatment. *CNS Drugs* 1997; 8: 293–322. (CII)

Research base is limited. There is evidence of only limited efficacy for a wide range of drugs. Fluoxetine is the most widely studied selective serotonin re-uptake inhibitor (SSRI). Phenelzine appears more effective than tricyclic antidepressants (TCAs) for re-experiencing symptoms. The most studied TCAs were imipramine and amitriptyline.

129 See reference 13a.

Concludes that the impact of psychological treatment on the primary symptoms of post-traumatic stress disorder (PTSD) may be limited, but it may reduce symptoms of depression and anxiety. The best evidence of efficacy is for exposure and other cognitive-behavioural methods.

130 Foa EB, Meadows EA. Psychosocial treatments for post-traumatic stress disorder: a critical review. *Ann Rev Psychology* 1997; 48: 449–480. (BII)

Shows that exposure — a behavioural treatment — and supportive counselling are equally effective at the end of treatment, but exposure is superior after 3 months.

131 Boolell M, Gepi-Atee S, Gingell C, Allen MK. Sildenafil: a novel effective oral therapy for male erectile dysfunction. *Br J Urol* 1996; 78: 257–261. (AII)

132 Padma-Natham H, Hellstrom WJG, Kaiser RE *et al*. Treatment of men with erectile dysfunction with transurethral alprostadil. *New Engl J Med* 1997; 336: 1–7. (AII)

133 Linet OI, Ogrine FG. Efficacy and safety of intracavernosal alprostadil in men with erectile dysfunction. *New Engl J Med* 1996; 334: 873–877. (AII)

134 McClusky HY, Milby JB, Switzer PK *et al*. Efficacy of behavioural versus triazolam treatment in persistent sleep-onset insomnia. *Am J Psychiatry* 1991; 148: 121–126. (BVplus)

This small trial found that triazolam had an immediate effect on persistent insomnia, and behavioural treatment took 3 weeks to have an equivalent effect. Behavioural treatment is more effective at 1-month follow-up.

135 Eisen J, MacFarlane J, Shapiro C. Psychotropic drugs and sleep. *Br Med J* 1993; 306: 1331–1334.

136 Rasmussen P. A role of phytotherapy in the treatment of benzodiazepines and opiate drug withdrawal. *Eur J Herbal Med* 1997; 3: 11–21 (CIV); as quoted in Wallcraft J. *Healing Minds: A Report on Current Research, Policy and Practice Concerning the Use of Complementary and Alternative Therapies for a Wide Range of Mental Health Problems*. London: Mental Health Foundation, 1998.

Refers to trials — some in animals — showing that valerian can improve the quality of sleep and without a hangover effect the next day. No studies of the long-term safety of valerian have been reported. The effect on sleep is weak.

137 Bootzin R, Perlis M. Non-pharmacological treatments of insomnia. *J Clin Psychiatry* 1992; 53(6 Suppl): 37–40.

This review found that sleep hygiene training during individual counselling and stimulus control instructions was more effective than relaxation training.

138 World Health Organization. *Insomnia: Behavioural and Cognitive Interventions*. Geneva: Division of Mental Health, WHO, 1993.

139 Goldberg R, Dennis H, Novack M, Gask L. The recognition and management of somatization: what is needed in primary care training. *Psychosomatics* 1992; 33: 55–61. (BV)

140 Smith GR, Rost K, Kashner M. A trial of the effect of a standardised psychiatric consultation on health outcomes and costs in somatising patients. *Arch Gen Psych* 1995; 52: 238–243. (BII)

141 Fishbain DA, Cutler RB, Rosomoff HL, Rosomoff RS. Do antidepressants have an analgesic effect in psychogenic pain and somatoform pain disorder? A meta-analysis. *Psychosom Med* 1998; 60: 503–509. (B1)

142 Pilowsky I, Barrow C. A controlled study of psychotherapy and amitriptyline used individually and in combination in the treatment of chronic intractable psychogenic pain. *Pain* 1990; 40: 3–19. (CIII)

143a Speckens A, van Hemert A, Spinhoven P *et al*. Cognitive behavioural therapy for medically unexplained physical symptoms: a randomized controlled trial. *Br Med J* 1995; 311: 1328–1332. (BII)

Six to 16 sessions of cognitive-behaviour therapy were conducted in medical out-patients. Intervention was effective and acceptable to patients, and gains were maintained at the 12-month follow-up.

b Kashner TM, Rost K, Cohen B *et al*. Enhancing the health of somatization disorder patients: effectiveness of short-term group therapy. *Psychosomatics* 1995; 36: 924–932. (BII)

Random controlled trial of 70 patients in primary care who were offered eight sessions of group therapy. Improvements, both physical and emotional, were maintained at 1 year.

c Guthrie E. Emotional disorder in chronic illness: psychotherapeutic interventions. *Br J Psychiatry* 1996; 168: 265–273.

This review includes eight studies of somatic presentation of psychological problems. Two studies show cognitive-behaviour therapy to be effective in atypical chest pain and functional dyspepsia, and hypnosis to be effective in two studies for irritable bowel syndrome. Compliance is poor, however. Patients with a long history of symptoms and marked abnormal illness behaviour are unlikely to respond to a brief intervention.

Mental disorders in adolescents — general issues

Introduction

While much of the information about the management of mental disorders in adults also applies to adolescents, there are significant differences. This section briefly describes these differences.

Prevalence

The rates of mental disorder in adolescents are similar to or higher than those in adults. The rates of all mental disorders (psychosis, depression, post-traumatic stress disorder, substance misuse) are substantially higher in young offenders than in young people in the community. This is to be expected as so many of them have experienced events in their lives that are known to increase the risk of mental disorder. Over one-third have been 'looked after' children in Local Authority care. The levels of previous physical, sexual and emotional abuse, school exclusion, low educational achievement and unemployment are all high and many are teenage parents. In addition, a significant group of young people are exposed to further victimisation (eg bullying, violence, unwanted sexual attention) while in prison.

The prevalence of antisocial, paranoid or emotionally unstable ('borderline') personality disorders (or combinations of these) in the 16–21-year group is also very high. The prevalence of mental retardation and pervasive developmental disorders (eg autism) in adolescents in prison in England and Wales is not known, but levels in delinquent populations are significantly higher than in the general population. Specific learning difficulties such as dyslexia (reading disorder) and difficulties with spoken communication are over-represented among young offenders in prison. Reading problems are strongly linked with psychiatric problems in general and behavioural problems in particular.

For a summary of the epidemiological information about psychiatric morbidity in young offenders, see page 117.

Issues in assessment

To identify what is abnormal, it is necessary to have an understanding of normal development. Adolescents are engaged in particular developmental tasks (eg becoming independent from others while still maintaining appropriate emotional closeness to them; developing a sense of identity, including a sexual and cultural identity, a body image and self-esteem). The behavioural problems that peak in the teenage years such as delinquency, substance misuse, deliberate self-harm and anorexia nervosa often involve exaggerated and unresolved versions of ordinary adolescent development. As a result, abnormal behaviour in adolescents is more likely to be interpreted or dismissed as a normal response to life events by healthcare professionals, teachers, parents and the patients themselves, resulting in missed or late diagnoses. A good working knowledge of adolescent development can help prevent this, as can a thorough assessment that includes information from a variety of informants.

Carrying out the assessment

Where a young person is thought to have a mental disorder, the assessment should include taking a history and an assessment of the mental state (see **Assessment**, page 165), in addition to the following.

- Explain the limits of confidentiality. Many adolescents want a promise of secrecy.
- Interview several informants if possible. The family, social services staff, educational staff and residential staff can all contribute important information from their different perspectives. Residential staff will have information about the individual's mood and behaviour, any incidents of self-harm, relationships with staff and peers, participation in association and education, whether the individual has a job, and the reasons for any adjudications and episodes in the segregation block.
- Expect and look for comorbidity. Emotional problems are often overlooked in the presence of aggressive and disruptive behaviour. Substance misuse may be a consequence of conduct disorder or a way of self-medicating for emotional disorders. Between 30 and 50% of individuals with early onset conduct disorder also have attention deficit hyperactivity disorder (ADHD)/hyperkinetic disorder. Systematically, you should ask about:
  — worries, phobias, obsessions
  — depressive symptoms
  — inattention, impulsivity, excessive activity
  — aggressive, delinquent and rule-breaking behaviour
  — problems with learning
  — bizarre or strange ideas and behaviour
  — use of substances and
  — relationships with parents, siblings and peers.
- Ask about suicidal thoughts and self-harming behaviours.
  — The principles of assessing and managing suicide and self-injury are generally applicable to young people (see page 204).
  — Suicide is a leading cause of death in people aged 15–24. Self-harm is most frequent during adolescence.
  — Ask direct questions.
- Ask about bullying/abuse/debt. Focus on current and recent abuse to prevent further harm.
- Assess the impairment in functioning (eg can the individual maintain former levels of self-care such as grooming and eating, as well as relationships with others and work/education).
- Identify the strengths and resources in the individual and their network of family, friends and staff. Ask if there is any adult in the young offenders' institute (YOI) who they trust and have a good relationship with. This is important for developing the management plan.

Which professional (or combination of professionals) carries out this assessment will vary according to the composition of the healthcare team. Where the team includes mental-health nurses, they are likely to be involved.

Tests of cognitive functioning and academic achievement

Developmental disabilities (eg learning disability, autism), specific learning difficulties (eg dyslexia, dyspraxia) and communication difficulties (eg stammering, getting words muddled) are all more common in young offenders. The appropriate tests are usually administered by clinical psychologists, education staff or speech and language therapists and may be conducted as part of the individual's initial screening. Where they have not been done and a problem in one of these areas is suspected, request an assessment from the local Learning Disability Trust (for developmental disabilities). Assessments for specific learning difficulties may need to be obtained under contract from Local Authority Educational Psychology Departments. Appropriate treatment can improve the outcome of any mental disorders.

Summary of the areas to consider in an assessment of young offenders

Psychiatric disorders, eg depressive disorder, substance misuse
Specific delays in development, eg dyslexia
Intellectual level, eg mild mental retardation
Medical condition(s), eg epilepsy
Psychosocial adversity, eg institutional upbringing
Functioning in day-to-day life, eg serious problems relating to others
Strengths and resources, eg enjoys art, has a trusting relationship with a probation officer in the home area

---

Issues in management

Emotional and behavioural disorders in young people are to a greater extent symptoms of disordered relationships within the family, peer group or wing/unit than symptoms of a disorder within the individual. Consequently, the following may be found.

- Medication plays a lesser role than in adult disorders (with the exception of ADHD/hyperkinetic disorder).
- Interventions that attempt to change the young person's environment and relationships or help him/her to cope better with them play a greater role. The larger part of management consists of helping others (residential staff, teachers, other staff) to develop and carry through a management plan. See the guidelines for particular disorders for details.
- Interventions that aim to increase the young person's emotional resilience or increase their self-esteem are protective against further deterioration of mental state and should always form part of the management plan.
- Although particularly difficult to achieve in the YOI context, the family should be involved in treatment wherever possible, especially with a younger adolescent who still lives at home. Contact with the youth justice worker, probation officer or social worker from the home area is also likely to be helpful.

Comorbidity

- Separate treatment is required for associated problems.
- Substance misuse by adolescents is less likely to require medical treatment for dependence and more likely to be a symptom of a behavioural disorder. Treatment, therefore, will be less substance-oriented and will involve a broader range of interventions.[1]

Medication

- There is generally less information about the efficacy and side-effects of drugs in adolescents than in adults.

- The dosage may need to be modified according to the adolescent's weight.
- Poor compliance and overdosing are common issues with adolescents. The stigma of being diagnosed and treated for a mental disorder is a major issue that needs discussion.

Informed consent

This is more complex with young people (see page 300).

Confidentiality

Adolescents are often particularly concerned about their privacy (for a discussion of the issue, see page 304).

Referral and aftercare

- Prepare the individual for a referral to a mental-health professional. Emphasise that referral does not mean that they are 'mental' or crazy. Emphasise the collaborative nature of psychological therapy.
- Generally, if the young person is at school or under the age of 17, the parents should be involved in the referral process where possible. Where there is a conflict of interest, the interests of the patient take precedence over those of the family.
- Where possible, seek to involve the NHS mental-health services in the area to which the young person is to be released at least 6 weeks before release.
- See the guidelines for specific disorders for referral criteria. In general, young people identified as being acutely psychotic, severely depressed and those with a severe personality disorder should, wherever possible, be swiftly transferred to and accepted by outside hospitals.
- For more information on liaison, referral and aftercare, including the Care Programme Approach, see page 151.

In-house mental-health services

Primary-care staff require the support of specialist services. To achieve equivalence with out-patient child and adolescent mental-health services in the community, the establishment would need the support of a multidisciplinary team including psychiatry, clinical psychology, nursing, and individual and family therapy. Strong links between these, the primary-care staff, drug project team, chaplain and probation officers are needed. Direct access by young prisoners and prison officers and other staff is desirable. The development towards this is likely to be incremental.

[1] Merrill J, Peters L. Substance misuse. In Gowers SG (ed.), *Adolescent Psychiatry in Clinical Practice*. London: Arnold, 2001.

Adolescent conduct disorder — F91#

Introduction

Many young offenders meet the diagnostic criteria for conduct disorder simply by virtue of their persistent criminal activities. Unless their behaviour is regarded as abnormal by the individuals themselves, their peers or family, healthcare intervention is unwelcome and cooperation unlikely. This guideline, therefore, aims to help primary-care staff to do the following.

- Identify and treat associated mental disorders.
- Support and advise other staff who form the mainstay of the management of these individuals.
- Identify those individuals who may benefit from further assessment and treatment for their behavioural problems by specialists.
- Participate effectively in the multidisciplinary management of individuals with more severe disorder, thus reducing or preventing associated problems such as psychiatric disorders, self-harm and violence, and reducing the probability of the individual developing lifelong personality disorder.

Presenting complaints

Most individuals present associated problems rather than the conduct disorder itself, eg depression, deliberate self-harm or repeatedly seeking psychotropic medication. Others, particularly prisoners on remand, may ask for help in controlling their anger. Staff or other inmates may express concern about the individual's behaviour, eg persistent disruptive behaviour ('something to calm him down'), social isolation, bullying or being the victim of bullying.

Diagnostic features

There is a pattern of persistently excessive antisocial behaviour lasting at least 6 months and usually much longer. Symptoms may include vandalism, cruelty to both people and animals, bullying, lying or cheating (to con others), starting physical fights, using weapons during fights, stealing outside the home, setting fires to cause damage, repeated truancy, and forcing others to perform sexual acts against their will.

Conduct problems involve three overlapping domains: defiance of authority, aggressiveness and antisocial behaviour that violates other people's rights, property or person. These behaviours, to a certain degree, are a part of normal child and adolescent development. A diagnosis should only be made when the behaviours are extreme and persistent or result in impairment in everyday functioning.

Two groups of young people with antisocial behaviour have been identified.[1]

- **Late onset**: antisocial behaviour begins during adolescence and is associated strongly with social factors such as a family history of criminality, the influence of peers and substance misuse. The early history is often unremarkable, with a conflict with authority, which may be normal within the delinquent subculture, becoming apparent as the child enters adolescence. Young offenders thought of by staff as 'normal' may fall into this category.

• **Lifetime persistent**: this group displays antisocial and disturbed behaviour often from early childhood. There is a much higher incidence of impaired social functioning, emotional problems, psychiatric illness, self-harm and substance misuse. The group is at particular risk of developing adult antisocial personality disorder.

Differential diagnosis

• Occasional antisocial acts do not warrant this diagnosis.

• Adjustment reaction (if antisocial behaviour lasts no more than 6 months and follows a stressor such as family breakdown, bereavement, trauma, abuse or adoption).

• Depression or bipolar disorder (where irritability and aggression are not part of a long-standing pattern of behaviour and other symptoms of depression are present).

• Early onset schizophrenia: behavioural disturbance that mimics conduct disorder may be part of the early (prodromal) phase of schizophrenia. Suspect the early stages of a severe mental illness where there is a clear change in social functioning (eg a decline in work or school performance) and any changes in thinking (eg a preoccupation with odd ideas, increased suspiciousness), behaviour (eg increased withdrawal) or mood (eg rapid mood changes, inappropriate moods) (see **Early onset psychosis**, page 131).

• Autism spectrum disorders, generalised learning disability (mental retardation) and other pervasive developmental disorders are frequently accompanied by behavioural problems. Autistic individuals may be identified by their lack of a capacity to socialise, severely restricted language or odd style of speech, and preoccupation or obsession with sameness (see **Learning disability**, page 255).

• Personality disorder: a diagnosis of 'personality disorder' is generally not appropriate in adolescents under the age of 18.

Essential information for the patient and the primary support group

• The way the institution is run affects outcomes for young people. The beneficial effects of incarceration may be derived from education and training that open up opportunities on release, from help for drug misuse, from a pro-social ethos with good relationships and role models, from encouraging strong, regular links with families, and from encouraging the young people to do things for themselves and to feel proud of any achievements they make.[2]

• In severe cases, the young person is likely to be temperamentally different from others and therefore cannot easily control his/her actions.

• Antisocial behaviour is in part learned and can be corrected (unlearned). However, this requires substantial motivation, effort and support — especially where the behaviours are long-standing, severe and persistent.

• Disruptive individuals tend to externalise distress and conflict. They may have trouble recognising fear or sadness in themselves. They also frequently have difficulties in using negotiation skills or problem-solving skills as alternatives to aggression. Adults who can model or teach these skills can be helpful.

• The long-term prognosis is not good without intervention. Individuals do not 'grow out of it'. However, there may be improvements with appropriate management. Some factors known to help protect against a poor outcome may be available within a young offenders' institute (YOI). They include:

— having a caring, supportive relationship with at least one adult
— having friends who do not get into trouble
— experience of achievement in some sort of activity (eg sport, any form of education or training, a responsibility within the institution)
— absence of (or successful interventions for) learning problems, such as dyslexia
— absence (or successful treatment) of other mental disorders (especially substance misuse and attention deficit hyperactivity disorder [ADHD])
— experience of establishing a stable work record and
— remaining at school until the age of compulsory school end or longer.

Identification and arrangement of treatment for associated conditions

Coexistent disorders are easily missed and should be carefully assessed.

- **Alcohol and drug misuse**: substance misuse appears not to cause conduct disorder (which usually precedes substance misuse), but it may exacerbate and perpetuate it. In most cases uncomplicated by more severe psychopathology, the successful treatment of drug and alcohol problems will probably do most to reduce the likelihood of problems persisting into adulthood.
- **Specific reading retardation (dyslexia)**: achievement and employment both predict good outcomes in conduct disorder, so referral for interventions for dyslexia is of great practical importance. Difficulties with spoken language (eg stuttering, getting words muddled) are also common in the young offender population and interfere with successes in work and education.[3,4]
- **Hyperkinetic disorder/ADHD**: rates of comorbid ADHD have been reported to be as high as 30% of boys and 59% of girls with conduct disorder.[5] ADHD is a developmental risk factor for conduct disorder.[6] The prognosis for young people with both disorders is poorer, so it is essential to diagnose and treat ADHD.
- **Depression**: rates of comorbidity are reported as being between 23 and 36%.[7] Depression requires treatment in its own right. Behaviour problems do not usually reduce after treatment of depression.

See the guidelines for relevant disorders for information on diagnosis and management.

Advice and support for the patient and the primary support group

Behavioural management is most likely to be effective where the individual is of a younger age and does not have a 'callous, unemotional' interpersonal style, and where the regime and staff behaviours consistently support appropriate behaviours and do not tolerate inappropriate ones. Staff should be encouraged to do the following.

- **Develop a regimen where staff model the appropriate behaviour**, eg dealing with aggression by 'talking down' in the first instance, bullying is not tolerated and opportunities for constructive activity and achievement are plentiful.
- **Encourage positive strengths**, eg work, sport, art, education, continued family contact, other relationships. Anything that allows achievement and raises self-esteem is likely to be helpful.
- **Where possible, develop a relationship with the young person**, eg identify a shared interest and spend a short time as often as possible discussing or doing the activity together (eg football). Aim to interact with the young person in ways other than giving orders.

- **Set clear rules and give short, specific commands about the desired behaviour, not prohibitions about undesired behaviour**, eg 'please walk calmly' rather than 'don't run'.
- **Where staff have a positive relationship with a young person, help him/her try to find alternative strategies to replace those that lead to trouble,** eg 'If someone else confronts you, rather than hitting him first, ask why he is angry or go and tell someone you trust.' Praise and reward any progress.
- **Provide consistent and calm consequences for misbehaviour**. The wing minor report system can be used to mark overstepping behavioural boundaries. Avoid getting into arguments or explanations with the individual as this only provides more attention for the misbehaviour. Conversely, ignoring minor problems such as defiant language may be effective.

Severe, long-standing behavioural problems

- Assess the risk to yourself, the individual and to others. Self-harm is common in this group (see **Assessing and managing people at risk of suicide** and **Dealing with aggression**, pages 204 and 282).
- Discuss the most challenging individuals with those delivering regimes in the prison to see if a package of activities can be organised to help the individuals structure their day.
- For further management advice, see **Antisocial personality disorder** and **Managing prisoners with complex presentations and very difficult behaviour**, pages 70 and 202).

Medication

No drugs have shown an effectiveness as treatments for antisocial behaviours in general or for aggression in particular. The psychostimulant methylphenidate is effective for comorbid hyperactivity and can reduce aggression[8] — but **only** if hyperkinetic disorder/ADHD is present. See the guideline on hyperkinetic disorder/ADHD.

Psychological treatment

There is no conclusive evidence about the effectiveness of any single intervention. The Thinking Skills programme offered under the Prison Service's Offending Behaviour programme has been shown to reduce the risk of re-offending among 'ordinary' young offenders. However, multimodal, well-structured, intensive, lengthy programmes that are cognitive-behavioural in orientation have proven most effective with adolescents who show severe antisocial behaviour and are at highest risk of developing adult personality disorder.[9]

Treatments that have shown the most promise are listed below.

- **Cognitive-behavioural programmes**, especially multimodal ones incorporating anger control, problem-solving, self-control and moral reasoning ability.[10]
- **Multisystemic therapy.**[11,12]
- **Family therapy.**[13]
- **Behavioural management training**: more appropriate for a younger age group or where the adolescent is actively involved in developing and agreeing the programme.[14]

Currently, thinking skills and problem-solving skills training may be available under the Prison Service's Offending Behaviour programme. Multisystemic therapy is not yet available in the UK. Family therapy and behavioural management training is often available from the adolescent mental-health services, both the general and forensic services.

Where symptoms are severe, the individual is motivated and the service exists, treatment may be offered in a residential setting. Results are best if the programme is structured, the atmosphere warm, there are high expectations, there are positive staff and adolescent relationships, and the programme lasts for more than a year.[15]

Referral and resettlement

Prisoners with conduct disorder come to the attention of wing staff, probation officers, education officers, and health and workplace staff. Sentence planning pulls all these threads together. Health staff should ensure that their skills are part of sentence planning. Where an individual's behaviour is leading to impairment and distress, regular multidisciplinary case conferences and a care plan are recommended.

Consider referring to in-house or local adolescent mental-health services

- suspected hyperkinetic disorder/ADHD
- comorbid severe psychiatric illness
- where there is serious risk to self or others.

Consider referring to the adolescent forensic services (if available) the most severe cases where there is evidence of sadism or sexually inappropriate behaviour or where there is severe social isolation. Interventions work best with patients who are willing to engage in therapy. In practice, choosing whether to refer the most severe cases or more motivated patients with less severe problems is a practical trade-off between the likely responsiveness to treatment and the seriousness of the disorder.

Consider referral to learning disability services where autism is suspected or where there is a learning disability and a change in behaviour (see **People with learning disability**, page 255). For those with specific learning or communication difficulties, consider organising a special package with the Education Department and with others.

If a release of individuals with severe behavioural problems is planned, contact the local youth offending team and enquire whether there are specific services within the local child and adolescent mental-health service that would be of help to the young person. If no service is available, notify the Public Health Department at the relevant Primary Care Trust. Liaison with a probation officer will also be important. For severely affected individuals, consider the risk to others. Prison Service Order 6450 and Probation Circular 27:2000 set out the arrangements to be made for the release of people who are considered dangerous.

Resources for patients and primary support groups

National Family and Parenting Institute: 020 7424 3460

Young Minds Trust: 020 7336 8445 (office)
102–108 Clerkenwell Road, London EC1M 5SA
(Produces a range of leaflets for young people and their parents. It also runs a **Parent Information Service:** 0800 0182138 (freephone), which provides information and advice for anyone concerned about the mental health of a child or a young person)

1   Moffitt TE. Adolescence-limited and life-course-persistent antisocial behaviour: a developmental taxonomy. *Psychological Review* 1993; 100: 674–701.

2   Rutter M, Giller Hand Hagell A. *Antisocial Behaviour by Young People*. Cambridge: Cambridge University Press, 1998.

3   Bryan K. Survey of speech, language and communication skills in young prisoners. In *HM Inspector's Report of Inspection at HM YOI Swinfen Hall*. London: HMSO, 2000.

4   Crowe TA. Speech and hearing status of prisoners. *Bulletin of the College of Speech and Language Therapists* 1991; 466: 2–4.

5   Szatmari P, Boyle M, Offord DR. ADDH and conduct disorders: degree of diagnostic overlap and differences among correlates. *Journal of the American Academy of Child and Adolescent Psychiatry* 1989; 28: 865–872. Reports the Ontario Child Health Study and shows that of young people aged 12–16 years, of boys 6.7% had pure conduct disorder, 3.8% had pure ADDH and 2.9% had both disorders; of girls 2.7% had pure conduct disorder, 1.6% had pure ADDH and 1.6% had both disorders.

6   Taylor E, Chadwick O, Heptinstall E, Danckaerts M. Hyperactivity and conduct problems as risk factors for adolescent development. *Journal of the American Academy of Child and Adolescent Psychiatry* 1996; 35: 1213–1226.

7   Kovacs M, Paulaskas S, Gastoris C, Richards G. Depressive disorders in childhood: III. A longitudinal study of comorbidity with and risk for conduct disorder. *Journal of Affective Diseases* 1988; 15: 205–217.

8   Hinshaw SP. Stimulant medication and the treatment of aggression in children with attentional deficits. *Journal of Clinical Child Psychology* 1991; 20: 301–312.

9   Bailey S. Responding to the needs and risks of young offenders. In Gowers SG (ed.), *Adolescent Psychiatry in Clinical Practice*. London: Arnold, 2001.

10 Baer RA, Nietzel MT. Cognitive and behavioural treatment of impulsivity in children: a meta-analytic review of the outcome literature. *Journal of Clinical Child Psychology* 1991; 20: 400–412.

11 Borduin CM, Mann BJ, Cone LT *et al*. Multisystemic treatment of serious juvenile offenders: long term prevention of criminality and violence. *Journal of Consulting and Clinical Psychology* 1995; 63: 569–578.

12 Henggeler SW, Schoenwald SK, Borduin CM, Rowland MD, Cunningham PB. *Multisystemic Treatment of Antisocial Behaviour in Children and Adolescents*. New York: Guilford, 1998.

13 Alexander JF, Barton C, Schiavo RS, Parsons BV. Systems behavioural interventions with families of delinquents: therapist characteristics, family behaviour and outcome. *Journal of Consulting and Clinical Psychology* 1976; 44: 656–664.

14 Patterson GR. *Coercive Family Process*. Eugene: Castalia, 1982; Dishion TJ, Patterson GR. Age effects in parent training outcomes. *Behaviour Therapy* 1992; 23: 719–729.

15 Harris DP, Cole JE, Vipond EM. Residential treatment of disturbed delinquents: description of centre and identification of therapeutic factors. *Canadian Journal of Psychiatry* 1987; 32: 527–583.

Hyperkinetic disorders — F90

Includes attention deficit hyperactivity disorder (ADHD)

Introduction

Attention deficit hyperactivity disorder (ADHD) and hyperkinetic disorder are disorders with a strong genetic component, characterised from an early age (before 7 years) by disturbances in the areas of attention, impulsiveness and hyperactivity.

The disorders are reputed to be more prevalent in the USA than in the UK, but this is largely the result of the use of less strict diagnostic criteria, which include people with less severe symptoms. Hyperkinetic disorder is the name given to the disorder diagnosed using the stricter ICD-10 criteria; 1.7% of primary school children meet these criteria. ADHD is the name given to the disorder diagnosed using the less strict DSM-IV criteria; 3–6% of primary school children meet these criteria. These disorders are more common in boys.

Contrary to what was previously thought, a significant proportion of children with ADHD continue to have the disorder in late adolescence and some still show symptoms 10 years later, though inattention is more frequently prominent in adults than is hyperactivity. The prevalence of ADHD in young offenders' institutes (YOI) and adult prisons is not known. However, the fact that ADHD is frequently accompanied by conduct disorder, substance misuse and specific learning difficulties means that the prevalence is likely to be significantly higher than in the community. Some young people and adults with the disorder will be unrecognised.

Presenting complaints

- The patient may have a pre-existing diagnosis of ADHD/hyperkinetic disorder.
- The patient may be referred by a member of staff concerned about the fact that his/her behaviour is extreme in some or all of the following ways:
  — cannot finish anything he/she starts doing
  — does not seem to listen
  — cannot sit still
  — runs everywhere
  — cannot wait for others
  — is distracted very easily
  — is very loud and noisy and
  — always answers when not asked and butts into conversations; the staff member may think the individual has 'taken something'.
- The patient may attend with frequent injuries: broken bones, falls, scratches.

Adults with ADHD usually have more symptoms of problems with attention than with hyperactivity. They may complain of being unable to organise and plan and of being irritable and fractious.

Diagnostic features

- **Severe and enduring difficulty in maintaining attention**, eg short attention span, has frequent changes of activity, is very easily distracted, is disorganised.
- **Abnormal physical restlessness**, eg fidgeting or whole body movements. These are often most evident in the classroom or at mealtimes, but movements often increase during sleep.

- **Impulsiveness**, eg the individual cannot wait his/her turn or acts without thinking.

Individuals with this disorder are frequently rejected by their peers and show a variety of difficulties in social relationships.

- **For a diagnosis of hyperkinetic disorder**, inattention, overactivity and impulsiveness must all be present, must be clearly excessive for the individual's age, produce significant impairment and be evident in all situations (in the home, young offenders' institute or prison, school, healthcare centre). The behaviours will have been present from before 7 years of age and frequently from before the age of 2 (though diagnosis is frequently made later).
- **For a diagnosis of ADHD**, inattention and/or some combination of the symptoms of hyperactivity and/or impulsivity must be present, must be excessive for the individual's age, must produce impairment and be evident in at least two situations.

Adults and older adolescents are more likely to show predominantly symptoms of inattention rather than of hyperactivity, though they may have been hyperactive when younger.

Where there is no previous diagnosis and ADHD/hyperkinetic disorder is suspected, note the following.

- Laboratory tests (eg electrocardiogram [EEG], tests of attention) are of little assistance in diagnosing this condition.
- In addition to interviewing the patient, ask the patient and staff to monitor the patient's behaviour over time.
- If possible, an informant (eg a family member) should be interviewed with the patient's permission. If this is not possible in the prison/YOI, it could perhaps be done by a professional in the community (eg a general practitioner) or over the telephone. Information about the age of onset and the development of symptoms is essential to diagnosis. The testimony of the patient about their own childhood is not always very reliable and a parent should be asked to describe the patient's behaviour as a child (by age 7). The list of diagnostic criteria provided on the disk may be helpful 💾.
- If on the basis of the available information there is good reason to suspect ADHD/hyperkinetic disorder, refer the patient to a specialist for more detailed assessment. Investigation for specific learning difficulties should be part of the assessment.

Differential diagnosis

The following may be the sole cause of the symptoms displayed. Alternatively, they may be comorbid with them.

- **Restlessness, agitation and impaired concentration due to depression, anxiety or mania** (where symptoms usually follow an episodic course and lack the early onset and chronicity of ADHD). Depression may also result from problems caused by ADHD.
- **Conduct disorder only** (the individual exhibits disruptive behaviour **without** inattentiveness). ADHD commonly coexists with conduct disorder.
- **Mild learning disability** (where poor educational achievement is due solely to low intelligence). ADHD may coexist with learning disability.
- **Severe problems in family relationships** (attachment disorders), where symptoms arose in reaction to or were made worse by, for example, neglect,

abuse and multiple care placements. A careful history and multiple informants are essential to identify this problem. It may coexist with ADHD.

- **Autism** (social/language impairment and stereotyped behaviour are also present). Autism may coexist with ADHD.
- **Brain injury** (if there is a history of head injury and symptoms of ADHD are evident following the injury and not before). ADHD may coexist with brain injury.
- **Specific rare physical disorders.**

Identification and arrangement of treatment for associated problems

See 'Differential diagnosis' above. The following are particularly common in association with ADHD/hyperkinetic disorder.

- Conduct disorder: ADHD can be understood as a developmental path to conduct disorder.
- Substance misuse: adolescents and adults with ADHD use tobacco, cannabis and multiple drugs at an earlier age two to three times more commonly and they become dependent more quickly than those without the disorder.
- Developmental disorders such as dyslexia-specific reading disorder and dyspraxia, developmental coordination disorder and educational underachievement.
- Tourette's syndrome (multiple motor tics and one or more vocal tics, eg grunts, swear words, throat clearing). Mild forms do not require treatment. Where impairment is significant, medication will be required. Seek advice from a specialist.

Associated conditions require management separately. The successful treatment of dyslexia and other specific learning difficulties can improve the outcome in both adolescents and adults. Successful treatment of ADHD can improve outcomes in substance misuse and conduct disorder.

Essential information for the patient and the primary support group

- Hyperkinetic behaviour is not the patient's fault. It is most likely that genetic factors play a very important role in this disorder as 70–80% of cases are estimated to be inherited.[1] The way that family, teachers, staff and others respond to the child is thought to interact with the behaviours and make more or less likely the development of associated problems such as delinquent and antisocial behaviour, substance misuse and underachieving at school.
- Many hyperactive children make a satisfactory adjustment, but some continue to have difficulties into adulthood. The outcome is better if parents, teachers and other adults can be calm, accepting, have realistic expectations of the individual and avoid reinforcing the individual's disruptive behaviour.
- Behavioural treatment is important and the role of parents, teachers and other adults/staff is central. It is important to persevere even though behavioural management is time-consuming and the results are not immediate. Medication may increase the effectiveness of other treatments such as for behaviour therapy.

Management advice for the patient and the primary support group

The patient's behaviour is likely to be causing problems in all areas — on the Residential Unit, in education and in the workplace. A consistent, multidisciplinary plan that the patient is actively involved in developing is essential. Staff can be assisted with the following.

- To understand that the patient's behaviour is due to a disorder and not to wilful misconduct.
- To expect problems with concentration and therefore to set short tasks the patient can handle. Hyperactive individuals require particularly clear instructions. Short, specific commands about the desired behaviour are best rather than prohibitions about undesired behaviour, eg 'please walk calmly' rather than 'don't run'.
- Focus on the immediate, consistent, positive response to desired behaviour rather than on critical comments or punishment for the undesirable behaviour.
- Create a predictable routine. The prison regime will be beneficial in this respect, but the individual will need help in planning activity during any long spells in their cell or association.
- Encourage staff (eg teachers, personal officers) to spend time with the individual engaged in activities that require attention (eg completing a jigsaw) and to give positive feedback or recognition when the individual pays attention.
- Minimise distractions (eg in education, have the individual sit at the front of the class, work one-to-one or in a small group).
- Keep the individual busy and encourage sports and other constructive activity.
- Where possible, ignore non-dangerous, disruptive behaviour, eg defiant language.
- Monitor progress, identify problem areas and consider the options for addressing them. (For example, if problems arise during association, consider ways of reducing stimulation, eg talk with only one friend at a time.) Progress charts can help with this.

There is some evidence that some patients are better when specific foods (eg artificial colourings and other additives) are excluded from their diet.[2] However, formal dietary exclusion programmes are only very rarely indicated. If the patient is motivated to explore possible links between food and behaviour, keeping a food diary can be helpful. The advice of a dietitian is important before instigating exclusion diets.

Adults may be helped by education about the disorder and with counselling that focuses on helping them to recognise and build on their strengths, and to develop ways of coping with difficulties and problem-solving. ADD information service (see **Resources** below) may be helpful.

Medication

For more severe cases, stimulant medication (methylphenidate, dexamphetamine) may improve attention, reduce overactivity[3,4] and reduce drug misuse. Medication may be one part of a comprehensive package of treatment. Stimulants have been most extensively studied in children under 16. In older adolescents and adults, the rates of improvement in symptoms may be lower and higher doses may be required.[5] The need for medication should be reassessed periodically. Individuals may respond to one drug but not to another.

Medication for ADHD/hyperkinetic disorder should be initiated by a specialist. General practitioners and generic mental-health services should use only methylphenidate and dexamphetamine, with the use of other drugs and combinations confined to specialist centres. If a patient enters prison/YOI on a combination of drugs and is under the care of a specialist centre, then this can be continued with monitoring and on-going advice from the specialist.

Stimulants are given orally two or three times per day and should be tailored to individual needs. The effects typically appear less than 1 hour after ingestion. The duration of effect is 3–4 hours, but there is considerable individual variation. If the individual is still growing, his/her height and weight should be measured at regular intervals.

The potential side-effects include the following.

- A mild loss of appetite, nervousness and insomnia (the most common side-effects). These usually diminish after 2–3 months. Dose readjustment or changing the time of day when the medication is taken is often enough to reduce sleep difficulties.

- Blood pressure changes (rare in adults): should be monitored carefully when treatment begins and then at regular intervals.

- Tics (more common in children than in adolescents and adults): if they occur, medication should be stopped. Stimulant medication does not seem to cause Tourette's disorder, but may trigger the onset in predisposed individuals.

- Allergic reactions such as rashes and psychotic reactions are unusual but sometimes occur. Psychotic reactions have not been reported in adults.

Whether or not the patient has a history of substance misuse, medication use should be regularly monitored and independent ratings of behaviour obtained to ensure that positive effects are being maintained.

Referral and resettlement

General: refer to the specialist mental-health services

- For confirmation of diagnosis and for detailed assessment (where a hyperkinetic disorder is diagnosed for the first time in an adolescent or adult).

- Where autism, Tourette's syndrome or brain injury are suspected.

- Before starting a drug treatment.

Other things to consider include the following.

- Where there is a pre-existing diagnosis of ADHD/hyperkinetic disorder, involve the community service in advising on treatment in the YOI/prison.

- Referral for specific cognitive-behavioural treatment,[6] if available, can improve attention and self-control. It can be particularly helpful if there are associated mood difficulties.

- If the patient is of school age, discuss with the education manager the involvement of the Educational Psychology services. Many affected children have special educational needs.

- Where possible, involve the adolescent community mental-health services in the patient's home area well before release. The services may undertake preparatory work with the patient's family.

Resources for patients and primary support groups

ADD Information Services: 020 8906 9068
(Extensive catalogue of books and videos on ADHD)

LADDER (National Learning and Attention Deficit Disorders Association):
01902 336272
(Parents' and family support group)

Young Minds Trust: 020 7336 8445 (office)
102–108 Clerkenwell Road, London EC1M 5SA
(Produces a range of leaflets for young people and their parents. It also runs a
Parent Information Service: 0800 0182138 (freephone), which provides
information and advice for anyone concerned about the mental health of a child)

Kate Kelly and Peggy Ramundo. *You Mean I'm Not Lazy, Stupid or Crazy?!: A Self
Help Book for Adults with Attention Deficit Disorder.* New York: Simon & Schuster,
1993. An American book written for people with ADHD. It is lengthy but may be
helpful for staff wishing to understand the disorder

1   Taylor E, Sergeant J, Doepfner M *et al.* Clinical guidelines for hyperkinetic disorder.
    European Child and Adolescent Psychiatry 1998; 7: 184–200. Suggests a heritability estimate of
    80% for hyperkinetic disorder.
2   Kavale KA, Forness SR. Hyperactivity and diet treatment: a meta-analysis of the Feingold
    hypothesis. *Journal of Learning Disabilities* 1983; 16: 324–330.
3   Spencer T, Biederman J, Wilens T *et al.* Pharmacotherapy of Attention-Deficit Hyperactivity
    Disorder across the life cycle. *Journal of the American Academy of Child Adolescence Psychiatry*
    1996; 35: 409–432.
4   National Institute for Clinical Evidence. Guideline on the use of methylphenidate (Ritalin,
    Equasym) for Attention Deficit Hyperactivity Disorder (ADHD) in childhood. October
    2000. Available on the NICE website: URL: http://www.nice.org.uk/ The guideline only
    considers evidence on children below 16 years of age.
5   Joughin C, Zwi M. Focus on the use of stimulants in children with attention
    deficit/hyperactivity disorder. In *Primary Evidence-based Briefing No. 1.* London: Royal
    College of Psychiatrists, 1999.
6   Miller A, Lee S, Raina P, Zupancic J, Olsen L. *A Review of Therapies for Attention-
    Deficit/Hyperactivity Disorder.* Ottawa: Canadian Coordinating Office for Health Technology
    Assessment (CCOHTA), 1998.

Emotional disorders in young people — F93

Introduction

Emotional disorders are often associated with conduct problems. Many young people detained in custodial settings have had poor experiences of parenting and have not developed skills in identifying and managing their own emotional states. They tend to be impulsive and, when distressed, frequently use maladaptive coping strategies such as:

- aggressive behaviour
- deliberate self-harm
- substance misuse and
- somatisation.

Such young people frequently find it difficult to cope even with minor events. This renders them at increased risk of developing emotional disorders such as depression and anxiety disorders.

Adults (officers, teachers, family, health professionals) often underestimate the degree of depression in young people.

There are many similarities in the presentation and treatment of emotional disorders in young people and adults. This guideline outlines the key differences. It is meant to be read in conjunction with the guidelines for adults, in particular **Depression, Generalised anxiety, Phobias, Panic disorder, Post-traumatic stress disorder** and **Suicide** and **Self-injury**.

Presenting complaints

Patients may present initially with one or more physical symptoms, eg 'tired all the time' or irritability. They may also present with panic attacks, sleep disturbance, nightmares, self-harm and social withdrawal. They may present with substance dependence, with the underlying emotional disorders becoming apparent following withdrawal.

Diagnostic features

The diagnostic criteria for individual disorders are the same for adults and adolescents, but presentation may vary. See the guidelines for individual disorders for details. Mixed presentations are the norm.

Depression

Differences include the following.

- Young people often appear irritable and grouchy rather than sad or unhappy.
- 'Atypical' presentations are more common, eg sleeping more than usual, increased appetite, agitation.
- Rates of comorbidity with other disorders are higher, especially anxiety disorders (38%), conduct disorders (15–30%) and substance misuse (20–50%).[1]

Adolescents with a depressive disorder usually have multiple problems.

Anxiety

Worries and self-doubt are more common in young people than in adults, eg most adolescents are concerned about being disliked, rejected or criticised by their peers. An anxiety disorder is likely if such worries become intense or pervasive and cause substantial impairment in functioning. Diagnostic criteria are as adult disorders. Differences include the following.

- The focus of anxiety in adolescents is often on the fear of social situations, on social embarrassment, on worrying about catastrophic events or on performance anxiety.
- Young people with an anxiety disorder may also be overly conforming, perfectionist and unsure of themselves. They may constantly seek approval and require excessive reassurance.
- Particularly in a custodial setting, a young person typically will seek to hide worries and associated physical symptoms from his/her peers.
- Obsessional thoughts and/or compulsive rituals (eg washing rituals, checking rituals) frequently start in childhood or adolescence. Sufferers may go to great length to hide their symptoms.

Differential diagnosis

- Certain physical conditions (eg thyrotoxicosis) can cause anxiety symptoms, especially symptoms of panic (for more details, see **Panic disorder**, page 67).
- Use of alcohol and drugs may cause symptoms of anxiety and depression. Alternatively, they may mask these disorders that emerge following withdrawal/detoxification.
- **Acute psychotic disorder — F23** (page 11) if hallucinations, eg hearing voices, or delusions, eg strange or unusual beliefs, are present. The most common age for psychotic disorders to develop is the late teens and early 20s. Some individuals develop transient psychotic disorders in response to stress. Never assume that psychosis in an individual who is also abusing substances is necessarily substance-induced. Review the symptoms at intervals following detoxification.
- **Bipolar disorder — F31**: if the patient has manic episodes (eg excitement, rapid speech, elevated mood), periods of depression or mood swings.

Essential information for the patient and the primary support group

- Reassure the patient that he/she is not 'going mad'. Emotional disorders are common and help is available for their symptoms.
- Treatment consists mainly of helping the patient to deal with the problems that have triggered the disorder (eg bullying) or are maintaining it (eg problems with relationships with peers or debt). The patient has an important role to play in this, as have any adults (eg staff) that they can trust. More severe disorders may require a form of psychotherapy or family therapy. Medication only has a limited role.

Advice and support for the patient and the primary support group

- Assess the risk of suicide and self-harm. Ask a series of questions about thoughts, plans and intent (eg Has the patient often thought of death or dying? Does the patient have a specific suicide plan? Has he/she made suicide attempts in the past? Can the patient be sure not to act on suicidal ideas? How sure/safe does he/she feel? For how long does he/she feel sure to be able to resist suicidal ideas?). Involve the mental-health team. Close supervision by officers or friends, moving the patient to a healthcare centre or the use of a care suite may be needed (see **Assessing and managing people at risk of suicide**, page 204).

- Especially where symptoms are severe or long-standing, obtain information from as many informants as possible (with the patient's permission) including their family, residential staff, teachers and workshop supervisors.

- Identify current life problems or social stresses, including precipitating factors. Ask about family relationships and peer/social relationships. Identify what help the individual needs to address them.

- Identify any appropriate positive or enjoyable factors in the patient's life and seek to help the patient to increase access to these. Exercise and opportunities to be creative (eg art) may be helpful.

- Identify someone the patient can confide in. Encourage him/her to seek practical and emotional help from others. Inform the patient about the role and availability of the prison healthcare team and any other support available (eg chaplain, listener/buddy). Consider supporting him/her in obtaining additional telephone calls to their family and friends outside.

- Support the development of good sleep patterns and encourage a balanced diet (see *Getting a Good Night's Sleep* on the disk 💾).

- Ask the patient if there is a staff member (eg personal officer, residential manager) who he/she trusts and seek permission to involve that person(s) in the management plan. Explain to the patient that as management is largely a matter of solving or ameliorating the relationship and environmental factors associated with the disorder, it will be carried out mostly by non-healthcare staff. Advise the residential staff:
  - to recognise and address bullying — many vulnerable young people with emotional disorders are 'easy targets' for bullies
  - to encourage the development of adaptive skills in coping with stress, eg talking to supportive staff members to elicit help in problem-solving, an activity to distract thoughts, relaxation skills, thinking skills courses
  - to avoid removing resources that can be used to cope, eg radios, telephone contact, association, as this will lead to more use of maladaptive coping
  - to encourage the young person to reflect on the links between stressors and their behavioural responses in debriefing sessions if possible: 'What were you feeling/thinking just before that happened'; 'Could it be that something has made you feel angry/stressed/sad before you did that'
  - to model appropriate problem-solving skills for them — generate a wide range of solutions, consider the pros and cons of each and choose the most appropriate solution and
  - to help in the development of an emotional vocabulary by labelling emotional states, eg 'I think you could well be feeling angry/sad/anxious/excited now.'

In addition, see the guideline for relevant adult disorder(s) for further management advice.

Medication

- Depressive symptoms in adolescence are frequently related to environmental stressors and the management described above is most helpful — antidepressants may not add anything. Psychological treatments, where available, should be tried before medication.

- If psychological treatment has been ineffective or depression is severe and persistent (especially with biological or psychotic symptoms), use antidepressant medication (see **Depression — F32#**, page 47). Avoid tricyclic antidepressants (TCAs), as they are known to be ineffective in adolescents.[2] Preliminary findings support the use of fluoxetine in adolescents.[3] There are no reported trials in adolescents of noradrenergic and specific serotonergic antidepressants. If there are psychotic symptoms, in addition to an antidepressant the use of an antipsychotic should be considered.

- If there is a good response to medication, the evidence in adults suggests a better outcome from continuing treatment for 4–6 months before a gradual monitored withdrawal.

- In general, both antidepressants and benzodiazepines have proved ineffective in treating anxiety in adolescents. However, in the absence of any large-scale trials, some clinicians support the use of selective serotonin re-uptake inhibitors (SSRIs) in the treatment of severe social phobia and panic disorder (see **Phobic disorders — F40** and **Panic disorder — F41.0**, pages 79 and 67).

- Benzodiazepines are contraindicated.

Referral (including for psychotherapy)

- Refer the patient for an urgent assessment if there are psychotic symptoms or if suicide risk results in the need for frequent observations.

- Refer the patient to specialist mental-health services for assessment if there is a lack of progress despite the above measures and for persistent self-harming behaviour.

- Adolescents with emotional disorders referred for specialist assessment are best assessed by child and adolescent mental-health professionals if possible as the developmental and systemic nature of the problems and the difficulties in communicating with these young people require specialist skills and experience.

- Cognitive-behavioural therapy may be useful for depression[4] and anxiety,[5] as may family therapy and interpersonal therapy. Most families will also benefit from sessions that provide general education and support. Access to these therapies may be limited.

- If possible, liaise in good time with providers of services in the community before release (see **Managing the interface with the NHS and other agencies**, page 149).

Resources for patients and primary support groups

Chaplains, listeners/buddies schemes

Who Cares? Linkline: 0500 564570 (helpline: Monday, Wednesday and Thursday, 3:30 pm–6 pm); 020 7251 3117 (administration)
Kemp House, 152–160 City Road, London EC1V 2NP
(Telephone information and support for young people who are or have been in care, and for carers)

Young Minds Trust: 020 7336 8445 (office)
102–108 Clerkenwell Road, London EC1M 5SA
(Produces a range of leaflets for young people and their parents. It also runs a **Parent Information Service:** 0800 0182138 (freephone), which provides information and advice for anyone concerned about the mental health of a child)

Youth Access: 020 8772 9900 (office hours: Monday–Friday, 9 am–1 pm, 2 pm–5 pm)

2 Taylors Yard, 67 Alderbrook Road, London SW12 8AD

(National umbrella for youth information, advice, counselling and personal support agencies [YIACs]. It gives information on and referrals to appropriate local YIACs, including youth counselling services that help with self-injury)

P Graham and C Hughes. *So Young, So Sad, So Listen.* London: Gaskell, 1995. £6.00

For more resources see the guidelines for particular disorders

1   Rohde P, Lewinsohn PM, Seeley JR. Comorbidity of unipolar depression: II. Comorbidity with other mental disorders in adolescents and adults. *Journal of Abnormal Psychology* 1991; 100: 214–222, as quoted in Stanway T, Cotgrove AJ. Affective and emotional disorders. In Gowers SG (ed.), *Adolescent Psychiatry in Clinical Practice*. London: Arnold, 2001.

2   Hazell P, O'Connel D, Healthcoat D, Robertson J, Henry D. Efficacy of tricyclic drugs in treating child and adolescent depression. *British Medical Journal* 1995; 310: 897–890.

3   Emslie G, Rush A, Weinberg W *et al*. A double bind, randomized placebo-controlled trial of fluoxetine in depressed children and adolescents. *Archives of General Psychiatry* 1997; 54: 1031–1037.

4   Harrington R, Whittaker J, Shoebridge P. Psychological treatment of depression in children and adolescents: a review of treatment research. *British Journal of Psychiatry* 1998; 173: 291–298.

5   Stanway T, Cotgrove AJ. Affective and emotional disorders. In Gowers SG (ed.), *Adolescent Psychiatry in Clinical Practice*. London: Arnold, 2001.

Psychosis in young people

See the **Acute psychosis** guideline. The information below consists only of supplementary information specific to the development of psychotic illness in a young person.

Healthcare staff in young offenders' institutes (YOI) and adult prisons are very likely to see patients who are developing a psychotic illness for the first time and do not have a previous diagnosis as:

- the median age for the experience of a first episode of a psychotic illness is 19 years in men and 22 years in women (with 80% falling within the range 16–30 years)[1] and
- there is some indication that psychosis is caused by a poorly understood combination of biological factors that create a vulnerability to experiencing psychotic symptoms. These symptoms often emerge in response to stress (eg the stress of imprisonment or bullying on the wing) or drug abuse in the vulnerable individual.

Often, there is a long delay before treatment begins for the first episode of psychosis. The longer the illness is left untreated, the greater the disruption to a person's family, friends, study and work. In addition, delays in treatment may lead to slower and less complete recovery.[2]

Presenting complaints

Staff may send the patient to healthcare because they are concerned about changes in behaviour such as withdrawal, suspiciousness or odd ideas. When the young person appears in the healthcare centre, he/she may deny that there is a problem.

Diagnostic features

The earliest phase of a psychotic disorder can last from a few weeks to up to 2 years. Initially, vague changes may occur that may be difficult to detect and can be mistaken for normal changes of adolescence. The early warning signs ('prodrome') are:

- changes in thinking: a difficulty in concentrating, a poor memory, increased suspiciousness and a preoccupation with odd ideas
- changes in mood: a lack of emotional response, rapid mood changes and inappropriate moods
- changes in behaviour: odd or unusual behaviour
- social changes: withdrawal or isolation (eg spending more time in a cell, not coming out for association) and
- changes in functioning: a decline in performance at school or work.

The onset may be insidious or acute. The disturbed patient with unmistakable hallucinations and delusions is only one mode of presentation (usually late). Just as common is the quietly psychotic patient who gradually slips backwards and whom people may dismiss is being just odd.

Assessment should include information from the family, residential staff, teacher and workshop supervisor as appropriate.

Differential diagnosis and comorbidity

The clinical presentation of psychotic depression, mania and schizophrenic disorders is often very similar in young people. Diagnosis can be complicated by comorbid conduct disorder, drug abuse or other issues, including differences in culture. While early recognition of these problems is essential, it is important to avoid making a definite diagnosis prematurely. The broader term 'psychosis' may be used to cover these disorders in the first instance.

A young person may both abuse substances and be experiencing the first episode of a psychotic illness. The assumption should never be made that a young person who presents with psychotic symptoms for the first time has a 'drug-induced psychosis', even if they abuse drugs. In some instances, the individual may be using substances to help them deal with the distress of the early symptoms of the illness (see **Comorbidity**, page 191).

Find out if there is a record of previous contact with health or other personal and social services' agencies. Take a history and examine the patient, including the nervous system. Look for evidence of endocrine disease (thyroid, pituitary, adrenal), genetic conditions (Huntington's chorea, Wilson's disease with a Kayser–Fleischer ring) or focal neurological abnormality, or other systemic disease (eg systemic lupus erythematosus). Consider puerperal psychosis and a hidden pregnancy.

Advice and support for the patient

- People experiencing a psychotic illness will often be distressed and frightened. Acknowledge that the patient may be nervous or wary and try to find some common ground for discussion, gradually building up towards more specific questions about their psychotic experiences.
- The patient may need time to build up trust and repeat appointments may be needed to reach a diagnosis.
- The patient initially may be willing to accept help for their 'confusion' or 'sleep difficulties' while you 'check things out further', but they may react badly to an abrupt announcement that he/she has schizophrenia.

Referral

- Refer all young people experiencing their first psychotic episode to the mental-health services.
- Where the young person is also abusing drugs, it is ideal for the specialist to have expertise in both areas. Psychiatrists may also make inappropriate assumptions about 'drug-induced psychosis'.
- There is strong evidence for the benefits to be gained from psychosocial treatment and work with the young person's family. The NHS is developing special services for young people who have had a first episode of psychotic illness. Put the individual and their family in touch with this service, if available, as soon as they are diagnosed and certainly before release.
- For patients on the age borders between services for adolescents and adults, it may be helpful for representatives from both services to meet to agree their respective responsibilities and which treatment facility the patient should be transferred to (if appropriate) both now and in the event of any future relapse when the patient will be older.

Medication

People experiencing their first psychotic episode are typically very sensitive to the pharmacological effects of the drugs and to their side-effects. Patients experiencing a first episode of psychosis require lower doses of medication and may benefit from an atypical (ie newer generation) drug. It is important to inform the young person about possible side-effects and build up very gradually to the appropriate dosage.

1   Birchwood M, McGorry P, Jackson H. Early intervention in schizophrenia [Editorial]. *British Journal of Psychiatry* 1997; 170: 2–5.
2   McGorry PD, Edwards J, Mihalopoulos C, Harrigan SM, Jackson HJ, Early Psychosis Prevention and Intervention Centre (EPPIC). An evolving system of early detection and optimal management. *Schizophrenia Bulletin* 1996; 22: 305–326.

Postnatal depressive disorder — F53.0

The information below consists only of supplementary information specific to postnatal depression (see also the **Depression** guideline, page 47).

Between 10 and 15% of women become depressed in the year following delivery of an infant.[1] Women at higher risk include those with a previous history of depression (especially postnatal depression), who had psychological problems during pregnancy, lack social support or someone to confide in, have marital problems, have had a recent negative life event (eg bereavement), have lost their own mother when young or are ambivalent about the pregnancy.[2]

Presenting complaints

The patient may present with multiple physical complaints, repeated minor concerns about the baby's health, exhaustion, problems sleeping, irritability, feelings of being overwhelmed and being unable to cope. Staff at the Mother and Baby Unit (MBU) may refer because of concerns about the mother's lack of interest in herself or the baby. The mother may resist reporting depression directly for fear of the baby being taken away from her.

Diagnostic features

There is usually a gradual onset, usually within 6 weeks of delivery, some within 6 months, and occasionally within 12 months.

Low mood and/or loss of interest and pleasure (including lack of pleasure in the baby) for most of the day for at least 2 weeks plus four of the following items.

- Sleep disturbance.
- Appetite disturbance.
- Frequent tearfulness.
- Tiredness and poor concentration.
- Feelings of guilt or worthlessness.
- Agitated behaviour (eg pacing).
- Slowing of movement or speech.
- Suicidal thoughts.
- Increased irritability and aggression.

The following symptoms are also common.

- Anxiety and/or panic, eg being afraid to be alone with the baby, having constant worries about the baby's health, having fears about losing the baby.
- Fear of having a heart attack or of going mad.

The more severe the depression, usually the greater number of symptoms and (most importantly) the greater the degree of interference with normal social or occupational functioning. Biological symptoms are more common in more severe depression.

The Edinburgh scale should be used in routine clinics, eg 6-week baby check, to screen for postnatal depression. However, this does not give an accurate assessment of severity (there is a copy on the disk). Women at a high risk of postnatal depression often score about 12, but clinical impression is more important and any positive score on the item relating to suicidal thoughts should be taken seriously.

Differential diagnosis

- **Maternity/baby blues**: symptoms of weepiness, unusual emotional sensitivity, crying spells, mood swings, insomnia, a feeling of rejection by carers occur around days 3–5 and resolve within a few days. Maternity blues are common and 50–80% of women experience them. Treat the symptoms with reassurance, sleep and arranging short-term support in caring practically for her baby.
- **Panic disorder — F40.0** (page 67).
- **Alcohol misuse — F10** or **Drug-use disorder — F11#** (pages 18 and 55). If heavy alcohol or drug use is present. Substance misuse may cause or increase depressive symptoms. It may also mask underlying depression (see **Comorbidity**, page 191).
- **Puerperal psychosis** where delusions and, less commonly, hallucinations occur.
- **Chronic mixed anxiety and depression — F41.2** (page 33).
- **Delayed maternal response** (see **Problems of the mother–baby relationship**, page 144).

Some medications may produce symptoms of depression. These include β-blockers, other antihypertensives, H_2-blockers, oral contraceptives and corticosteroids.

Comorbidity

Depression frequently coexists with anxiety and panic, unexplained physical complaints and problems in the mother–baby relationship (such as delayed maternal response). Specific treatments are indicated for each set of problems. See the relevant guidelines.

Essential information for the patient and the primary support group

- **Feelings of helplessness, hopelessness, anxiety and emotional swings are all symptoms of the illness.** They do not mean that you are going mad. Postnatal depression is very common and anyone can get it.
- **Learning to care for a new baby is hard and tiring work.** Mothering takes time to learn. Practical help is needed.
- **Not feeling the way you expected to towards the baby.** This does not make you a bad mother, nor does it mean that you will harm your baby.
- **You will get better, but it may take time.** Arrangements must be made for you to be supported until you have recovered. There are several different treatments that may speed your recovery.
- **The illness may recur in subsequent pregnancies.**
- **Asking for and accepting help with the depression will increase the chances of the baby being allowed to stay in the MBU.** Babies are only separated from their mothers if there is imminent risk to the baby or if, for health reasons, the mother can no longer look after the baby.

Advice and support for the patient

For advice on management, including suicide risk assessment, see the **Depression** guideline (page 47). In addition:

- **Assess the risk of harm to the baby**: ask: How do you feel about the baby? Have you had any unusual thoughts? Have you been worried that harm might come to your baby, or even that you might harm him/her?:
  - If there are signs of harmful intent towards the baby, involve the mental-health services and the liaison social worker, following the prison child-protection procedures. Consider transfer to an in-patient unit, preferably one with an MBU.
  - Where there is no sign of harmful intent to the baby but the depression is chronic and the mother cannot meet the baby's emotional needs (eg the baby appears flat and avoids eye contact with his/her mother), treat the depression and involve the social services. Involving the liaison social worker should be seen as a way of obtaining additional support for the mother and baby.
  - Be aware that if the mother is admitted to the prison healthcare centre or an NHS hospital, arrangements will be made to hand her child to outside carers, except where the NHS hospital has an MBU.
- Encourage steps to get more sleep, eg rest during the day as much as possible; learn the art of cat napping.
- Encourage the woman to find some time for herself, eg 30 minutes for an uninterrupted bath.
- Encourage the woman to eat regularly even if she does not feel like it and to aim for a balanced diet including plentiful fluids.[3] This is not the time to try and lose weight. If appropriate, advise a reduction in caffeine intake.[4]
- Identify someone the patient can confide in. Encourage her to seek practical and emotional help from others. Inform her about the role and availability of the prison healthcare team, the health visitor and any other support available. Support her in obtaining additional telephone calls to family and friends outside. If appropriate, discuss support for a possible application for a temporary licence (see also **Types of release on licence** on the disk🖫). Give her a copy of *Coping with Depression*.

After improvement, plan with the patient the action to be taken if signs of relapse occur. As psychiatric morbidity remains high during the second postpartum year, regular follow-up and monitoring should continue.

Liaison and advice for the health visitor, MBU staff and other carers

Ask the mother's permission to discuss the following with the other staff caring for her. Inform her that you will only do this with her permission, except where there is a risk of harm to herself or others.

- Inform them of the outcome of the assessment of risk to the mother herself or the baby and discuss risk management, including the level of monitoring required. Discuss the location, including a shared room, if possible.
- The support of staff and family is an important element of treatment. Support to depressed women by caregivers may help the depression resolve more quickly.[5] Discuss increasing the level of practical support to the mother, eg help with feeding and bathing the baby, institute a routine, arrange a break from the baby to allow sleep.
- Discuss ways they can support the mother (eg helping her break routine tasks down into manageable bits, praising her when she completes even a small task, avoiding additional stresses). Give them a copy of *Working with Mothers and Babies: The Psychological Aspects* 🖫 .

- Inform staff of the likely impact of the illness on the mother's functioning (eg irritability and aggression can cause an increase in arguments between the mother and carers, and between the mother and their partner and family during visits). If possible, explain this to the patient's partner or family and encourage their additional patience and support for the mother.

Psychological treatments

Psychological treatments, where available, are often preferred to medication by women. Such therapy allows the woman to review her relationship with her baby, partner and family. The best evidence of effectiveness in the treatment of depression is available for cognitive-behavioural therapy and interpersonal therapy.[6] Marital/couple and family therapy may have a particular role where there are problems in these relationships.[7] Person-centred counselling by specially trained health visitors[8] and psychodynamic psychotherapy[9] may also be useful.

Professional and/or social support may also help postpartum depression.[5] Parenting-training programmes may be helpful for mothers with mild depression or those recovering from more severe depression.[10] Patients with chronic, relapsing depression may benefit more from cognitive-behavioural therapy (CBT) or a combination of CBT and antidepressants than from medication alone.[11,12]

Medication

For advice about prescribing for depression, see the **Depression** guideline (page 47). In addition, check thyroid function and treat it if found to be abnormal.[13]

Choice of medication

- In general, non-sedating antidepressants (a tricyclic such as lofepramine or a selective serotonin re-uptake inhibitor [SSRI]) are preferred, especially if the mother is breast-feeding. If the woman cannot sleep, a sedative tricyclic (eg trazodone) may be used. If this is not sufficient, consider the use of hypnotics **in the short-term**, except where breast-feeding. If either type of sedating drug is used, provision must be made for adequate supervision of the baby.

If the patient is breast-feeding

- Decisions about safety are difficult: all psychotropic drugs pass into breast milk, and while concentrations are normally much lower than those that pass through the placenta during pregnancy, infants are poor metabolisers of drugs.
- All drugs should be avoided if the infant is premature or has renal, hepatic, cardiac or neurological impairment. The infant's renal and hepatic function should be checked before it is breast-fed by a mother who has been prescribed psychotropic medication.
- In general, older drugs are preferred, as more is known about their effects on the baby.[14] Prefer tricyclic antidepressants (TCAs) (**except doxepin**). If SSRIs used, prefer those with short half-lives. **Avoid monoamine oxidase inhibitors (MAOIs) and lithium.**
- It is best to avoid sedating drugs and those with long half-lives.
- Avoid polypharmacy.
- If possible, give the drug as a single daily dose before the infant's longest sleep period. Breast-feeding should occur immediately before the dose is due. If

possible, avoid breast-feeding when drug concentrations peak in milk where this is known (eg amitriptyline 1.5 hours, imipramine 1 hour).

- Monitor the infant for adverse effects, eg sedation, irritability. If these occur, take appropriate action (eg dose reduction, drug change, referral for advice).
- Treat the mother with the lowest effective dose as adverse effects in the infant are often dose-related.

Referral

Refer for weekly listening visits by a specially trained health visitor if the depression is mild and there is no significant suicide risk.[8] Referral to the secondary mental-health services is advised:

- as an emergency if there is a significant risk of suicide or danger to the baby, or if there are psychotic symptoms, severe agitation or retardation with impaired food/fluid intake or
- as a non-emergency if:
  — significant depression persists despite treatment in primary care. Antidepressant therapy has failed if the patient remains symptomatic after a full course of treatment at an adequate dosage. If there is no clear improvement with the first drug, it should be changed to another class of drug
  — there is a history of severe depression, especially of bipolar disorder.

If drug or alcohol misuse is also a problem, see the guidelines for these disorders. If the mother has used alcohol or drugs during pregnancy, the baby will require close monitoring physically. There is increased risk of foetal alcohol syndrome, neonatal withdrawal syndrome and low birth weight. Problematic alcohol or drug use after pregnancy may reduce the parent's ability to provide adequate care for the infant due to unpredictable, inconsistent and ineffective patterns of behaviour.

Involve non-healthcare support (eg chaplain, counsellor, voluntary support group) in all other cases where symptoms persist, where the patient has a poor or non-existent support network, or where social or relationship problems are contributing to the depression.[15]

Severely depressed adolescents are difficult to assess and manage, and referral is recommended.

Throughcare and prerelease planning should include advice on services available to support mothers who have psychological problems and their babies (such as Homestart and Newpin, see below), as well as close liaison with medical and socialcare staff in the community (for more details, see **Managing the interface with the NHS and other agencies**, page 149).

Resources for patients and primary support groups

Association for Postnatal Illness: 020 7386 0868
145 Dawes Road, Fulham, London SW6 7EB (SAE needed)
(Can put you in touch with other mothers who have come through PND)

BM CRY-SIS: 020 7404 5011
London WC1N 3XX
(For parents of crying children)

Depression Alliance: 020 7633 0557
35 Westminster Bridge Road, London SE1 7JB
(National network of self-help groups for people experiencing depression)

Homestart UK: 0116 233 9955
2 Salisbury Road, Leicester LE1 7QR
(Volunteers offer support, friendship and practical support to young families
with at least one child under 5 who are experiencing difficulties and stress)

Meet a Mum Association (MAMA): 020 8768 0123
26 Avenue Road, South Norwood, London SE25 4DX
(Self-help groups for pregnant women and mothers of small children)

Newpin: 020 7703 6326
Sutherland House, 35 Sutherland Square, London SE17 3EE
(Promotes the protection and preservation of mental health among parents and
children. It supports families with emotional difficulties and mental distress)

National Childbirth Trust: 020 8992 8637
Alexandra House, Oldham Terrace, Acton, London W3 6NH
(Advice, support and counselling on all aspects of childbirth. Many local groups)

Pen Pal Project for Mothers in Prison: Tel: 001 805 967 7636; Fax: 001 805 967
0608; URL: http://www.chss.iup.edu/postpartum
Jane Honikman, Founding Director and Coordinator, PSI, 927 N. Kellog Avenue,
Santa Barbara, CA 9311, USA. E-mail: jhonikman@earthlink.com
(The US-based non-profit organisation Postpartum Support International [PSI]
runs a support network for new mothers in prison often as the result of
infanticide. Mothers write to each other)

Resource leaflet:
Coping with Depression

Books:
Erika Harvey. *The Element Guide to Postnatal Depression: Your Questions Answered.*
Shaftesbury: Element, 1999

J Douglas, Richman N. *My Child Won't Sleep.* London: Penguin, 1988

Whiteford B, Polden M. *The Postnatal Exercise Book.* London: Penguin, 1992

[1] O'Hara MW, Swain AM. Rates and risks of postpartum depression: a meta-analysis. *International Review of Psychiatry* 1996; 8: 37–54.
[2] Kumar R. Postnatal mental illness: a transcultural perspective. *Social Psychiatry and Psychiatric Epidemiology* 1994; 29: 250–264.
[3] Wallin M, Rissanen A. Food and mood: relationship between food, serotonin and affective disorders. *Acta Psychiatrica Scandinavica* 1994; 377 (Suppl): 36–40. (CV)
[4] Greden JF. Anxiety or caffeinism: a diagnosis dilemma. *American Journal of Psychiatry* 1974; 131: 1089–1092. (AV)
[5] Ray KL, Hodnett ED. Caregiver support for postpartum depression. Cochrane Library, Oxford 1998, issue 3. Update software.
[6] Department of Health. *Treatment Choice in Psychological Therapies and Counselling.* London: Department of Health, 2001.
[7] Sandberg JG, Johnson LN, Dermer SB *et al.* Demonstrated efficacy of models of marriage and family therapy: an update of Gurman, Kniskern and Pinsof's chart. *American Journal of Family Therapy* 1997; 25: 121–137.

8   Holden JM, Sagovsky R, Cox JL. Counselling in a general practice setting: controlled study of health visitors' intervention in treatment of postnatal depression. *British Medical Journal* 1989; 298: 223–226.

9   Murray L, Cooper PJ (eds). *Postpartum Depression and Child Development*. London: Guildford, 1997.

10 Barlow J, Coren E. Parent-training programmes for improving maternal psychosocial health. Cochrane Library, Oxford 2001, issue 1. Update software. States that parenting programmes may make a substantial contribution to the improvement of maternal psychosocial health. However, further research is required to identify whether this is so, irrespective of the level of pathology present in the mother.

11 Thase M, Greenhouse J, Frank E *et al.* Treatment of major depression with psychotherapy or psychotherapy–pharmacotherapy combinations. *Archives of General Psychiatry* 1997; 54: 1009–1015.

12 Evans M, Hollins S, De Rubeis R *et al.* Differential relapse following cognitive therapy and pharmacotherapy of depression. *Archives of General Psychiatry* 1992; 49: 802–808.

13 Harris B, Othman S, Davis JA *et al.* Association between postpartum thyroid dysfunction and thyroid antibodies and depression. *British Medical Journal* 1992; 305: 152–156.

14 Yoshida K, Kumar R. Breastfeeding and psychotropic drugs. *International Review of Psychiatry* 1996; 8: 117–124, as quoted in World Psychiatric Association. *Depressive Disorders in Physical Illness*. New York: NCM Publications, 1998.

15 Ostler KJ, Thompson C, Kinmonth ALK *et al.* Influence of socio-economic deprivation on the prevalence and outcome of depression in primary care: the Hampshire Depression Project. *British Journal of Psychiatry* 2001; 178:12–17.

Puerperal psychosis

See the **Acute psychosis** guideline. The information below consists only of supplementary information specific to puerperal psychosis.

Presenting complaints

The mother may have experienced extreme and labile emotional states (manic or depressed), abrupt-onset hallucinations, delusions or confusion.

Between 0.1 and 0.2% of newly delivered women suffer from a postpartum psychosis. Women with previous episodes of postpartum psychosis or bipolar disorder or who have had a family history of bipolar disorder are at very high risk,[1,2] and where there has been a previous episode of bipolar disorder or postpartum psychosis planned psychiatric referral during pregnancy is advised.

Diagnostic features

Postnatal psychosis usually appears suddenly within 2 weeks of the birth.
- Marked mood swings: severely depressed or mixed/elated mood.
- Over-preoccupation or abnormal interaction with the baby.
- Severe anxiety or agitation.
- Perplexity and confusion.
- Suicidal and infanticidal ideation may occur (eg that the mother and baby would be better off dead).
- Less commonly, schizophrenia-like symptoms may occur (eg hallucinations such as hearing voices and experiencing strange smells or delusions, eg that the baby is evil).

Differential diagnosis

- Non-psychotic postnatal depression.
- Organic brain syndromes (eg consequent on infection, metabolic disturbance or haemorrhage).

Essential information for the patient and the primary support group

- Withdrawal, agitation, strange behaviour and thoughts are symptoms of the illness.
- The mother's mental state and symptoms will fluctuate daily.
- The prognosis for recovery from puerperal psychosis is very good.
- There is an increased risk of recurrence with further pregnancies.
- Medication is central to treatment and will help resolve the symptoms. Inform the mother about side-effects.
- In the acute stage, the illness will affect the mother's capacity to look after her baby:
  — A severely depressed mother may experience slowed movement and speech, a difficulty in concentrating and persistent exhaustion.
  — An agitated, manic mother may not be able to respond sensitively to her baby.

— Mothers who have severe psychosis may experience suicidal thoughts or impulses to kill their baby. They may require someone with them at all times.

— When the mother is less acutely ill but still recovering, she may require close supervision as her mental state may make her vulnerable to making dangerous errors of judgement, eg giving the baby feeds that are boiling hot.

Advice and support for the patient and the primary support group

- Ensure the safety of the patient, the baby and those caring for them. Postpartum psychosis in the acute stage (especially where delusions involve the baby) may necessitate separating the mother and baby until the mother's mental state has improved, unless adequate supervision and support is provided, usually in an in-patient Mother and Baby Unit (MBU). Contact the liaison social worker in accordance with prison child-protection procedures.

- The subjective experiences of a mother suffering from puerperal psychosis are bizarre and often terrifying. Avoid confrontation or criticism, unless it is necessary to prevent harmful or disruptive behaviour.

- Arrange support for the patient from carers and family to help her comply with treatment and, when appropriate, to re-establish sensitive mothering.

Referral

Refer **as an emergency** to the secondary mental-health services. It is essential that a mother suffering from postpartum psychosis is treated in a specialist psychiatric hospital, usually in an MBU.

Planned psychiatric referral is advised for women who have had a previous episode of puerperal psychosis and are pregnant again, as prophylactic interventions may significantly reduce the risk of recurrence. As the pattern of any subsequent relapse is remarkably similar to the original illness, it is essential that there is continued psychiatric monitoring, especially around the expected time of onset of the illness.

Medication

Medication for postpartum psychosis will vary according to the clinical picture (depressive, schizophrenic, manic, mixed) and should be prescribed by a specialist. If diagnosis is clear, however, and there is a delay in specialist consultation, commence antipsychotic medication acutely to manage disturbed behaviour or severe distress (see **Acute psychosis**, page 11).

If the patient is breast-feeding, consider the following.

- Decisions about safety are complex: all psychotropic drugs pass into breast milk, and while concentrations are normally much lower than those that pass through the placenta during pregnancy, infants are poor metabolisers of drugs.

- All drugs should be avoided if the infant is premature or has renal, hepatic, cardiac or neurological impairment. The infant's renal and hepatic function should be checked before it is breast-fed by a mother who is prescribed psychotropic medication.

- In general, older drugs are preferred, as more is known about their effects on the baby.[3] **Avoid monoamine oxidase inhibitors (MAOIs), lithium and clozapine.**

- As a general rule, the mother should not breast-feed if she requires a dose of haloperidol > 20 mg day^{-1} or chlorpromazine > 200 mg day^{-1}.

- Monitor the infant for adverse effects, eg sedation, irritability. If these occur take appropriate action (eg dose reduction, drug change, referral for advice).
- Treat the mother with the lowest effective dose as adverse effects in the infant are often dose-related.
- It is best to avoid sedating drugs and drugs with long half-lives.
- Avoid polypharmacy.
- If possible, give the drug as a single daily dose before the infant's longest sleep period. Breast-feeding should occur immediately before the dose is due. If possible, avoid breast-feeding when drug concentrations peak in milk where this is known (eg chlorpromazine 2 hours after oral administration).

Resources for patients and primary support groups

See the organisations listed under **Postnatal depressive disorder** (page 134)

1   Kendell RE, Chalmers JC, Platz C. Epidemiology of puerperal psychoses. *British Journal of Psychiatry* 1989; 150: 662–673.
2   Marks MN, Wieck A, Checkly SA, Kumar R. Contribution of psychological and social factors to psychiatric and non psychiatric relapse after childbirth in women with previous histories of affective disorder. *Journal of Affective Disorders* 1992; 29: 253–264.
3   Yoshida K, Kumar R. Breastfeeding and psychotropic drugs. *International Reviews in Psychiatry* 1996; 8: 117–124, as quoted in World Psychiatric Association. *Depressive Disorders in Physical Illness*. NCM Publications New York, 1998.

Problems with the mother–baby relationship

The quality of the relationship between a mother and her baby influences the child's emotional, cognitive and physical development. It is important, therefore, that staff look out for and try to ameliorate problems in the mother–baby relationship.

Why mothers may have problems

- A woman who has herself experienced poor parenting or who has spent some or most of her childhood in Local Authority care may have limited parenting skills.
- A person who has suffered poor or abusive parenting herself is more likely to be neglectful or abusive of her own children.
- A woman may develop postnatal depression, which has an impact on her ability to respond emotionally to her baby (see the **Postnatal disorders** guideline, page 134).
- A woman may have mental-health problems for other reasons.
- A woman who gives birth while imprisoned does not have access to her partner, family or friends for emotional and practical support as non-imprisoned women do.
- The experience of pregnancy and childbirth may bring back (possibly painful) memories and feelings from a woman's own childhood. She may feel more than usually hurt and needy.

Diagnostic features

Signs that the mother–baby relationship is at risk

The mother can show any of the following.
- Irritable with the baby most of the time.
- Avoids holding and looking at the baby.
- Repeatedly unresponsive to crying or obvious distress.
- Does not show any pleasure in the baby over time.
- Does not handle the baby in a gentle or tender way.
- Repeatedly over-stimulates the baby, eg vigorous and prolonged games with a very young baby.
- Makes repeated critical remarks towards or about the baby.
- Attributes malicious intent to the baby, eg believes that the baby deliberately cries to annoy her or to get attention that it does not need.

A lack of sensitivity to the baby's signals, if it continues over time, results in the baby becoming increasingly withdrawn. When the mother's response is repeatedly unexpected and inappropriate (eg sometimes hostile, sometimes ignoring the baby, sometimes loving, but with no pattern to the responses), the baby becomes confused and eventually avoids his/her mother and other people — not responding to them. If this goes on for a long period, the child grows up to have problems with attention, concentration and behaviour.

Differential diagnosis

- 'Maternity blues'/'baby blues'.

- If there are significant symptoms of depression (see the **Depression** guideline, page 47).
- Anxiety states (see **Panic disorder** and **Mixed anxiety and depression,** pages 67 and 33).
- **Puerperal psychosis** (page 141) where avoidance of a baby is related to delusional beliefs (eg that the baby is evil or dangerous).
- Faltering growth or failure to thrive. Only a very small minority of babies have faltering growth because of abuse or neglect.[1,2] However, mothers may feel an acute sense of failure if they cannot ensure adequate food for their child, especially if they have been told by medical staff that there is nothing wrong physically with their child. The mother may feel that it has been implied that she is a bad mother. This can greatly increase the stress and anxiety felt by the mother. Refer to health visitor in the first instance. The Children's Society publishes useful information on this topic (see **Resources Directory** page 316).

Disorders of the mother–baby relationship often coexist with depression and anxiety states.

Essential information for the patient and the primary support group

- Feelings of love for the baby do not appear immediately and automatically. For many women, it can take weeks or even months to develop closeness and mothering feelings.
- Learning to care for a new baby is hard and tiring work. Mothering takes time to learn.
- Crying is a communication that means the baby needs the mother. It is not hostile.

Advice and support for the patient and the primary support group

- Sympathise with the stress of being the mother of a young child.
- Demonstrate how to respond when the baby is upset or wants to play.
- Encourage the mother to find some time for herself (eg 30 minutes for an uninterrupted bath).
- Encourage her to get enough sleep, eg rest during the day as much as is possible and learn the art of cat napping.
- Do not criticise the mother directly. This will undermine her confidence and self-esteem still further. Try phrases like: 'Some mothers find that … works well'; 'All babies are different. Why don't you try … or … and see if it works for you?' Encourage her to experiment with ways of satisfying the baby. Praise her.
- Try not to take sides against the partner or baby when the mother is critical of them.
- Encourage the mother to identify and take up anything that helps her feel good about herself (eg art, exercise, education) or that will help her get a job or social contacts when she is released.
- Encourage the mother to attend parenting classes, if available.
- Arrange a follow-up appointment to monitor the problem and the effect on the child.

Liaison and advice with MBU officers and other staff

Seek patient permission to do the following.

- Discuss with Mother and Baby Unit (MBU) officers and nursery nurses the provision of practical help for the mother, eg help with feeding and bathing the baby, instituting a routine, a break from the baby to allow sleep.
- Inform them that good social support can lessen the stress of the early years of motherhood even in vulnerable women. This means that staff in prison can be important to the health of the mother and the long-term emotional health of the baby.
- Consider setting up a befriending scheme whereby older and more experienced mothers from the community pair up with and support mothers in the MBU. This will help relieve pressure on staff and can be a very helpful resource for the mothers. A local Volunteer Bureau, Council for Voluntary Service, Mothers' Union or National Childbirth Trust branch may be willing to help with this (see **Resources** below).
- Consider setting up an education and support group for MBU officers, nursery nurses and other staff to help deal with the stress of managing difficult or distressed mothers. For example, a monthly group session could be arranged with in-house and outside speakers that discusses topics such as normal child development and how to manage particular problems. The health visitor may be able to suggest suitable outside speakers.

Medication

Medication is only appropriate for comorbid disorders, eg depression, panic (see the relevant guideline).

Referral

- Refer to the health visitor for routine support and monitoring.
- Refer to the general adult psychiatrist if an underlying or comorbid severe mental disorder (eg psychosis or severe depression or anxiety) is suspected in the mother.
- Refer to the child and adolescent psychiatrist for advice if you are unsure about whether the mother–baby relationship is damaging to the baby.
- Parenting programmes have been shown to make a significant contribution to the psychosocial health (eg self-esteem, mood, stress) of mothers in general.[3]

Child protection

If signs of poor mother–baby attachment continue for more than a month or do not resolve when a mental disorder is treated and the quality of the relationship is deteriorating, discuss your concerns with the mother, involve the liaison social worker in accordance with prison child-protection procedures and explore obtaining further support for the mother and baby (see **Child protection**, page 276).

Resources for mothers and primary support groups

Association for Postnatal Illness: 020 7386 0868
145 Dawes Road, Fulham, London SW6 7EB (SAE needed)
(Can put you in touch with other mothers who have come through PND)

BM CRY-SIS: 020 7404 5011
London WC1N 3XX
(For parents of crying children)

Council for Voluntary Service (CVS): 0114 278 6636 (find via the National
Association of Councils for Voluntary Service)
(Most local areas have a CVS that coordinates and supports local voluntary
organisations. Some have a Volunteer Bureau [see below] as part of their
organisation)

Depression Alliance: 020 7633 0557
35 Westminster Bridge Road, London SE1 7JB
(National network of self-help groups for people experiencing depression)

Meet a Mum Association (MAMA): 020 8768 0123
26 Avenue Road, South Norwood, London SE25 4DX
(Self-help groups for pregnant women and mothers of small children)

National Childbirth Trust: 020 8992 8637
Alexandra House, Oldham Terrace, Acton, London W3 6NH
(Advice, support and counselling on all aspects of childbirth. Many local
groups)

Pen Pal Project for Mothers in Prison: Tel: 001 805 967 7636; Fax: 001 805 967
0608; URL: http://www.chss.iup.edu/postpartum
Jane Honikman, Founding Director and Coordinator, PSI, 927 N. Kellog Avenue,
Santa Barbara, CA 9311, USA. E-mail: jhonikman@earthlink.com
(The US-based non-profit organisation Postpartum Support International (PSI)
runs a support network for new mothers in prison often as the result of
infanticide. Mothers write to each other)

Volunteer Bureau: (see the telephone directory or local library reference section)
(Most local areas have a Volunteer Bureau that recruits volunteers and matches
them with organisations that need volunteers)

Resource leaflet:
Coping with Depression

Books:
Erika Harvey. *The Element Guide to Postnatal Depression: Your Questions Answered.*
Shaftesbury: Element, 1999

J Douglas, Richman N. *My Child Won't Sleep.* London: Penguin, 1988

Whiteford B, Polden M. *The Postnatal Exercise Book.* London: Penguin, 1992

Faltering Growth — Taking the Failure Out of Failure to Thrive and *My Child Still
Won't Eat.* Available from: The Children's Society, Edward Rudolf House,
Margery Street, London WC1X 0JL. Tel: 020 7841 4400;
URL: http://www.the-childrens-society.org.uk

1   Boddy J, Skuse D. Annotation: the process of parenting in failure to thrive. *Journal of Child Psychology and Psychiatry* 1994; 35: 401–424.

2   Wright C, Talbot E. Screening for failure to thrive — what are we looking for? *Child Care Health and Development* 1996; 22: 223–234.

3   Barlow J, Coren E. Parent-training programmes for improving maternal psychosocial health. Cochrane Library, Oxford 2001, issue 1. Update software. States that parenting programmes may make a substantial contribution to the improvement of maternal psychosocial health. However, further research is required to identify whether this is so irrespective of the level of pathology present in the mother.

Managing the interface with the NHS and other agencies

This section is intended to be used in conjunction with the guidelines on the diagnosis and management of particular disorders.

Developing effective liaison with the NHS and other agencies

Effective liaison with the NHS and other agencies is crucial to good-quality care and may be necessary at various points during a stay in custody.

- When prisoners first come into custody.
- On first suspecting that a prisoner is suffering from a mental disorder.
- During the course of a sentenced prisoner's career — 'throughcare' or 'resettlement' and sentence planning.
- When a prisoner is about to be released.
- In the week following release.

Certain structures and systems may make liaison with other agencies more effective. For example:

- Service agreements with local mental-health services.
- Designated liaison worker within the prison.
- Use of the Care Programme Approach (CPA).
- Agreements for sharing information while respecting patient confidentiality.

Service agreements

It will be important for some establishments to have a service agreement with local mental-health services that include the following.

- Provision of psychiatric assessments.
- Standards for the speed of response to emergency, urgent and routine requests for assessments. Scottish Prison Service specifications for mental-health services include the following standards: response to emergencies (within 24 hours), to urgent referrals (within 7 days) and routine referrals (within 4 weeks).
- Advice on the management of patients in prison who are refused transfer to hospital. This advice should include:
  — immediate and long-term management of the patient within prison
  — arrangements for liaison before release and
  — risk management and guidelines on when to re-refer, if the situation changes
- Advice on management, including medication.
- Where appropriate, the local service will also provide some services within the prison, eg daycare or clinics on the wings.

Liaison worker

Effective liaison with health services in the community takes time and effort. A designated member of staff can speed liaison and referrals when an individual first comes into prison or is first diagnosed with a serious mental disorder, during their prison career and before release. The liaison worker could ensure that each individual with a serious mental illness has a care plan and a designated care coordinator in the community before release, as stipulated in the NHS plan. Establishments with experience of such mental health liaison staff include the following.

- HMP Liverpool. Contact: Merseyside Criminal Justice Mental Health Liaison Service. Tel: 0151 255 0040; Fax: 0151 236 4799.
- HMP Belmarsh. Contact: Julliet Telfer (Forensic Mental Health Liaison Nurse) or Jo Fox (Psychiatrists PA), HMP Belmarsh, Western Way, Thameswade, London SE28 0EP. Tel: 020 8317 2436 ext. 338.

Participating in the joint Prison Service–NHS partnership work

Very useful personal links may be developed and maintained by participation in joint projects, eg needs assessments, continuing professional development opportunities, and local or regional Joint Planning Groups.

Agreements for sharing information while respecting patient confidentiality

There are several ways to maximise the sharing of information that is required for multidisciplinary care while maintaining the requirements of confidentiality and the trust of the patient. These are outlined in **Ethical issues** (page 300).

Where there is a grave risk of serious harm to the individual or to others, but the individual refuses consent to disclose information to avert such harm, the duty of confidentiality can be overridden by the duty to prevent the serious harm. In this case, information relevant to managing that risk should be shared on a 'need to know' basis. Unless doing so risks serious harm, the individual should be informed about who has been told what and why. For more details, see **Ethical issues** (page 300).

Assessment

Before making a referral, it is important to carry out an assessment with the following steps.

- Take a history and do a Mental State Examination (MSE) of the patient, including:
  — previous mental-health problems and treatment
  — recent drug or alcohol abuse
  — current symptoms and
  — observation and documentation of the sleep pattern, eating, speech, behaviour and interaction with others. (This will require information from residential staff or observation within the health centre).
  A brief overview of the MSE is provided on the disk 💾.
- Obtain the previous inmate medical records (if any).
- Carry out a physical examination and investigations as required.
- Perform a urine drug screen.
- **With the patient's consent**, and where possible obtain more information from the following:
  — past psychiatric records (if any)
  — CPA key-worker (if appropriate)
  — general practice notes

— sentence planning assessments and reviews (available from the sentence planning officer or probation officer)

— relative or close friend and

— solicitor.

It is always good practice to seek the patient's consent. However, if in the judgement of the responsible medical officer (RMO) previous records are needed to make proper and informed treatment decisions, then the patient's consent is not required to obtain information from previous health professionals, or to obtain a list of previous convictions or pre-sentence reports. Wherever appropriate, the patient should be informed if records are obtained without their consent. If records are obtained without consent, the reasons for doing so must be documented. It would be highly undesirable to contact a relative or close friend without the person's consent.

Care Programme Approach (CPA) and Section 117

All people who have previously been patients of secondary mental-health services and who have complex and continuing needs should have a care programme (an on-going care plan based on an assessment of their health- and socialcare needs) and a key-worker. The key-worker, most usually a community psychiatric nurse (CPN) or social worker, coordinates the care and should maintain some contact or knowledge of the patient even during his/her prison sentence. Patients who were on CPA when they entered prison should continue to be treated in accordance with their care plan — suitably amended to reflect their change in circumstances.

In addition, where an individual has previously been treated under Section(s) 3, 37, 47 or 48 of the Mental Health Act 1983, they are entitled to on-going aftercare under Section 117, whether or not they are in prison. Their previous care coordinator should stay in contact with the individual while they are in prison and be involved in planning their care.

• Assess the risk to self or others (for information on assessing risk to self, see **Assessing and managing the risk of suicide**, page 204).

Psychiatric assessment of risk to others

History:

• Previous violence and/or suicidal behaviour.

• Evidence of rootlessness or social restlessness, eg few relationships, frequent changes of address or employment.

• Evidence of poor compliance with treatment or disengagement from psychiatric aftercare.

• Presence of substance misuse or other potential disinhibiting factors, eg a social background promoting violence.

• Identification of any precipitants and any changes in mental state or behaviour that have occurred before violence and/or relapse.

Are these risk factors stable or have any changed recently?

• Evidence of recent severe stress, particularly of loss events or the threat of loss.

• Evidence of recent discontinuation of medication.

Environment:

- Does the patient have access to potential victims, particularly individuals identified in mental state abnormalities, eg those who figure in the patient's delusional system?

Mental state:

- Evidence of any threat/control override symptoms: firmly held beliefs of persecution by others (persecutory delusions) or of the mind or body being controlled or interfered with by external forces (delusions of passivity).
- Emotions related to violence, eg irritability, anger, hostility, suspiciousness.
- Specific threats made by the patient.

Conclusion:

A formulation should be made based on these and all other items of history and mental state. The formulation should, so far as possible, specify factors likely to increase the risk of dangerous behaviour and those likely to decrease it. The formulation should aim to answer the following questions.

- How serious is the risk?
- Is the risk specific or general?
- How immediate is the risk?
- How volatile is the risk?
- What specific treatment, and which management plan, can best reduce the risk?

Source: with permission of Royal College of Psychiatrists Special Working Party on Clinical Assessment and Management of Risk. *Assessment and Clinical Management of Risk of Harm to Other People*. Council Report CR, April. London: Royal College of Psychiatrists, 1996

A brief risk indicator checklist is provided on the disk 💾. These are examples of risk assessment tools that may be useful.

Liaison with wing staff will often be a useful source of information.

Where the patient is admitted to a healthcare centre, observations by the nurse or health care officer in charge of their care form a valuable part of the in-patient assessment. An initial assessment form to be completed by a nurse or other staff member is provided on the disk 💾.

Consider referral to the psychiatric services

After the assessment, decide whether a referral is needed and, if so, how urgently. See also the criteria for referral in the guidelines for specific disorders.

Criteria for non-urgent referral

Non-urgent referral will be required for a number of reasons including the following.

- Danger of harm to self or others and the patient is or may be mentally disordered.
- Treatment in hospital is likely to be required. If mental illness is suspected, the patient should be referred for assessment, and the solicitor notified, with patient permission. Do not rely on the patient coming to psychiatric notice by other means (eg through the court).

- Patient is so disabled by their mental disorder that they cannot be managed on an ordinary location or fulfil activities of daily living.
- An individual on hunger strike should be referred for assessment at an early stage, before the individual's physical health has deteriorated, even where mental illness is not thought to be present (see **Food refusal and mental illness**, page 292).
- General practitioner requires the expertise of secondary care to confirm a diagnosis or to implement specialist treatment.
- There is a need for care and/or treatment beyond the capacity of primary-care services in prison, eg particular psychotropic medication such as clozapine or lithium.

Criteria for urgent referral and possible transfer

Urgent referral will be required for a number of reasons including any one of the following:
- Serious psychotic symptoms causing severe distress, dangerous behaviour or major disruption to functioning.
- Patient cannot be looked after safely in the prison because of his/her mental illness.
- Patient is not accepting treatment and may, if left, deteriorate to the point of requiring emergency treatment under common law or has needed this already.
- Severe physical deterioration of the patient (eg ceasing to eat and drink because of mental illness).
- Patient is at high risk of suicide (eg requires 'within eyesight' or 'within arms length' observation.
- Stupor.

Vigorous steps should be taken to remove such patients urgently (within days not weeks) to a more appropriate setting.

Making a referral

Making an urgent referral for possible transfer to the secondary mental-health services. A number of steps are required when making a referral to such services.

Consider where to refer

Refer to dedicated or sessional mental-health services within the prison, if they exist. If not, refer to the mental-health service covering the patient's original catchment area.

To locate the catchment area service, do the following:
- If the last address and a pre-custody general practitioner are available, the catchment area can usually be traced.
- If the prisoner is of no fixed abode and/or not registered with a general practitioner, then the place of offence or magistrate's court is used as a proxy for the last address. In some areas, there may be a 'no fixed abode rota' between all the main psychiatric hospitals within a defined area.
- If the person is an immigration detainee with no place of residence, contact the Director of Public Health (or equivalent) at your Primary Care Trust for advice on the most up-to-date procedure.

Consider to whom to refer

Obtain the names, telephone numbers, fax numbers, emergency availability (eg bleep or mobile) of the following key personnel:

- Senior consultant psychiatrist in the catchment area.
- Manager of the community mental-health team.
- CPA key-worker (if the person is previously known to the psychiatric services).
- Manager of the mental-health service of which the community mental-health team is a part (eg Director of Mental Health in the NHS Mental Health Trust). Ask if they are currently available or on leave. Ask who to contact if they are not available. This senior manager may help resolve differences or problems that arise with the clinical staff.

Should you refer to general or forensic psychiatric services?

Psychiatrists visiting prisons may be general psychiatrists (adult or adolescent) or forensic psychiatrists (adult or adolescent) according to local arrangements.

In addition to local arrangements, considering the following factors may be helpful in deciding between referral to a general or forensic psychiatrist.

- Offence.
- Clinical picture.
- Assessment of risk.

A forensic psychiatrist is more likely to be required if the following apply.

Offence:

- Offence involves homicide, a serious sexual assault or serious violence.
- Prisoner has offended while within a treatment setting and that environment is no longer considered suitable or safe.

Clinical picture:

- Prisoner is sentenced and likely to need a Section 47 transfer to hospital for treatment or remanded for a serious offence and is likely to need transfer to hospital under Section 48.
- Assessment is required for treatment of a major personality disorder.
- Prisoner or court is asking for an opinion about treatment for sexual offending.
- There is a past history of treatment in a medium secure unit or special hospital.
- There is a history of serious violence whether or not convictions have ensued.
- The presentation of their illness is such that, after assessment by local generic services, they could not be managed by these services.

Risk assessment: there is a risk of serious violence or this risk needs to be assessed.

A local directory of services can be useful. Further advice may be obtained from administrators, medical records' departments, clinical team leaders in local hospitals or from community mental-health teams.

Exchange all relevant information

With due regard to patient consent and confidentiality, obtain the names and addresses of the individual's general practitioner, solicitor and any friends or relatives that the individual nominates to act on their behalf.

Contact the senior consultant psychiatrist or CPA key-worker in the first instance. Give as much information as possible about the current problem including severity, provisional diagnosis, current management, problems in managing the person, pending court appearances and the urgency of transfer required, eg 1 day, 1 week, 2 weeks, 1 month, etc. with reasons. Be able to give the index offence and any relevant previous convictions. This will help to assess the risk and to decide which service may be appropriate (eg forensic, high dependency, open ward).

Check that the person you are talking to has the same understanding as you do of terms such as 'severe', 'urgent' or 'very ill'. If there is any doubt, describe the behaviours; be explicit.

If you are familiar with the services, indicate where you think the person is likely to need to be placed, if transferred out of prison (eg open in-patient ward, locked ward, medium secure unit, maximum security). If not, say that you are not familiar with how the services are organised and ask the mental-health service to re-refer to a more appropriate person or service, if necessary. It is their responsibility to do so.

Negotiate the timetable for assessment

Ask how soon the service can assess the individual. Indicate to them if you feel the delay is unacceptable. If the service cannot offer an earlier date, ask the contact person if they can advise an alternative service and agree who will refer to this service. Ensure both general and forensic services are considered. If the catchment area service has no beds available anywhere, ask the contact person to seek alternative beds in other hospitals or services. It is their responsibility to do so, not yours.

Document all actions and conversations

Use both telephone and fax and follow up any verbal discussions with a record of what is discussed. Send this record to the person involved so that they can identify discrepancies or misunderstandings. Diligently copy into the inmate medical record (IMR) at all times.

Consider involving the Home Office Mental Health Unit

It is often helpful to involve the Home Office Mental Health Unit at an early stage. It has a database of hospitals. Contact:

- Mental Health Unit, Home Office, 50 Queen Anne's Gate, London SW1H 9AT.
- Tel: 020 7273 3394 in office hours for prison transfers to hospital for remand and sentenced prisoners. In case of difficulty, ask switchboard on 020 7273 4000 for an officer of the Mental Health Unit, quoting the patient's surname.
- Fax nos: 020 7273 3411/2937/2172.
- On-call, out-of-hours service for emergencies. **Tel: 020 7273 2069**.

If transfer under Sections 47 or 48 of the Mental Health Act 1983 is planned, write a letter to the Home Office Mental Health Unit indicating what action is planned and has been taken, soon after referral to the catchment area service (see **Use of the Mental Health Act 1983**, page 163).

Take further action if no progress is made

If there is still no acceptable resolution, contact the senior manager of the NHS Trust. Most senior managers try to resolve disputes before recourse is made to outside agencies. If the problem is not resolved at this stage, do the following.

- Inform the patient's solicitor, general practitioner, relatives or nominated representatives and, in the case of a patient on remand, write to the local court clerk that the patient is scheduled to attend, indicating what is happening.
- Telephone and write to the Mental Health Lead in the Strategic Health Authority that serves the catchment area. This is the person with lead responsibility to identify suitable placements for those who need secure mental health services, including prisoners and to intervene if necessary in cases that are difficult to resolve. Copy the letter/fax to the Prison Lead in the catchment area Primary Care Trust. Ensure you have up-to-date contact details of the relevant person(s) for your establishments.
- At this stage, where the prisoner is on remand, write a full letter/report detailing the difficulties encountered in transferring the person to hospital, to the local clerk of court so that information is available to magistrates, judges and the patient's legal representatives.
- Advise patients of other parties that they could contact (eg Community Health Council or its equivalent, European Court of Human Rights).

An up-to-date list of the contact details of Primary Care Trusts, Strategic Health Authorities and other NHS agencies can be obtained from: Prison Service Health Task Force, Wellington House, 133–155 Waterloo Road, London SE1 8UG. Tel: 020 7972 2000.

Making an urgent referral for acute medical treatment

Where a patient requires medical treatment as an emergency (eg for an overdose or acute confusional state that may be delirium), but, because of mental disorder or otherwise (eg unconscious after a fall), does not have capacity to give or refuse consent, such a patient may be taken to a general hospital for treatment under common law. In such a case, a medical doctor may make this decision without the involvement of a psychiatrist. The Mental Health Act does not come into play for treatment for a physical disorder, including an overdose. Transfer the individual under escort, by ambulance if necessary, to the nearest A&E and inform the relevant consultant that the patient is on his/her way (for more information, see **Consent and capacity**, page 300).

Where the patient's physical condition has deteriorated as a direct consequence of mental illness (eg patients with anorexia nervosa and reduced insight who require special forms of feeding, and patients with severe depressive illness who stop eating or drinking), treatment for these direct consequences of mental illness may be provided under the Mental Health Act. In this situation, obtain an urgent (on-call) assessment in the prison, stating that transfer to an NHS psychiatric hospital under Sections 47 or 48, or to an NHS general hospital under common law, will be needed, depending on the urgency of the need for treatment. If the urgent need is for a psychiatric bed and there are difficulties obtaining one, telephone the Home Office Mental Health Unit: 020 7273 3394 (office hours) or 2069 (out of hours emergencies).

Arranging the assessment visit

When the date of the assessment visit is agreed, give the visiting team as much information as possible about how to arrange a visit, how to find the prison, when it is possible to see inmates, security arrangements, etc. (a leaflet may be useful here) and smooth their entry at the gate.

Try to arrange for a healthcare worker who knows the inmate to be available to discuss the problem and to deal with feedback after assessment.

Consider treatment

See the relevant disorder-specific guidelines. In addition:

- Discuss with the catchment area team whether to start treatment before assessment.
- Find out what has been effective before.
- Initiate the CPA if specialist care is involved. Request that the mental-health specialist documents the assessment and the care plan, agrees who the key-worker is and sets a date for the review of the care plan. Ensure that you have a copy of the care plan in the medical notes. Write the name and contact details of the key-worker clearly on the front of the notes. Copies of CPA documentation should be provided by the local NHS Trust.

Other issues

Other issues may need to be considered, for example:

- **Consider opening a 2052SH form** (in Scotland, an Act to Care form).
- **Consider the most appropriate location for the patient.** Discuss between the healthcare team and other relevant staff whether the prisoner needs to be located in the healthcare centre and the levels of observation (see **Observing a patient at risk of suicide**, page 220). Consider a single/shared cell/care suite. If the prisoner is to be on ordinary location, give the wing manager as much advice about the appropriate management of the patient as is consistent with patient confidentiality. One of the information leaflets for prison officers on the disk may help 💾.
- **Consider who needs to be informed**:
  - **Court**: it may be necessary to make the prisoner 'unfit for court'. Write/fax the court, explaining the reasons for this.
  - **Next of kin**: consider informing the next of kin and/or the solicitor if the patient gives permission.
  - **Health services**: where the prisoner has had previous contact with the health services, support the maintenance of contact wherever possible. For example, ask if the patient had hospital appointments booked and, if so, what for.
  - **Sentence planning**: where the patient is a sentenced prisoner, consider informing the sentence-planning officer and a probation officer if the patient gives permission. It is in the patient's best interests for healthcare input to be made to the process for planning multidisciplinary care to the individual while in prison and following release (for more details, see **Throughcare** below).
- **Consider the need for 'medical hold'.** To ensure continuity of treatment, consider placing the prisoner on 'Medical Hold' to complete assessment or a course of treatment.

Participation in prison multidisciplinary care planning

Where prisoners have mental-health needs, it is in their interests for these to be considered alongside their social, psychological and offending behaviour needs, within existing prison multidisciplinary assessment and care-planning procedures. Such multidisciplinary health- and socialcare is a requirement of community mental healthcare outside prison and of mental healthcare in all Scottish prisons. For some prisoners, it is appropriate for their key-worker to continue to oversee their care plan and to provide follow-up care under Section 117 while they are in prison. This is easier to arrange when the prison is near the catchment area.

Sentence planning

Sentenced prisoners already receive a multidisciplinary assessment of their needs and a plan is developed to meet these needs, as far as possible. Interventions that may form part of the sentence plan include educational courses, substance misuse courses, offending behaviour courses, including anger management, sex-offender treatment and enhanced-thinking courses. The aim is to reduce future offending, provide support to the individual and his/her family, help towards better social functioning and prepare for release. The sentence-planning process may be coordinated by a probation officer/prison social worker or by a prison officer.

Further multidisciplinary assessments are also made in order to plan the release of the prisoner, either permanently or under **supervision on temporary licence**, on **life licence** or on **discretionary conditional release (also known as parole)**. Psychiatric reports for these purposes should ideally be written by a psychiatrist with catchment area responsibility for the locality to which the prisoner is likely to be released.

Providing healthcare input to throughcare processes

In Scotland, arrangements to ensure healthcare input are made to throughcare processes and they are mandatory. In England and Wales, if it is not yet routine for healthcare input to be made to throughcare processes in a prison, consider a regular meeting between the healthcare manager, senior medical officer, mental-health staff, probation staff, chaplain, psychologist, education manager and sentence-planning manager to discuss how best to achieve this. The discussion should include the issue of confidentiality.

An appropriate member of the healthcare team should attend multidisciplinary care-planning meetings.

Benefits of healthcare input

Information about mental-health needs, prognosis and the likely pattern of relapse (if known) is relevant to the following.

- Assessments of risk.
- Planning an appropriate location, eg moves between wings, especially healthcare centre to wings and 'respite' stays in the healthcare centre; management, eg need for quiet, lack of confrontation; and activities, eg varying activities to match varying patterns of symptoms arising from depot medication. Jointly consider a mixed location (eg education centre or sheltered work during the day; healthcare centre at night, or daycare centre during the day, normal wing location at night).
- Identifying and responding appropriately to signs of relapse.
- Planning a response to a crisis. This can be particularly helpful in cases of chronic self-injury in the presence of a personality disorder, where several disciplines may be involved.
- Appropriate goals for substance misuse interventions.
- Integrating treatment of mental-health needs with offending behaviour needs; eg an individual might make better use of offending behaviour groups if he/she first attended an anxiety management group.

- Planning aftercare following either temporary release on licence or permanent release.

What information to provide

Provide information, with the patient's permission, to the sentence-planning team on the patient's:

- mental health history
- previous contact with the mental-health services
- current presentation and treatment
- prognosis
- early warning signs of relapse
- guidelines for further management within the system and
- recommendations, as appropriate, for further assessments.

Ensure that staff in areas where the individual spends time (eg wing manager, workshop supervisor, teacher) have a copy of the appropriate information 💾.

If attendance at meetings is not possible

- Ask to be kept informed in good time of discussions about possible release dates, including temporary licence or home detention curfew.
- Ask for a summary of planned throughcare, including care after release.
- Send a letter outlining the patient's mental-health needs and giving clear guidelines for further management within the system. This may include a recommendation that a further opinion be sought, eg from a clinical psychologist or drug/alcohol services.

Liaison with residential and other staff about all patients

Whether or not the individual is in prison for long enough to have a sentence plan, residential and other staff will need information to provide appropriate management and support to the patient on ordinary location. With patient permission, consider providing advice, where appropriate, on the following:

- Location (eg single or shared cell).
- Risk of suicide, self-harm or harm to others.
- Suitable work placements.
- Signs of relapse (eg becoming very withdrawn or verbal content becoming strange or out of context), when the health centre should be contacted again.
- Reducing noise and stress.
- Promoting increased family contact, extra visits, telephone calls.
- Facilitating a safe environment, eg concerns about bullying or debt.
- Provision of activities in a cell, eg art materials, reading materials.
- How to respond to difficult behaviours.

Prerelease planning and liaison

Arrangements for appropriate on-going care in the community need to be put in place, wherever possible, before a prisoner is released. This should be done before release of any kind (eg on temporary licence, for home detention curfews and before permanent release) and should be done, wherever possible, as part of a multidisciplinary plan (see the disk for a description of different types of temporary release 💾).

Unplanned release

When prisoners are released unexpectedly (eg criminal proceedings discontinued, bail) and the individual is in need of admission to hospital, consider contacting the following:

- General practitioner.
- Mental Health Crisis Service.
- General mental-health services.
- Probation Service.
- Court Liaison Service.
- Police mental health liaison officer.

Alternatively, consider contacting the Police so that they can alert the relevant Local Authority. They may then consider the use of Part II of the Mental Health Act.

Planned release 1

Notify the individual's general practitioner that release is planned, with patient permission. Give the release date if known. If the individual gives permission, give the general practitioner sufficient information to enable him/her to coordinate quickly the services required should problems arise. Include as many of the following as possible.

- Patient's name, date of birth, address and telephone number.
- Brief personal and social history.
- Past psychiatric history.
- Current mental state.
- Current medication and details of any medication tried in the past.
- Drugs and alcohol history.
- Details of carers and significant others.
- Recommended involvement of other services, eg socialcare, housing.

If the individual does not have a general practitioner, support him/her in registering with one. If possible, obtain from the local Primary Care Trust/Local Health Group a list of practices whose lists are open (still taking new patients). Give the individual information about how to register with a general practitioner. If there is a primary-care service in the area that provides walk-in treatment for homeless or unregistered people, give its details. Inform the individual that if an acute injury or illness occurs before they register, they may ask for short-term treatment at any practice. All general practitioners must provide such treatment that is 'necessary and immediate' and may claim payment for doing so from the Primary Care Trust, without the patient being registered.

Planned release 2

Where the release date is known, refer as soon as possible and at least 4–6 weeks before release to the mental-health services in the appropriate area. Prisoners with serious mental illness should have a designated care coordinator and care plan agreed before release. The referral letter (or fax) is best written by a mental-health worker or psychiatrist and sent to the mental-health services, with a copy to the individual's general practitioner. Include the following information.

- Background circumstances of referral.
- Index offence.
- Forensic history.
- Personal history.
- Social circumstances (eg housing).
- Psychiatric history.
- Substance misuse.
- Current mental state.
- Current treatment and progress.
- Details of other services that have been put in place to tackle other areas of the individual's needs (eg probation, substance misuse). Where healthcare staff have not already had input into the plans of both probation and sentence-planning staff, liaise now to ensure you are fully aware of plans.
- Where the individual has both psychiatric and substance misuse needs, ensure that services (if separate) are aware that the individual needs both services concurrently. Where you are certain that symptoms of mental illness are not substance-induced (eg where successive drug screens have shown an individual to have psychotic symptoms while drug free), state this clearly.
- If the individual has previously been treated in hospital under Sections 3, 37, 47 or 48, include the information and send a copy of the letter to the Local Authority concerned. Health Authorities and Local Authorities have a duty to provide aftercare for these individuals under Section 117.
- Where the individual does not have a general practitioner, make sure that the care coordinator is aware of this fact and include help for the individual in registering with a general practitioner as part of the care plan.

Planned release 3

Where the individual has a range of complex needs and is likely to find it difficult to access or maintain contact with the appropriate statutory services in the community (eg someone with some mental illness plus personality disorder who also abuses substances and is of no fixed abode), request an assessment visit before release by the catchment area psychiatrist or other team members. Establishing personal contacts increases the chance of successful follow-up.

In some areas, voluntary agencies may operate services that specialise in supporting this group of patients in making and maintaining contact with statutory services, eg Revolving Doors, which operates a service in HMPs Pentonville, Holloway, Woodhill and Wormwood Scrubs, and the Mental After Care Association (MACA), which operates in the Inner London area. Access to MACA's schemes is via the London Probation Service. The relevant specialist commissioning group (now based in Strategic Health Authorities) will have details.

Consider the need for practical help to ensure that the individual can get from the prison, when released, to the first of his/her appointments.

Follow-up

Where possible, the care coordination plan should include an appointment with both the general practitioner and the mental-health service within 5 days after release. There is a need for partnership work between the health, prison, probation and social services to ensure continuity of care.

Liaison when a patient is transferred back to prison from hospital

Someone who has been transferred to a secure hospital under Sections 37, 47 or 48 may be returned to prison. Such patients **are entitled to on-going care under Section 117 of the Mental Health Act**. This section obliges Primary Care Trusts and Local Authorities to provide aftercare for those treated under the Mental Health Act in hospital and then discharged. Prison healthcare staff should expect, before transfer of the patient from hospital to prison:

- to be invited to a case conference along with in-house or sessional mental-health services if available, or the appropriate Health Trust and local social services to agree Section 117 needs and arrange suitable CPA and aftercare services
- to receive a copy of a discharge plan that includes risk factors for relapse, a crisis plan and what to do if the patient relapses after transfer to prison and
- to receive the results of the assessments and advice on how the person's behaviour should be managed, if the patient is to be returned as 'untreatable'.

For more information about the use of the Mental Health Act 1983, see page 163.

Use of the Mental Health Act (England and Wales) 1983: a basic guide for general practitioners working in prisons

Relevant sections of the Mental Health Act

The Mental Health Act (England and Wales) 1983 currently provides the legal framework for compulsory admission and treatment of patients suffering from mental disorder. The sections of the Act most relevant to general practitioners and medical officers working in a prison setting are the following.

- **Section 48**: transferring an unsentenced prisoner (including civil prisoners and those detained under the Immigration Act 1971) from prison to hospital. A civil prisoner is one detained for non-criminal acts, eg non-payment of debt.
- **Section 47**: transferring a sentenced prisoner who has become mentally disordered after entering prison or whose mental disorder was not identified before sentence to an NHS hospital.
- **Section 37**: this is a hospital order (a sentence of the court) imposed as an alternative to sentencing that individual to prison. The prisoner may remain in the prison for 28 days while awaiting a bed in hospital.

Less frequently, a general practitioner or medical officer in prison may be involved in arranging assessments under the following:

- **Section 35**, where a court remands an individual to hospital rather than to prison for psychiatric assessment and report.
- **Section 36**, where a crown court remands a defendant to hospital for psychiatric assessment and report. Psychiatric treatment can be given.
- **Section 38**, which is an interim hospital order where a court orders a convicted person to be detained in hospital temporarily to test if a hospital order is appropriate.

Principles of treatment under the Mental Health Act

The Mental Health Act code of practice stresses the following:

- Mentally disordered people who are subject to criminal proceedings have the same right to psychiatric assessment, treatment and care as anyone else.
- Anyone in prison who needs medical treatment that can only satisfactorily be given in a hospital should be admitted to an NHS hospital or appropriate registered mental nursing home. Prison 'hospitals'/healthcare centres do not qualify as hospitals under the Act, so compulsory treatment under it may not be given in them.
- If it is essential to give medication without the patient's consent, this can only be administered under common law and where the patient lacks 'capacity' (see **Emergency treatment under common law**, page 168).

General points about the Mental Health Act

In the Act, mental illness is not defined and is a matter for clinical judgement. Decisions about whether to seek to transfer a prisoner under the Act require that the statutory criteria are met.

163

Sections 47 and 48 are used to transfer to hospital a patient in need of hospital treatment without the involvement of a court. The Home Secretary's consent is rarely refused if it can be demonstrated that the level of security at the receiving hospital is adequate. If in doubt, refer.

If a defendant on remand is mentally disordered but does not require urgent transfer to hospital under Section 48, refer the defendant for psychiatric assessment and, with patient consent, notify his/her solicitor that you have done so. This may prompt the court to consider a hospital order. Never rely on notice of a mental disorder coming to the court by other means.

Criteria for the use of the Mental Health Act, Sections 48, 47 and 37

- **Section 48**: applications to the Home Secretary to direct the transfer of an unsentenced, civil or Immigration Act prisoner can only be made when:
  — the person is suffering from mental illness or severe mental impairment
  — the nature and/or degree of the mental disorder makes it appropriate for the person to be detained in a psychiatric hospital for treatment and
  — the person is in urgent need of such treatment.
  A sentenced civil prisoner is someone not convicted under criminal law, eg someone imprisoned for debt.

- **Section 47**: applications to the Home Secretary to direct the transfer of a sentenced prisoner can only be made when:
  — the prisoner is suffering from mental illness, psychopathic disorder, severe mental impairment or mental impairment
  — the nature and/or degree of the mental disorder necessitates detention in a psychiatric hospital for treatment and
  — in the case of psychopathic disorder or mental impairment, such treatment is likely to alleviate the condition or prevent further deterioration.

- **Section 37**: magistrates and crown courts can impose a hospital order on a person convicted of an imprisonable offence other than murder, if they are satisfied that:
  — the same criteria governing use of Section 47 are met (see above) and
  — a hospital order is the most appropriate way to deal with the case.

How to arrange a Mental Health Act assessment for Sections 47 or 48

The medical officer/senior medical officer, in consultation with the prison governor, is responsible for making the arrangements. For a transfer application to be successful, the following are required.

- Two doctors, one Section 12-approved (usually a psychiatrist) and one who, wherever possible, has prior knowledge of the individual (often the medical officer), complete a form (No 218 or 218a), recommending to the Secretary of State that the patient is suffering from one of the appropriate categories of mental disorder. The doctors must state if a special hospital would be appropriate.
- Home Secretary agrees.
- Hospital has accepted the patient (this may occur after the order is made)
- Transfer is enacted within 14 days of the assessment. Otherwise, a further transfer direction must be sought.

Refer to the catchment area mental-health service for assessment. Indicate that use of Sections 47 or 48 is likely.

Discuss with the psychiatrist or hospital manager the availability of a bed and the level of security required at a suitable hospital. Ideally, a psychiatrist with beds at this hospital should be one of the assessing doctors.

Write to the Home Office Mental Health Unit as soon as possible after referral to the catchment area psychiatric service indicating what action has been taken and what is planned. Discuss the level of security required with the Mental Health Unit.

In the case of a remand prisoner, notify the court in relation to fitness to plead.

Following the assessment, write again to the Home Office Mental Health Unit, enclosing the medical reports. These must specify the form of disorder that the person is suffering from and the hospital to which the person will be transferred.

To ensure that transfer occurs within 14 days of the assessment, maintain close contact with the Home Office Mental Health Unit to make sure that a bed becomes available. If problems or delays are experienced, telephone the unit for help (for more information, see **How to refer urgently**, page 153)

Arrangements for a Mental Health Act assessment for Section 37

Hospital orders are made by the court.

Refer to the catchment area mental-health service for assessment under Section 37.

Discuss with the psychiatrist or Care Programme Approach (CPA) key-worker the availability of a bed at a suitable hospital. A psychiatrist employed at this hospital should be one of the assessing doctors.

The individual may be admitted to a 'place of safety' (usually the remand prison) for 28 days pending admission to hospital. Inform the court of any difficulties in admitting the patient within this period or if the hospital subsequently withdraws its undertaking to admit the individual. During these 28 days, even though the individual has been placed under a hospital order, he/she cannot be treated against their will in the prison except under Common Law (see page 155).

If the transfer arrangements break down, contact the individual's Health Authority and ask it to find another hospital within the 28 days. If this is not possible, the individual must be returned to court within the 28 days and resentenced.

Before the assessment

Information is a very important part of the assessment. Ensure that the information already gathered with the patient's permission is available: old psychiatric notes, general practice notes, care programme approach key-worker, family or close friend, solicitor. This will speed the assessment and allow a better decision to be made about what sort of treatment is needed and where it is best provided (see 'Assessment' in **Managing the interface with the NHS and other agencies**, page 137).

Assessment

A multidisciplinary assessment is preferred if possible. For possible admission to hospital, the presence of a doctor and nurse is usual. If psychological treatment is a prominent issue, the presence of a psychologist is valuable. Make sure that the gate lodge staff know who to expect and that escorts are available. Ensure that the patient is available. Ensure that any staff member who knows the patient is available to speak to the visiting assessment team. If the doctor who made the referral is not on-site at the time of the assessment, ensure that he/she is readily available for discussion by telephone.

If the patient is not accepted for admission

The fact that a patient is not accepted does not mean that he/she is not seriously mentally ill. In most cases, on-going psychiatric treatment will be required with possible re-referral in the future.

If the decision is felt to be reasonable, request advice on the following, as appropriate.

- How to manage the patient in the short and longer term within the prison.
- Risk management.
- Arrangements for liaison before release.
- Clear guidelines on when to re-refer if the situation changes.

Ensure that the provision of such advice in all assessments forms part of any service agreements drawn up by the prison and local mental-health services.

If it is felt that the non-acceptance is unreasonable, do the following:

- Communicate this in a doctor-to-doctor telephone conversation.
- Follow-up the telephone conversation with a letter.
- Ask for a second opinion, preferably a local one.
- Notify the patient's solicitor, with patient consent, of all actions taken. The solicitor may help in arranging a second opinion.
- For more actions to take, see **How to make an urgent referral** (page 153).

If the criminal proceedings are discontinued

Refer to 'Unplanned release' in **Managing the interface with the NHS and other agencies** (page 149).

On admission to hospital

The following information must be sent to the hospital at the time of transfer (if it has not already been sent).

- An up-to-date medical report sent by the medical officer to the patient's responsible medical officer (RMO).
- Any relevant social inquiry reports prepared by the Probation Service (addressed to the principal hospital social worker).
- Patient's inmate medical record (IMR) (hospital staff may copy relevant parts of the IMR and return it to the prison).
- Any relevant risk information from the health or security records.

In addition, for patients transferred under Sections 47 or 48, it is important to do the following:

- Identify by name the psychiatrist and key-worker who will be responsible for the care of the prisoner while in hospital.
- Write their contact details on the prisoner's file.

- Make personal contact (by telephone) with the psychiatrist and/or key-worker. Ask them to let you know when possible transfer back to the prison is being considered and (at that time) any information about treatment, the recommended follow support and the risk assessment.

If the individual is returned to prison from hospital

Someone who has been transferred to a secure hospital under Sections 47 or 48 may be returned to prison. Such patients, and any others who have previously been in hospital under sections of the Mental Health Act, eg Sections 3 and 37), **are entitled to aftercare under Section 117 of the Act**. This section imposes on Primary Care Trusts and Local Authorities the duty to provide aftercare for persons treated under the Act in hospital and then discharged. Before transfer of the patient from hospital to prison, prison healthcare staff should expect the following:

- To be invited to a case conference along with in-house or sessional mental-health services if available, or the appropriate Health Trust and local social services to agree Section 117 needs and arrange suitable CPA and aftercare services. This may not be possible in the case of emergency transfers.
- To receive a copy of a discharge plan that includes risk factors for relapse, a crisis plan and what to do if the patient relapses after transfer to prison.
- If the patient is to be returned as 'untreatable' to receive the results of assessments and advice on how the person's behaviour should be managed.

If this does not happen.
- Ask for a discharge plan to be sent, covering the areas outlined above.
- Consider arranging a case conference at the prison. Invite staff from the secure hospital and in-house or sessional mental-health services, if available, or request a visit from Catchment Area Services and local social services. Inform the hospital and the catchment area services and Local Authority that the individual is entitled to aftercare under Section 117 of the Act. Consider including staff from other areas of the prison who will be involved in the patient's care (see **Confidentiality**, page 304).

This is not intended to be a comprehensive guide to the Mental Health Act. Consultation of the most recent Code of Practice and with Home Office and Department of Health guidance relating to mentally disordered offenders, including Home Office Circular 12/95, is recommended.

Treatment for mental illness without consent under common law

Use of compulsory powers under the Mental Health Act 1983 is not allowed in prison. This applies equally to patients in prison awaiting transfer to a psychiatric hospital for assessment or treatment under the compulsory powers of the Act. Treatment without consent for mental illness may be provided in prison under common law under certain circumstances.

In what circumstances may treatment for mental illness without consent under common law in England and Wales be considered?

If a patient is refusing treatment and you have done all you can to transfer him/her to a mental hospital, you can provide treatment without consent for mental illness under common law if the following conditions are met.

(1) Patient has a mental illness and treatment is 'in their best interests'

Key principles are the following.

- Treatment without consent is for treatment of an illness and not for control of aggressive behaviour in the absence of mental illness (for advice on managing aggressive prisoners, including criteria for use of medication for that indication, see **Managing aggression and violence**, page 282).
- Patient's best interests are not confined to what is in his/her best medical interests. Case law has established that other factors that may be taken into account include the patient's values and preferences when competent, their psychological health, well-being, quality of life, relationships with family or other carers, spiritual and religious welfare and their own financial interests.
- A doctor has a duty of care under common law to provide treatment in the patient's best interests where the patient lacks a capacity to consent to or refuse treatment and there is no valid advance statement.

and

(2) Treatment is in accordance with a practice accepted at the time by a reasonable body of medical opinion skilled in the particular form of treatment in question

This is why it is essential to obtain an opinion from a specialist.

and

(3) Patient lacks 'capacity' to accept or refuse treatment

To have capacity, the patient must:

- understand what in broad terms is the nature of the treatment and that somebody has said that he/she needs it and why the treatment is being proposed
- understand its principal benefits, risks and alternatives

- understand what will be the consequences of not receiving the proposed treatment and
- retain the information for long enough to make an effective decision.

For more details, see **Consent and capacity** (page 300).

In what circumstances may treatment for mental illness without consent under common law *in prisons* be considered?

The criteria set out under (1) above must be met in all places in which compulsory treatment for mental illness under common law is given. Meeting those criteria is an essential legal requirement. There are **in addition** important considerations that arise because of the nature of prisons and of prison healthcare facilities. These are outlined below.

Whenever possible, prison healthcare centres are advised to restrict themselves to treatment that addresses only those medical needs which most urgently need to be met

In a prison context, it is important for the healthcare team to distinguish between the following:

- Treatment that might be needed urgently in the incompetent patient's best interests.
- Treatment in the patient's best interests that can wait until he/she has been transferred to a mental hospital.

Usually treatment needed urgently that cannot wait until the patient has been transferred to a mental hospital will be where:

- the patient's life is endangered
- serious harm or distress may otherwise come to the patient or others and
- a failure to treat would result in an irreversible deterioration in the patient's condition.

In any emergency, the doctor should not exceed the treatments needed to sustain life and health. Other, less urgent, treatments considered to be in the patient's best interests should be clearly specified in the patient's care plan. The care plan should also specify which member of the healthcare team is taking action to arrange for these remaining healthcare needs to be met.

Emergency treatment under common law should only be provided if the appropriate equipment and trained staff are available

Administering emergency treatment without consent is usually dangerous. For example, aggression and hyperexcitability may increase the risk of sudden death and injury.

Staff competencies required

Staff need to be competent in the following:

- Assessment of the risks and benefits involved in intervening with patients who may be highly aroused, have been using illicit drugs or are physically ill.
- Identification of the likely complications of these interventions.
- Resuscitation and the regular monitoring of such patients (Airways, Breathing and Circulation — ABC).

Equipment required

Appropriate resuscitation and patient monitoring equipment must be available (manual ventilation, cardiac resuscitation, pulse oximeter). Emergency medication and equipment should be checked regularly to ensure it is maintained and in date.

Protocols and care pathways required

Protocols required by Prison Health Care Standards on treatment without consent, emergency treatment, restraint, seclusion and transfer of prisoners to a treatment facility should be known, accessible, up to date and regularly reviewed.

Local Trusts will have a protocol on emergency treatment. The *Bethlem and Maudsley Prescribing Guidelines* contain a regularly updated section on rapid tranquillisation and may be a useful resource.[1]

Important action to take before giving compulsory treatment under common law

If you are contemplating treatment without consent, you should, if time allows, do the following:

- Urgently refer for an assessment for possible transfer to a psychiatric hospital under the Mental Health Act. Nearly all patients likely to require emergency treatment under common law should be transferred as soon as possible to an appropriate psychiatric hospital. Mental-health services should work towards meeting a standard of assessing and, where appropriate, admitting such patients within 24 hours.
- Obtain a specialist opinion from a consultant psychiatrist not connected with the case.
- Hold a multidisciplinary meeting involving the doctor, nursing and/or other healthcare staff and the duty governor. The meeting should be recorded in the inmate medical record and the care plan.
- Reconsider the diagnosis. The cause of what appears to be a psychosis may be alcohol-induced hallucinosis, post-epileptic confusion, infectious or febrile illness or other physical disease (for other possible physical causes, see **Delirium — F05**, page 41). These possibilities should be considered before, during and after treatment.

Before giving repeat treatments without consent, you should follow the same procedure as above. It is not acceptable to give recurrent top-up medications without holding a case conference, where viable and possible, for each top-up dose. Care should be taken to avoid an overdose by repeating treatments without consent. If there is fever, rigidity and/or labile blood pressure, stop antipsychotic medication and refer immediately to the on-call physician for investigation for neuroleptic malignant syndrome.

How to administer treatment without consent in an emergency

See the local guidelines. The following does not give full details of medications, dosages and routes of administration (see **Acute psychosis**, page 11).

- Document the clinical state and discuss it with colleagues.
- Explain the situation to the patient.
- Try talking down, distraction.

- Move spectators away to avoid audiences and ensure privacy and dignity.
- Obtain a drug history (types and amounts given in the previous 24 hours) and a history of the effective treatment in the past. Carry out a physical examination, including an electrocardiogram (ECG) if possible.
- Use doses at the lower end of the recommended range unless you are certain that the patient is currently taking psychotropic drugs. Do not exceed the *BNF* limits in any 24 hours. The senior prison doctor present should administer the medication.
- Try oral therapy. Benzodiazepines are safer than antipsychotics, but beware of accumulation.
- Use benzodiazepines alone if there is any cardiac disease.
- Low potency antipsychotics such as chlorpromazine or sulpiride are preferred.
- Never give Clopixol Acuphase to a struggling patient or to those who have not built up some tolerance to antipsychotics.
- Procyclidine IV/IM must be available. Consider its use as prophylaxis.
- If IM therapy is required, give the injection deeply into either the middle third of the outer aspect of the thigh or the upper outer quadrant of the buttocks. The patient may need to be restrained using approved techniques. Restraint should be done under health supervision and by staff currently trained in control and restraint techniques.
- Monitor the patient's vital signs every 5 minutes until peak concentrations have been reached (up to 2 hours, or longer in the elderly or physically ill). Give flumazenil if the respiratory rate drops below 10 per minute. After 2 hours, continue to monitor less frequently in case of adverse reaction.
- Consider converting to oral medication soon.
- A record of treatment, dosage and procedure should be made and signed by the senior prison doctor in the drug chart and the inmate medical record.

Action to take after the incident

- It is good practice to debrief those involved after emergency treatment.
- There should be on-going regular reviews of the patient's condition and treatment:
  — Review the patient's competence as this may fluctuate.
  — Review the extent to which any of the unmet needs start to become more urgent.
  — Arrange for newly urgent needs to be treated in the prison if the patient is still not competent.
  — Arrange for consent to treatment for all remaining healthcare needs to be discussed with the patient if he/she becomes competent.
  — Pursue proactively the referral to hospital if unacceptable delays are occurring.
- Incident should be recorded in the inmate medical record (IMR) and also in a document separate to the IMR.
- Significant event audit should take place. The policies, relationships and management may need reviewing. Questions to consider include the following:
  — Could the incident have been avoided and, if so, how?
  — Was the treatment appropriate and effective?
  — Were staffing levels and skills appropriate?

— Was the treatment given with as much consideration of the patient's dignity and privacy as possible?

Consider with the relevant NHS service what occurred, the severity of the situation and how it might support the prison in avoiding a repetition on future occasions.

- All significant event records should be collated and reviewed from time to time.

---

[1] The Bethlem & Maudsley NHS Trust. *2001 Prescribing Guidelines*, 6th edn. London: Martin Dunitz, 2000. 224 pages, ISBN 1-85317-963-9. Telephone orders can be made with credit cards on 020 7482 2202.

Nursing a patient with a severe psychotic illness — for general nurses and healthcare officers

Nurses play a central role in the assessment and treatment of patients with severe, psychotic mental illnesses. Nursing such patients is a skilled job that requires special training. Sometimes, general nurses or healthcare officers without mental-health training may augment the care provided by mental-health nurses. This section provides information to help them to do that. It covers two topics.

- Information about psychotic illness.
- What a generalist nurse can do to contribute to assessment and treatment.

It does not cover specialist topics such as how to assess hallucinations and delusions.

Information about psychosis

What is psychosis?

The word **psychosis** is used to describe a broad range of mental disorders that affect the mind, where there has been some loss of contact with reality. These types of disorders can vary greatly, though certain types of symptoms are characteristic. They include unusual and often extremely distressing experiences such as the following.

- **Disturbances of thinking**: thoughts become confused and may seem to speed up or slow down. Sentences are unclear or do not make sense. Patients may feel as if their thoughts are being put into their head and are not their own thoughts. They may have difficulty concentrating, following a conversation or remembering things. They may then appear to be unresponsive or uncooperative.
- **Delusions**: false beliefs that seem real to the patient and are not amenable to logical argument. They are often very frightening. For example, a person may believe that their food is being poisoned. Common themes for delusional beliefs are persecution, punishment, grandiosity and religiosity. For example, someone acutely ill may believe that he is Jesus.
- **Hallucinations**: patient sees, hears, feels, smells or tastes something that is not actually there. For example, they may hear voices that no one else can hear. Food may taste or smell as if it is bad or poisoned. Hearing voices is a very common symptom of schizophrenia. The hallucinations can range from occasional voices through to an almost constant barrage of derogatory comments from a large number of different voices.
- **Changed feelings**: patients may feel strange and cut off from the world. Mood swings are common and patients may feel unusually excited or depressed. Their emotions may seem dampened — they feel less than they used to or show less emotion to those around them.

Different types of psychotic disorder

There are different types of psychotic illness. These include the following.

- **Substance-induced psychosis**: use of, or withdrawal from, alcohol or drugs may be associated with the appearance of psychotic symptoms. Sometimes the symptoms remit as the effects of the substances wear off. Sometimes the illness lasts longer. It is possible for a patient to both have a more long-term psychotic illness **and** to misuse substances. It is not possible to tell from the symptoms alone whether someone has a substance-induced psychosis or whether they have another psychotic disorder. It is a mistake to think that because a prisoner is a drug user they cannot also have a severe psychotic illness such as schizophrenia.
- **Brief reactive psychosis**: psychotic symptoms arise suddenly in response to a major stress in the patient's life. The patient makes a quick recovery in a few days.
- **Organic psychosis**: physical injury or illness, such as a brain injury, encephalitis, AIDS or a tumour, may cause psychotic symptoms.
- **Schizophrenia**: psychotic illness in which the symptoms have been continuing for at least 6 months. The symptoms and the length of the illness vary.
- **Bipolar disorder (manic depression) and psychotic depression**: psychotic symptoms appear as part of a more general disturbance of mood. When psychotic symptoms are present, they tend to fit in with the person's mood. For example, someone who is depressed may hear voices telling them they should kill themselves. Someone who is unusually excited (manic) may believe that they have special powers and can perform amazing feats.

What causes psychosis?

Schizophrenia is probably caused by a combination of biological factors (such as a family history of schizophrenia) that create a vulnerability to experiencing psychotic symptoms. The symptoms often emerge in response to stress (eg breakdown of a relationship, being held in solitary confinement, bullying), drug abuse or social changes in vulnerable individuals. This theory of causation is known as the 'stress–vulnerability model'. It helps to explain why psychosis is usually an episodic problem, with episodes triggered by stress and patients often quite well between episodes. It also helps to guide management. International studies show that once a person has schizophrenia, the environment in which he/she lives can help them to stay well or can make them worse. In a calm environment and one where people provide plenty of support and encouragement, those with schizophrenia will suffer fewer psychotic episodes than if they are surrounded by people who push, frighten or criticise them.

Prognosis: do people get better?

Schizophrenia usually begins in early adult life but may occur at any time in an individual's life. Those who develop schizophrenia at a very early age do not tend to do as well as those whose illness begins in middle or old age. Although for some schizophrenia will be a life-long concern, others experience only one episode of the illness and never have a further episode. Generally, 20% of people recover completely, 35% are stable for long periods but have some further episodes of psychosis, and 45% experience long-term problems requiring continuing care. One-quarter of the latter group deteriorate more severely and rapidly and need very high levels of care and support.

When someone is in a very distressed, acutely ill state, it can be hard to believe that they will ever get better. Realistic hope is one of the most important treatments a nurse or healthcare officer has to offer.

What are the treatments?

- **Assessment**: first stage of treatment involves assessment, usually over some time. Mental-health specialists need to develop an understanding with the patient of how and why these symptoms affect them. A range of measures may form part of the assessment, eg the 'Delusion Rating Scale' and the 'Belief about Voices' questionnaire.
- **Medication**: along with other forms of treatment, medication plays a fundamental role in recovery from a psychotic episode and in the prevention of future episodes. The monitoring of side-effects is critical to avoid or reduce distressing side-effects that can lead to a patient being unwilling to accept the medication central to their recovery. Information about the medications used in mental illness is given on page 166.
- **Counselling and psychological therapy**: having someone to talk to is an important part of treatment. A person with acute psychotic symptoms may need to know that there is someone who can understand something about their experience and provide reassurance that they will recover. As recovery progresses, different forms of psychological therapy can:
  — help the patient and those caring for them (on ordinary location) learn how to keep stress levels low in order to prevent further episodes
  — help the patient and those caring for them (on ordinary location) recognise early warning signs that a further psychotic episode is developing and
  — help the patient learn ways of reducing the impact of hallucinations and delusions.
- **Practical assistance**: treatment often also involves assistance with employment, education, finances and accommodation.

What the generalist nurse or healthcare officer can do

Communication (engagement)[1]

In order for the healthcare team to help the patient, the patient has to feel that the team is on their side and be prepared to communicate and, at least to some extent, to cooperate with the team. A trusting relationship with any member of the healthcare team is therefore important to the success of the treatment. Building such a relationship is especially hard with a patient who is psychotic as, at least in the acute stage, they may believe that you intend to harm them. When you talk to the patient, it is likely that you will have to adapt your usual communication style as the patient's memory, concentration and tolerance levels may all be reduced.

- Talking with someone with a severe mental illness:
  — Never leave someone who is mentally ill to guess your intentions or the intentions of other members of the healthcare team. Their imagination will run riot. Always explain why you, the doctor or other person wants to talk with them.
  — Try to ensure that the environment is comfortable and safe for both you and the patient. Ask where in the healthcare centre the patient feels safe/OK to talk.
  — Remember that social interaction can be very stressful for the patient and be prepared to acknowledge this: 'I can see how hard this is for you. I appreciate you making the effort to talk to me'.
  — Be warm and friendly but also prepared to spend time in silence.
  — Always be aware of cultural issues. If you are not sure, ask. Finding out as much as you can about the patient's culture will help communication.

- Talking with someone who is hearing voices. If you are not sure someone is hearing voices at this particular time, ask them. If they are, do the following:
  — Acknowledge the difficulty and distress that voices cause. For example, 'It must be really difficult for you having this conversation. I really appreciate you making the effort'.
  — Do not challenge the fact that the patient can hear voices. They are real to the patient. However, you can say in a gentle and matter-of-fact way something like, 'It's your brain playing a trick on you just now'.
  — Talk clearly and slowly if necessary and be prepared to repeat questions.
  — Be prepared to take longer even for a simple matter.
  — If someone is obviously in distress, ask them if they have had enough. Be prepared to come back later.
- Talking with someone who mentions their delusional beliefs:
  — Show some understanding of the person's feelings, eg 'It must be really scary to think that someone else is controlling your thoughts'.
  — Do not argue about the strange ideas but do not pretend to agree with them either. Focus instead on how the delusions make them feel and then change the subject to something neutral or pleasant in real life (eg what is for dinner?).
  — If the conversation is distressing to the patient or to you, it is OK to say, 'I'll talk to you later when you're feeling a bit better'.
- Relating to someone who is withdrawn or isolated:
  — Be prepared to sit with the patient in silence.
  — Doing practical tasks close to the patient can be comforting. Sharing activities without talking can also be helpful.
  — Gently encourage other activities which are not too demanding (eg watching television, washing dishes, playing a board game).
  — Be prepared to keep trying. It can take a long time for some people to respond.
- Talking with someone who is angry or aggressive. People with schizophrenia are usually shy and withdrawn. However, they may also become aggressive, especially when they are experiencing fear or paranoia (feeling that they are being persecuted and that other people are out to get them) or voices (voices can, rarely, command a person to injure others).
- Information about dealing with aggression can be found in **Aggression** (page 282). To reduce patient fears and the potential for aggression, it may be helpful to do the following:
  — Give the patient space. Do not crowd them.
  — Inform the patient about what you are doing and intend to do.
  — Tell the patient that you do not mean them any harm.
  — Talk calmly and evenly.
  — Talk to the patient in a quiet environment.
  — Continually reassure them.
  — Keep your hands in view.
  — Keep your movements to a minimum.
  — Ask them why they are upset.

Observation: contribution to assessment

Nurses and healthcare officers may spend long periods with patients. Your observations of the patient's behaviour are a very valuable part of the assessment. General information about conducting observations is provided in **Observation** (page 200). In psychotic illness, helpful observations include the frequency, intensity and duration of 'positive symptoms' and the extent of 'negative symptoms'.

Positive symptoms include:	Negative symptoms include:
• Hallucinations. • Delusions. • Thought disorder. • Paranoia.	• Lack of motivation. • Social withdrawal. • Emotional withdrawal. • Difficulty in forming relationships. • Lack of spontaneity.

Make your observations as concrete and objective as possible, eg 'Spent all morning in bed. Appeared to watch television in afternoon but showed no reactions to the programmes or to changes of channel by others. Unresponsive to efforts to hold conversation' (rather than 'withdrawn').

Reassure, encourage and support the positives

People with a psychotic illness are likely to feel confused, distressed, afraid and lacking in self-confidence, both during the acute phase and for a long time afterwards. The illness has probably caused them to lose control of their thoughts and to feel overwhelmed by the world around them. As they recover, it is common for patients to:
- sleep for long hours every night (or during the day) for 6–12 months after the psychotic episode
- feel the need to be quiet and alone more often than other people and
- be inactive and feel that they cannot or do not want to do much.

It is helpful to explain to the patient what is happening to them, eg that psychotic symptoms usually appear as a response to severe stresses (see **What causes psychosis** above) and that additional sleep and inactivity is the body's natural way of slowing down to allow the brain to recover following the shock of an acute episode.

It is also helpful, as the patient recovers from the most acute stage of the illness, to encourage them to resume activities gradually that they have been able to do and have enjoyed in the past. Encourage the patient to help with simple jobs around the healthcare centre or to chat with you or to join in any art or other therapeutic activity on offer. If the patient refuses, do not pressure them but make it clear that they are welcome to come when they feel able to join in. Make it clear that they are welcome simply to sit in the company of others and watch or listen to people without joining in more actively. You may find that the patient likes to listen to loud music a lot of the time. This may be a way of drowning out distressing voices or thoughts. Earphones or a Walkman may be helpful.

Most importantly, it is helpful to relate to the patient as a human being who has interests and strengths separate from his/her psychotic symptoms or lack of them. This may be crucial in rebuilding some self-esteem and hope for the future. Find out what the patient's interests are and, if you can, discuss them with the patient. If the patient has contact with family members who are supportive, try to arrange a visit. It may be very helpful for the family members to have information about psychosis. This can be provided by an organisation such as the National Schizophrenia Fellowship (for details, see **Resource directory**, page 316).

Reduce stress and conflict

Because environmental stress plays such a prominent part in triggering episodes of psychosis, reducing such environmental stress is an important part of both treatment and prevention. The particular kind of stress that studies have found to be detrimental to patients with schizophrenia consists of high levels of 'expressed emotion'. This means:

- hostility: not only just bullying or physical aggression, but also angry shouting
- emotional over-involvement, eg 'Can you tidy your cell for me?' and
- criticism, eg calling a patient 'lazy', blaming him/her for being uncooperative.

Staying calm and using the communication tips in **Communication/engagement** above will be helpful. Ensuring that the patients are in an environment safe from bullying is also important. If the patient returns to normal location when the acute episode is over, residential managers should be aware that the way the patient is treated by staff and prisoners will significantly affect the likelihood of relapse. Additional patience and 'giving leeway' may be required.

Look out for depression and suicidal thoughts

People who have psychotic illnesses are at significantly higher risk of depression and suicide. They tend to have low self-esteem, to feel hopeless about their lives, to misuse drugs and alcohol, to lose their social role and be unable to attain their personal goals. In addition, some may hear voices telling themselves to kill themselves.

If the patient expresses depressed or suicidal thoughts to you, do the following.

- Listen to their feelings, but also point out that help is available.
- Express appreciation of the patient's feelings and the fact that he/she confided in you.
- Let the doctor and mental-health nurse know and consider opening a 2052SH form (in Scotland, an Act to Care form).
- Distract the patient by involving him/her in pleasant, low-key activities.
- Help them to be with someone by whom they feel accepted.
- Let the patient know that you accept and care about them.
- Consider whether any stressors can be removed that might be depressing the patient (eg worries about going back to a location on which he had been bullied).

Medication

Information on psychotropic drugs is provided on page 188. If you become aware that a patient is not taking the medication, do the following:

- Remind them calmly that the medication helps to keep them well.
- Ask if they are having any side-effects.
- Let the doctor or mental-health nurse know that the patient is refusing to take the medication.

---

[1] The section on communication was adapted from 'The guide to communicating with people who have serious mental health problems', developed by Katie Glover when she was at START, a Homeless Mentally Ill Initiative Project in London.

Medications used for mental-health problems
Information for non-specialist nurses

General nurses may be involved in administering psychotropic medication. This section is a brief guide to the main types of drugs used to treat mental disorders. The aim is to help you answer simple questions that patients may ask, and to know what to do if the patient does not turn up to collect their medicine. Further training is needed to help you recognise and deal with the side-effects of medication.

The things to remember are the following:

- A patient can only be given medication they have agreed to take (consent).
- Consent must be voluntary and reflect a continuing agreement to take the medication.
- Patients can change their mind about taking medication.
- When information is given to a patient about their illness and medication, it can increase the chance of consent being given.
- If a patient refuses to take the medication, you should record their views in the notes and report the fact to the prescribing doctor.

Anxiety and insomnia

Benzodiazepines

What are they?

Benzodiazepines are drugs used primarily to treat symptoms of the following.

- **Severe anxiety,** eg tension, feeling shaky, sweating and a difficulty in thinking straight. The drugs, known as anxiolytics and (misleadingly) minor tranquillisers, include diazepam (Valium), lorazepam (Ativan), oxazepam (Serenid) and chlordiazepoxide (Librium).
- **Short-term problems with sleeping.** Drugs known as hypnotics include loprazolam, nitrazepam (Mogadon) and temazepam (Normison).

Benzodiazepines also have muscle-relaxing properties and some (eg diazepam) can help the following:

- **Epilepsy**: particularly 'status epilepticus'.
- **Symptoms of alcohol withdrawal** (usually chlordiazepoxide). When someone has been heavily dependent upon alcohol, giving benzodiazepines during withdrawal may help prevent very serious, even life-threatening symptoms such as delirium tremens.

Side-effects

Common side-effects
Drowsiness, sleepiness and an inability to concentrate during the day.

Rare but important side-effects
- Patient becomes aggressive, excitable, talkative or disinhibited. Ask the doctor to review the medication.
- Rash: if this occurs, patients should stop the drug and see the doctor.

When are they not helpful?

Benzodiazepines are not ideal for the treatment of anxiety and insomnia because they only give symptomatic relief, do not treat the underlying illness and are addictive.

They should not be taken regularly for more than 4–6 weeks. Taking them once per day or every other day (for insomnia) or irregularly, eg for 1 or 2 weeks for panic attacks, reduces, but does not eliminate, the risk of addiction (for more efficacious and longer-term treatments, see the guidelines on **Sleep problems**, **Panic** and **Generalised anxiety disorder**, pages 91, 67 and 64). Benzodiazepines should be avoided wherever possible during pregnancy, childbirth and breast-feeding. They can sedate the baby and cause breathing problems. They should not be used routinely to deal with sudden stress (eg bereavement, imprisonment) (see the guidelines on **Bereavement** and **Adjustment disorders**, pages 23 and 15).

Important notes about benzodiazepines

General

- They are commonly traded illicitly on the street and in prison. Ensure that the drug goes to, and is taken by, the person for whom it is prescribed.
- If a patient misses a dose, do not give two or more doses together next time.
- They add to the effect of alcohol. Advise patients who may be released that alcohol is best avoided.
- Many people become addicted to benzodiazepines because of legal prescribing by their doctor.

Withdrawal

- Benzodiazepines should not be stopped suddenly if they have been taken regularly for more than 4–6 weeks.
- Withdrawal should never take less than 6–8 weeks — and often much longer
- Withdrawal symptoms can include anxiety, tension, panic attacks, poor concentration, difficulty in sleeping, nausea, trembling, palpitations, sweating, and pains and stiffness in the face, head and neck.
- The risk of suicide and self-injury increases during withdrawal and the regular monitoring of the suicide risk is required.
- During withdrawal (especially if it occurs quickly), the patient may behave unpredictably and pose a management problem. Advise officers that this may be part of the withdrawal syndrome. They should deal with the patient as calmly as they can. It may be possible to postpone adjudications until after the withdrawal is complete so that any improved behaviour can be taken into account.

Individuals withdrawing from benzodiazepines may benefit from help with anxiety-coping skills. Helplines and organisations providing support for those wishing to withdraw from benzodiazepines is provided below.

Resources for people addicted to tranquillisers

Battle Against Tranquillisers (BAT): 0117 966 3629 (helpline: Monday–Sunday, 9 am–8 pm)
PO Box 658, Bristol BS99 1XP
(Counselling and support for those considering stopping their tranquillisers and those who have succeeded in doing so)

CITA (Council for Involuntary Tranquilliser Addiction): 0151 949 0102
(Monday–Friday, 10 am–1 pm)
Cavendish House, Brighton Road, Waterloo, Liverpool
(Confidential advice and support)

Drugline: 020 8692 4975
(Advice and counselling for drug-related problems)

Helping You Cope: A Guide to Starting and Stopping Tranquillisers and Sleeping Tablets. Available from: Mental Health Foundation, UK Office, 20/21 Cornwall Terrace, London NW1 4QL. Tel: 020 7535 7400; Fax: 020 7535 7474; E-mail: mhf@mhf.org.uk; URL: http://www.mentalhealth.org.uk

Making Sense of Treatments and Drugs: Minor Tranquillisers. Available from: MIND, 15–19 Broadway, London E15 4BQ. Tel: 020 8519 2122; Fax: 020 8522 1725; E-mail: contact@mind.org.uk; URL: http://www.mind.org.uk/

β-Blockers

What are they?

β-Blockers include oxprenolol (Trasicor) and propranolol (Inderal). In lower doses, they can help treat the physical symptoms of the following.

- **Anxiety**, eg palpitations, sweating, shakiness. They do not affect the psychological symptoms (eg worry, tension and fear).
- **Heart conditions** such as hypertension (high blood pressure), angina and arrhythmias.

Side-effects

Common side-effects
Fatigue, cold extremities.

Rare but important side-effects
Rash or itchy skin, dry eyes, very slow pulse. Advise the patient to consult the doctor immediately.

Important notes about β-blockers

People with asthma should not take them.

- There is no evidence that they are addictive but they should be stopped gradually because of the likelihood of rebound tachycardia.
- If the patient misses a dose, do not give two or more doses at once. This may cause more side-effects.

Hypnotics

What are they?

Hypnotics are used as a short-term treatment for insomnia.

- **Non-benzodiazepine hypnotics** include chloral hydrate, chloral betaine (Welldorm), clomethiazole (Heminevrin), promethazine (Phenergan), diphenhydramine (Nytol), zaleplon (Sonata) and zopicline (Zimovane).

Promethazine and diphenhydramine are antihistamines. Chlormethiazole (Heminevrin) can help agitation and restlessness as well as alcohol-withdrawal symptoms.

Side-effects

Common side-effects
All hypnotics: drowsiness, dizziness, reduced reaction times during the day.

Rare but important side-effects
- Chloral: rashes/blotches, wheeziness (especially if the patient has asthma).
- Antihistamines: wheeziness (especially if the patient has asthma), palpitations/fast heart beat.
- If any of the above occur, advise the patient to stop the drug and consult the doctor immediately.

Important notes about hypnotics
- They are commonly traded illicitly on the street and in prison. Ensure that the drug goes to, and is taken by, the person for whom it is prescribed.
- They may cause addiction if taken regularly for longer than 4–6 weeks and should be taken in as low a dose as possible for the shortest time possible. Taking them only when required or every few days (eg on alternate nights) can be a useful way to use the drugs safely.
- It is recommended that chlormethiazole is taken for no longer than 9 days if used to help alcohol withdrawal.
- If dependence occurs, withdrawal symptoms can include anxiety, tension, poor concentration, difficulty in sleeping ('rebound insomnia'), palpitations and sweating.

Antidepressants

What are they?

Antidepressants are used to improve mood in people who are feeling low or depressed. Certain antidepressants may also be used to help the symptoms of panic disorder, obsessive-compulsive disorder, social phobia, bulimia nervosa, post-traumatic stress disorder (PTSD) and chronic pain syndrome. All these drugs seem to be equally effective for depression at the proper dose, but they have different side-effects. If one drug does not suit a patient, another may be tried. There are three main types of antidepressants.
- **Tricyclics (TCAs)**: include amitriptyline (Typtizol), amoxapine (Asendis), dothiepin or dosulepin (Prothiaden), Imipramine (Tofranil) and lofepramine (Gamanil).
- **Selective serotonin re-uptake inhibitors (SSRIs)**: include citalopram (Cipramil), fluoxetine (Prozac), fluvoxamine (Faverin), paroxetine (Seroxat) and sertraline (Lustral).
- **Irreversible monoamine oxidase inhibitors (MAOIs)**: include isocarboxazide (Marplan), phenelzine (Nardil) and tranylcypromine (Parnate). A special kind of MAOI is known as a reversible inhibitor of monoamine oxidase type A (RIMAs). These include moclobemide (Manerix).

There are, in addition, a number of other antidepressants, such as venlafaxine (Efexor), mirtazapine, nefazodone, reboxetine and trazodone.

Side-effects

Common side-effects

- TCAs: sedation, dry mouth, blurred vision, weight gain, constipation, sweating.
- SSRIs: insomnia, stomach upsets, sexual dysfunction.
- MAOIs: blurred vision, dizziness, drowsiness, dry mouth, constipation.
- RIMAs: dry mouth, nausea, headache, dizziness, insomnia.

Rare but important side-effects

- TCAs: skin rashes: stop medication and consult the doctor immediately.
- SSRIs: skin rashes: stop medication and consult the doctor immediately.
- MAOIs: urine retention: refer to the doctor immediately. Sweating, blurred vision, skin rashes, headache: stop medication and consult the doctor immediately.

Important notes about antidepressants

- If a patient misses a dose, seek them out and ask how they are. Ask the staff too. It is possible that the patient has not come to collect the medication because he/she has become more depressed, with increased lethargy, hopelessness and an increased risk of suicide.
- If a patient misses a dose, **do not** give two or more doses next time as this may increase side-effects.
- They may require at least 2 weeks before their mood starts to lift and 6 weeks before a full effect is achieved. Some changes (eg increased appetite, energy levels) may occur before this. Inform the patient about this lag in effectiveness. The risk of suicide may rise during this time. Careful monitoring is required.
- With TCAs, overdose attempts are serious and often fatal due to cardiac complications. The symptoms of overdose include: agitation, confusion, drowsiness, difficulty in breathing, convulsions, bowel and bladder paralysis, dilated pupils, and disturbances with the regulation of blood pressure and temperature.
- Tranylcypromine (a MAOI) by virtue of its amphetamine-like properties has a high abuse potential. Take extra care to ensure that the drug is given to, and taken by, the right patient.
- With MAOIs, dietary restrictions are necessary to prevent a tyramine-induced and potentially fatal hypertensive crisis. Tyramine is found in many common foods. Patients should not take any other drug at all (including over-the-counter cough and cold remedies) without consulting a doctor. **If a throbbing headache develops, medical attention should be sought immediately.**
- Most people may need to continue taking antidepressants for at least 4 months and some may need to continue for 12 months or more, especially if they have been depressed more than once, to reduce the chance of relapse.
- Antidepressants should not be stopped suddenly, even if the patient feels better. Their depression may return. In addition, they may experience 'discontinuation' symptoms. At worst, these could include headache, restlessness, diarrhoea, nausea, 'flu-like symptoms, lethargy, abdominal cramps, sleep disturbance and mild movement disorders. These are usually short lived and can even occur with missed doses.
- Despite the discontinuation symptoms, antidepressants are not addictive because they do not produce craving for the drug, or tolerance (ie needing more of the drug to get the same effect).

Antipsychotic medication
What is it for?

Antipsychotic drugs are called neuroleptics or, misleadingly, major tranquillisers. They are usually used only for the treatment of severe psychotic illnesses such as schizophrenia, mania and major depression with psychotic features. Their side-effects are common and often serious. They can also be used to help manage confusion, dementia, behaviour problems and personality disorders, or, in smaller doses, to help treat anxiety, tension and agitation. They have an initial, rapid, tranquillising (calming) effect.

Their effect on psychotic symptoms, such as delusions and hallucinations, may not appear for several weeks. There are two main groups of drugs.

- **'Typical' or classical antipsychotics**: include 'low-potency' drugs, such as chlorpromazine (Largactil), which are used in hundreds of milligrams per day, and 'high-potency' drugs, such as haloperidol (Serenace) and fluphenazine (Moditen), which are used in tens of milligrams per day.
- **'Atypical' antipsychotics**: such as risperidone (Risperdal), olanzapine (Zyprexa) and clozapine (Clozaril). Clozapine is an 'atypical' antipsychotic that has, to date, a unique effectiveness with patients who have not improved with other antipsychotics (drug-resistant schizophrenia).

Some typical antipsychotics are available as long-acting 'depot injections', such as fluphenazine decanoate (Modecate) and haloperidol decanoate (Haldol). Antipsychotic drugs have different side-effects to each other. If one drug does not suit a patient, another may be tried.

Side-effects

There is a wide range of side-effects. Many are common. They can cause significant impairment in functioning and may be the reason why some people stop taking their medication. They occur most commonly with the high potency typical antipsychotics. With appropriate advice and management, side-effects can be minimised. If a patient is distressed by side-effects, advise them to have a discussion with the doctor or mental-health nurse.

Common side-effects
- Constipation, dizziness, drowsiness, dry mouth, appetite increase, blurred vision. Movement disorders, known as 'extrapyramidal' side-effects, include shaky hands, feeling shaky, involuntary movements of the face, neck, eyes and tongue. Also, akathisia (acute feeling of restlessness in the legs, constant pacing).

Rare but important side-effects
- **Fever and muscle stiffness** could be 'neuroleptic malignant syndrome', which is rare but potentially fatal. Stop medication and call the doctor urgently. The patient should be cooled, and the body fluids and serum electrolytes monitored. Anticholinergic medication will be needed.
- **Skin rashes**: stop medication and consult the doctor immediately.

Depot injections

It is sometimes necessary or helpful for antipsychotics to be given as 'depot' injections. A depot injection is a long-acting injection usually given into a buttock.

The injection releases drug over several weeks, so the patient does not have to remember to take tablets at regular times each day. Depot injections are no more or less effective than tablets or capsules. They should only be given where essential, as they are painful to receive. The administration of depot injections should be preceded by an assessment of the patient's mental state and general physical health, including side-effects.

Important notes about antipsychotic medication

- It is essential that medication is taken regularly to avoid a recurrence of psychotic symptoms. If patients fail to turn up for their medication, make contact with them to assess why they have not taken their medication. Report this to the prescribing doctor or mental-health nurse.
- Sedative antipsychotics may impair mental abilities. If alertness is impaired, advise the patient to avoid operating machinery or driving.
- Remind patients, especially anyone who is taking clozapine (Clozaril), to report the sudden appearance of signs of infection (sore throat, fever). A complete blood count should be done immediately to check for the development of agranulocytosis.

Anticholinergic medication

What are they for?

Anticholinergic medication includes procyclidine (Kemadrin) and orphenadrine (Disipal). These drugs are used to reduce some of the extrapyramidal side-effects of antipsychotic medication. Acute dystonia and Parkinsonism respond quite well, tremor responds less well, akathisia responds poorly and tardive dyskinesia can be made worse by the drugs. These drugs should not be prescribed routinely for all people taking antipsychotic medication, but only after symptoms arise. Withdrawal of anticholinergic drugs should be attempted after 2 or 3 months without symptoms, as the drugs are liable to misuse and may impair memory.

Side-effects

Common side-effects
- Dry mouth, constipation, blurred vision.

Rare but important side-effects
- Urine retention: contact the doctor.

Important notes about anticholinergic medication

- Patients may trade them and may try to obtain an extra dose.
- Drugs have a mood-elevating effect and, when taken on their own, in the absence of antipsychotic medication, may also cause muscles to become stiff or, if enough is taken, to go into spasm.
- Take steps to ensure that the drug is given to and taken by the individual for whom it is prescribed.

Mood stabilisers

What are they for?

Mood stabilisers are drugs used to help prevent mood swings (feeling 'high' or 'low') in people who suffer from a bipolar illness (sometimes called manic depression). They include lithium carbonate (Camcolit), sodium valproate (Epilim) and carbamazepine (Tegretol). Lithium is also used in severe, recurrent depressive illness and in aggression. Carbamazepine and sodium valproate are also used to help control epilepsy. Carbamazepine is also used to relieve the symptoms of trigeminal neuralgia (a painful condition of the face) and in a number of other illnesses such as alcohol withdrawal or alcohol dependence, schizophrenia and withdrawal from benzodiazepines.

Side-effects

Common side-effects

- **Lithium**: nausea, diarrhoea, metallic taste in the mouth, weight gain, increased thirst, difficulty in concentrating.
- **Carbamazepine**: drowsiness, dizziness, stomach upset, visual symptoms (eg seeing double).
- **Sodium valproate**: nausea and vomiting, sedation, diarrhoea/nausea.

Rare but important side-effects

All three drugs can cause serious disorders. A range of blood tests is required for monitoring.

- **Lithium**: blurred vision, shaking and trembling, confusion, slurred speech, nausea and vomiting, diarrhoea, skin rashes. Advise the patient to stop taking the medication, to drink water and to see the doctor immediately.
- **Carbamazepine**: leucopenia, aplastic anaemia and agranulocytosis. Advise patients to report any symptoms of fever, rash, sore throat, infections, mouth ulcers, easy bruising, paleness of skin, weakness, bleeding or small purple spots on the skin.
- **Sodium valproate**: rash, impaired platelet function (patient bruises without reason and bleeds easily), impaired liver function (the patient feels sleepy, is sick, loses appetite, the skin may look yellow). Stop taking the medication and see the doctor immediately.

Important notes about mood stabilisers

- It is essential that these drugs are taken regularly. If lithium is stopped suddenly, there is a very high chance that the illness will return. If the patient misses several doses, they may need a new blood test to check their blood levels. If carbamazepine or sodium valporate is being given to help control fits or blackouts, missing a dose can cause the fits to return.
- If the patient does not turn up to collect their medication, seek them out and ask how they are. Ask the staff too. It is possible that the patient has not come to collect the medication because he/she has become more depressed, with increased lethargy, hopelessness and an increased risk of suicide.
- If a patient misses a dose, do not give two or more doses next time, as this may increase side-effects. If a patient misses two or more doses, refer them to a doctor for blood level checks.
- Remind the patient of the importance of reporting and responding to early symptoms of lithium toxicity. Make sure he/she has a copy of the information sheet on lithium toxicity (it is on the disk ▣). The most common cause of lithium toxicity is dehydration, which may occur during hot weather or physical exertion. Other causes are urinary tract infection and illnesses that cause vomiting and diarrhoea. These may occur despite regular blood tests.

- Remind patients taking carbamazepine of the importance of reporting immediately any fever, sore throat, infections, mouth ulcers, easy bruising, paleness of skin, weakness, bleeding or small purple spots on the skin.
- Remind patients taking sodium valproate of the importance of reporting immediately any jaundice and abdominal pain.

Drugs used for treating attention deficit hyperactivity disorder (ADHD)

The most commonly used drug in ADHD is methylphenidate (Ritalin). It is a stimulant and should be used along with educational, social and psychological help. Methylphenidate can help a young person's abilities to concentrate and reduce over-activity and destructive behaviour. It is usually available from specialist centres only, and from general practitioners under 'shared care' agreements with specialist centres. It is also sometimes used to help narcolepsy (a sleep disorder), depression in the elderly and for ADHD in adults.

Side-effects

The main side-effects are nervousness, lack of sleep, lack of appetite and stomach-ache. These can sometimes be reduced by changing the dose or changing the times of the doses. Sometimes the drug can slow down the rate of growth, although the young person will still end up the height they would have done. Less often, side-effects such as feeling sick and skin rashes can occur.

Important notes about medications for ADHD

- Methylphenidate is a stimulant drug. It can be addictive, especially in adults. Take especial care that the drug goes to and is taken by the person for whom it is prescribed.
- As methylphenidate is a stimulant, it is best not to give it after 4 pm as it may interfere with sleep.

Coping with common side-effects of medication

Some side-effects occur commonly with more than one type of drug. It is important for patients to know that all drugs have unwanted effects, that these vary from individual to individual and depend on the type of drug and dose being given. Sometimes the side-effects disappear after a few days or weeks, while other side-effects are more troublesome and persistent. It is very important that the patient reports any unwanted effects the drug seems to be having to his/her doctor. The unpleasant effects can often be eliminated, reduced in severity or made more tolerable by a range of simple strategies. The strategies the doctor may suggest include the following.

- Changing to a different medication.
- Decreasing the dose.
- Taking the drug in several, smaller doses spread through the day.
- Taking the medication with appropriate food.
- Taking extra medication to counteract the side-effects.

Strategies that you can advise to help patients deal with side-effects include the following:

Side-effect	Strategy for coping with it
Appetite (increase)	Eat a diet low in fat and high in fibre. Avoid sugary or fatty foods. Drink low-calorie soft drinks.
Constipation	Increase exercise. Increase fibre in diet. Increase fluid intake.
Dizziness	Get up slowly from lying or sitting. Avoid excessively hot showers or baths. Avoid alcohol, sedatives or other sedating drugs (eg marijuana).
Drowsiness	Take medication in a single dose before bedtime (talk to the doctor about this first). If you feel sleepy during the day, you should not drive or work with machinery.
Dry mouth	Ensure a regular fluid intake. Limit alcohol and caffeine (both enhance water loss). Use sugarless gums, fruit pastilles and lollies (sugar will promote dental decay). Suck on ice cubes. If it is very bad, ask your doctor about artificial saliva (Luborant).
Stomach upset	Take medicine after food. Consult with the doctor.
Sensitivity to sunburn	Avoid the midday sun. Regularly use sunscreen and wear a hat, sunglasses and shirt. Ask your doctor for a prescription for sunscreen.

A patient information sheet is available on the disk 💾.

Administering medication: general issues

The main issue in administering medication in a prison setting is how to make sure that the right medication goes to, and is taken by, the right patient at the right time. All psychotropic medications and many medicines used for physical conditions (eg analgesics) also may be used as currency on the wing. Patients may sell or give them to other prisoners or be pressured/bullied into doing so. There is also the possibility that patients may save medication and then use it to overdose.

Other issues, common to administering psychotropic medication in any setting, include the following:

- How to provide information about the medication and its side-effects to all patients, and also those with communication difficulties who may not understand the instructions. Information tends to increase compliance.

- What to do about those patients who are not capable of managing their own medication, eg those with learning disability.

- How to encourage 'compliance' or concordance without infringing the rights of patients to refuse medication they do not want. This is a particular issue with antipsychotic medication especially depot injections.

Possible solutions

A major response to the problem of reducing trading and the hoarding of medication is to supervise consumption of medication — giving it only 'in sight' and not 'in possession'. This solution may, however, bring its own problems. For example, giving medication in sight rather than in possession may:

- mean that the dose is given at the wrong time. For example, a sedative could be given at 4.00 or 5.00 pm and so be ineffective in helping the individual sleep at night
- turn medication into a battle ground between patients and healthcare staff and
- make it difficult or impossible to give medication twice or three times per day.

The decision about whether any particular medication should be given in possession or not is an individual one. It will depend upon the timing of the dose, the number of doses needed per day, the patient's ability to understand his/her medication, the risk of abuse, etc. Whether medication is to be given in possession or not and the reasons for the decision should be documented in the notes.

Systems and policies about medication

Effective programmes for administering medication include the following:

- Tracking and monitoring system that records whether patients are turning up for and taking their medication. Actively seeking out those patients who are considered to be at risk without their medication (including those on antipsychotics, mood stabilisers and some on antidepressants) who do not take it.
- Regular reviews of medication. Reviews will ideally take place in a clinic, be multidisciplinary, and include the prescribing doctor and administering nurse/HCO who together review compliance, the behaviour of the patient with regard to medication and the patient's own report of his/her progress.
- Regularly scheduled patient educational groups related to the use of psychoactive medications. These are important and can reduce the need for in sight administration of medications, with all its attendant problems. They also increase compliance.
- Policy on 'in possession' medication including flexibility within the policy.
- Awareness by all who are involved in administering medication of the need to obtain patient consent and of what to do if a patient refuses to take the medication.

The pharmacist responsible for the prison will be a valuable source of advice in setting up such medication systems.

Resources for patients and primary support groups

Mental Health Drugs Helpline: 020 7919 2999 (Monday–Friday, excluding Bank Holidays, 11 am–5 pm)
(The helpline, run by the UK Psychiatric Pharmacy Group and staffed by experienced mental-health pharmacists, provides independent advice and information about drugs to patients and professionals. The Chair of the Group also runs the **Drug information website for mental-health service users**, which contains detailed, user-friendly information on psychiatric drugs:
URL: http://www.nmhc.co.uk)

Prison Service Health Policy Unit: 020 7972 2000
Department of Health, Wellington House, 133–155 Waterloo Road, London
SE1 8UG
(Pharmacy and pharmacy-related information related to the Prison Service)

Comorbidity of substance abuse and mental disorders

May be known as 'dual diagnosis'

What is it?

Many prisoners have complex multiple disorders.[1] Polydrug users may be simultaneously dependent upon alcohol, benzodiazepines and opiates, with a history of self-harm and other more overt attempts at suicide.[2] Many of the prisoners using illegal substances also have a mental disorder — most commonly, depression, anxiety and/or personality disorder; less commonly, a psychotic disorder. It is not possible to place most patients into **either** substance misuse **or** mental disorder categories so it is essential to identify and treat both types of problem in their own right.

Effects

Having a diagnosis of both substance misuse and another mental disorder is associated with increased rates of homelessness, imprisonment, violent behaviour, suicide, premature death and an increased use of emergency psychiatric hospital admission and other services.

The information in this section is meant to be read in conjunction with the guidelines on specific mental and substance disorders.

For further information on substance misuse and detoxification, see the Department of Health Guidelines on *Clinical Management of Drug Misuse and Dependence* and Prison Service Order 3550: Clinical Services for Substance Misusers.

Different types of comorbidity

- **Primary mental disorder with subsequent/consequent substance misuse,** eg depression leading to the use of drugs to deal with anxiety and distress related to early childhood trauma.
- **Primary psychoactive substance use disorder leading to psychiatric symptoms,** eg prolonged use of amphetamines or cocaine causing psychotic symptoms.
- **Withdrawal from substances leading to psychiatric symptoms,** eg 'uppers' (amphetamines, cocaine, ecstasy) can cause acute depression when 'coming down'.
- **Concurrent diagnoses such as opiate dependence and major depression.** In this case, withdrawal from the substance can result in the need for active management of the depression.
- **Common aetiological underlying factors,** such as post-traumatic stress disorders (PTSDs) leading to both substance misuse and mood disorders.

Which disorders are associated with each other?

The strongest associations between disorders in a prison setting are the following.

- **Personality disorder** (especially antisocial personality disorder) and **drug dependence** (especially dependence on stimulants and opiates).

- **Depression and anxiety that underlie substance misuse** but are also significantly aggravated by it. Most people will show a marked improvement on completion of withdrawal, but a significant minority may experience severe anxiety or depressive disorder and should be assessed and managed for that condition.
- **Psychotic disorder and psycho-stimulant use.**

This section deals with comorbidity of substance misuse and mental disorders only. Other disorders commonly found together include transient psychotic disorder occurring when someone with a personality disorder is under stress. Information about managing someone with a severe personality disorder and mental disorder can be found at **Prisoners with complex presentations and very difficult behaviours** (page 202).

Presenting problems

- **Self-harm and suicide** during and after detoxification or withdrawal. This is a particular problem with psycho-stimulants, eg cocaine and amphetamines. Rates of use among those entering prison are high. Cocaine has a short half-life in the blood stream, does not have a specific medication for treatment and patients often fail to disclose their habit. Sleeplessness is a consequence of withdrawal from some substances (eg opiates, alcohol, hypnotics) and exacerbates the risk of self-harm, suicide and relapse. It is a particular problem in prisons.
- **Chaotic, high-risk taking and self-harming behaviour.** This is associated with polydrug use with mixtures of opiates, alcohol, psychostimulants and benzodiazepines. Self-harming behaviour is very common among women, but also occurs frequently among male prisoners.
- **Unpredictable, agitated, irritable/aggressive behaviour** may occur during and after withdrawal.
- **Primary sleep problems.**
- **Depressive symptoms.**
- **Symptoms of anxiety.**
- **Psychotic symptoms.**

Assessment

This is aimed at establishing:
- the chronology of the disorders
- the interrelationship (if any) of the disorders and
- whether the disorders need independent treatment or whether treating one will help alleviate the other.

It is not possible to tell in advance from the symptoms alone whether psychiatric symptoms are drug-induced or whether the patient has a mental disorder and is also abusing drugs.

History

To establish the above, take a history of the following:
- **Drug use**: type of drug(s), dose (weight, cost), how often, route of administration, effects, complications (physical, psychological, social), level of tolerance, withdrawal experience, dependence syndrome, history of drug use.

- **Recent history of alcohol use**: type and amount drunk where possible, effects, complications (physical, psychological, social) (see **Alcohol**, page 18).
- **Psychiatric history**: nature of illness, where treated and with what, any relationship with drugs or alcohol.
- **Mental State Examination (MSE)**: more information is provided on the disk, including an MSE form that can be printed out 💾.
- Corroborate information as much as possible (friends, relatives, other staff, old psychiatric reports, Drug Unit notes). Obtain a urine drug screen and liver function tests. Remember that use of drugs or alcohol may lead to blurring of historical events and facts, or a rationalisation to justify use.
- Where a patient has a previous diagnosis of psychotic illness, involve mental-health staff in the assessment and treatment (eg liaise with a mentally disordered offenders team or the equivalent). Confirm previous treatment if possible.
- When conducting the initial assessment, take care to distinguish between alcohol withdrawal and opiate withdrawal. Inappropriate use of opiates in alcohol withdrawal could result in death if the patient has no neuro-adaptation to opiates.
- Identify those patients with a history of delirium tremens or withdrawal seizures and ensure an appropriate active management. Be aware that the sensation of 'insects crawling under the skin', hallucinations and delusions are symptoms both of cocaine use and of delirium tremens in alcohol withdrawal. The patient may be unaware of the cause of the symptoms. Delirium tremens may be diagnosed by a history of alcohol use, the appearance of symptoms in the first 48–72 hours of withdrawal, the presence of the shakes and with tachycardia. Severe delirium tremens is an acute emergency. Transfer immediately to an NHS hospital to ensure safe management (for more information, see **Alcohol misuse** and **Drug misuse**, pages 18 and 55).

Assessment might require observation over an extended period. Careful recording of the time of resolution of symptoms following withdrawal will provide useful diagnostic clues. Periodic reassessment may be appropriate.

It is frequently not possible to establish which disorder is 'primary'.

Management

Key management principles

- Never assume that all mood and behavioural symptoms are solely caused by the substance abuse, even in the absence of a previous psychiatric diagnosis. It is important to identify and treat both types of disorder in their own right.
- Establish a provisional diagnosis but maintain an open mind and use on-going assessment to confirm the diagnosis.
- Attend to the substance-misuse problem if dependence is suspected and stabilise on a regimen, eg with opiate substitution therapy or benzodiazepine detoxification if appropriate.
- Reassess the individual in 1–2 weeks.
- If the psychiatric symptoms persist, initiate the appropriate treatment.
- Be aware that during and after detoxification is a time of high risk for self-harm and suicide. Supportive counselling is needed at this time, eg counselling, assessment, referral, advice and throughcare services (CARATS) staff, chaplains, befrienders, peer-support workers. Assessments from mental health-trained nurses or doctors should be available as required.

- Detoxification must be done under medical and nursing supervision.
- If management takes place under primary-care supervision, ensure that both psychiatric and substance misuse expertise/advice is available — ideally someone with expertise in both areas.

Advice and support to the patient and provision of physical care

- Advise patients that the use of alcohol or drugs exacerbates mental-health problems and in some cases causes them. Only by reducing or stopping alcohol or drug use will it be possible to assess the mental-health problem fully. It is important, however, to do this safely and to provide support for the patient during a time of increased emotional vulnerability.
- Assess and manage physical health problems (eg abscesses, thromboses, chest infections and other respiratory tract infections such as tuberculosis, subdural haematomas) and nutritional deficiencies (eg vitamin B_1).
- Offer hepatitis B vaccination to all injecting drug users and consider its use for non-injectors who are smoking heroin, polydrug using, or involved in other forms of risk behaviour. Rates of hepatitis C are estimated to be at least 50% among injecting drug users. An estimated 20% of hepatitis C-positive individuals develop chronic liver disease, including liver cancer.[3]

Monitoring for mental-health problems during and after detoxification

- Monitor for suicidal ideation (see **Suicide assessment and management**, page 204).
- Monitor for depression and anxiety (see **Depression and generalised anxiety disorder**, page 47 and 64). Where there is a well-substantiated history of prolonged and dependent use of benzodiazepines and they are being withdrawn, anxiety levels may increase to intolerable levels. Consider slowing down the detoxification programme and supporting the patient to learn alternative ways of managing anxiety, eg refer to mental-health services for anxiety management work.
- Monitor for psychotic symptoms. If psychotic phenomena emerge or get worse as detox progresses, check the patient's history of prescribed and non-prescribed drug and alcohol use. Worsening psychotic symptoms may be associated with:
  — withdrawal from major or minor tranquillisers. Consider gradual medicated withdrawal if appropriate and
  — alcoholic hallucinosis or previously unidentified Wernicke–Korsakoff syndrome. Wernicke's encephalopathy should be assumed where any one of ataxia, confusion, memory disturbance, hypothermia and hypotension, ophthalmoplegia or unconsciousness are present. Transfer immediately to a hospital where parenteral vitamin supplements may be safely administered.

Psychotic illness

If psychotic symptoms remain, involve the mental-health services. Anyone who has been in custody for a more than a few days without access to drugs and remains psychotic is likely to have a primary psychotic disorder. If self-harming behaviour emerges in the context of withdrawal, the patient's mood state should be assessed and support offered (see **Assessment and management following an act of self-harm**, page 211). There is a need for caution, however, to ensure that withdrawal regimens are not manipulated through self-harming behaviour. Hyperarousal associated with acute benzodiazepine withdrawal can significantly aggravate self-harming behaviour.

Personality disorder

Borderline personality disorder may be associated with disturbed behaviour during withdrawal, including dissociation and transient psychotic symptoms. It may also be associated with polydrug misuse as well as polypharmacy. In this situation, gradual withdrawal may be preferable, together with efforts to rationalise polypharmacy and reduce the overall number of medications prescribed. There is a high prevalence of personality disorder among prisoners with alcohol and drug dependence. Practitioners should ensure that patients with personality disorder can access the same treatment as those without and are not disadvantaged because of negative predictions about their response to treatment. Those providing services require expertise in both substance misuse and mental disorders (see **Personality disorder**, page 70).

Medication

Where the patient has a history of seizures, be cautious when using medication that will lower seizure threshold, eg tricyclic anti-depressants (TCAs), phenothiazines. Benzodiazepines during the withdrawal period will help reduce the risk of seizures.

Patients should not be initiated on to benzodiazepines except under exceptional crisis situations and only in the short term. Patients previously maintained in the community on benzodiazepines for anxiety-related indications, however, should not necessarily have this treatment withdrawn.

All types of psychotropic medication (and other medication, eg analgesics) may be used as currency in the prison. Non-pharmacological methods of managing anxiety, sleep problems and mild depression should be available. Appropriate pharmacotherapy for depression and anxiety should also be available to patients with a history of drug misuse, but caution should be exercised. Treatment should be monitored and reviewed regularly to assess progress, the suicide risk, the continuing need for medication and any problems with administering the medication.

Opiate maintenance programmes

Be aware that methadone levels can be raised by some antidepressants (fluvoxamine) and reduced by anticonvulsants, anti-tuberculous medication and combination therapy for HIV.

Depression

- The risk of suicide is particularly high in the period that follows starting antidepressants (as slowing of thought and movement may improve before mood lifts), so close monitoring will be required during this critical period. At first, the patient may only notice side-effects. Explain to them that these show the medication is beginning to work and that he/she will feel better soon.
- Be aware that the sedating effects of prescribed sedating antidepressants (eg amitriptyline, dothiepin, trazodone) will be enhanced by 'downers' such as opiates and benzodiazepines. There have been a number of deaths where

methadone and TCA medication interactions have resulted in respiratory depressions. TCAs should be avoided in combination with methadone prescribing. Selective serotonin re-uptake inhibitors (SSRIs) and similar compounds are not devoid of interaction with other drugs, but have the advantage of being safer in overdose.

- If the patient misuses alcohol and is about to be released, SSRI anti-depressants are preferred to TCAs because of the risk of tricyclic–alcohol interactions (fluoxetine, paroxetine and citalopram do not interact with alcohol) (see *BNF* Section 4.3.3).
- Avoid monoamine oxidase-inhibiting (MAOI) antidepressants. These can have potentially fatal interactions with 'uppers' (eg amphetamines, cocaine, ecstasy). Signs include high blood pressure, chest pain, neck stiffness, rigid muscles, flushing, vomiting and severe headache.

Psychosis

- **Antipsychotic medication makes seizures more likely during detoxification.** Confirm previous treatment if possible. Caution is required in the introduction or increase of anti-psychotic medication. Ensure an appropriate and active medication of withdrawal symptoms to reduce the risk.
- Be aware that the sedating effects of prescribed antipsychotics will be enhanced by 'downers' such as opiates and benzodiazepines. In mild cases, this will cause increased drowsiness, but in severe cases it may cause confusion, ataxia and reduced respiration.

Sleep problems

Profound sleep deprivation is a part of the experience of major drug withdrawal. Consider a **strictly short-term** use of a hypnotic in the very early stage of withdrawal. Explain the risk of developing dependence on these medications to the patient. For longer term or less severe insomnia, advise sleep hygiene rather than drugs (see the patient leaflet *Getting a Good Night's Sleep* on the disk 💾).

Administering medication

Take steps (eg supervised consumption) to ensure that the patient is not persuaded/bullied into passing his/her prescribed medication on to others, thereby placing themselves at risk of withdrawal symptoms.

After detoxification and withdrawal

Where psychiatric symptoms remain after detoxification

- Make regular appointments to review mental state. This may be done by the Detoxification Unit, with input from the mental-health services, or by primary-care staff with input from the mental-health services.
- Depressive symptoms improve in over 80% of individuals after detoxification. If major symptoms persist after alcohol, stimulant or opiate withdrawal, assess and treat for depression (see **Depression**, page 47).
- **If anxiety and agitation remain or increase after detoxification**: check for a history of benzodiazepine dependence. If benzodiazepine dependence is established and a decision is made to prescribe a benzodiazepine, use a long-acting one (eg diazepam) and consider instituting a programme of gradual

withdrawal. Such prescribing should be combined with anxiety management treatment.

- Assess and treat anxiety with appropriate non-pharmacological strategies (eg anxiety management) as a first-line intervention. Alcohol/substance use can also mask disorders such as panic disorder, social phobia and generalised anxiety disorder (see **Generalised anxiety**, **Panic** and **Phobias**, pages 64, 67 and 79).

If psychotic symptoms remain after detoxification

- Refer for psychiatric assessment (if possible to a psychiatrist with expertise in substance misuse and mental illness) and treat (see **Acute psychosis**, page 11).
- Observe closely while awaiting assessment or transport. Depression, with a high risk of suicide, is common in a patient with a psychotic illness during the weeks following withdrawal.
- Be aware that a psychotic illness may emerge for the first time or as a result of severe stress.
- Ensure that any antipsychotic medication prescribed is not causing unacceptable side-effects (eg akathisia).
- Be aware that the presence of complex problems with poor social support greatly reduces the chances of the patient successfully remaining drug free. Take all steps possible to maximise the chance of the individual staying in on-going treatment, both within the establishment and the community. In some instances, supervised maintenance treatment will help keep the patient in treatment after release.

Stimulants: where problems emerge on ordinary location

Cocaine withdrawal
There is no specific medication to treat cocaine withdrawal and prisoners often fail to disclose their use at reception. Withdrawal after heavy stimulant use over several days may produce a 'crash' that lasts hours or several days. Cocaine withdrawal begins with depression, agitation, anorexia and craving, during which time the suicide risk is high. This is followed by fatigue and insomnia accompanied by an intense desire to sleep. In the later stages of the crash, there is exhaustion and excessive sleeping. For several weeks afterwards, there may be variable craving, anxiety and other symptoms.[4]

Amphetamine withdrawal
This is longer but may be less severe than cocaine withdrawal. Prison officers may assume that prisoners who sleep excessively have taken an overdose as they may be unaware of the 'crash' that can occur following stimulant use. Officers need to be made aware of this issue so that they can bring those who seem to be showing stimulant withdrawal symptoms to the attention of the health-care and substance misuse staff.

Support for a prisoner withdrawing from stimulants

- Make basic observations (pulse, blood pressure [BP], temperature), which will usually distinguish between overdose or non-tolerance of methadone and heavy sleep. If the BP is very depressed, the patient extremely tachycardic or they are difficult to rouse, or there is any serious doubt about the level of intoxication, refer the patient to the local A&E for full assessment. A clear joint protocol on this process should be drawn up between the prison and the local NHS service and best practice standards jointly agreed (see **Management of poisoning**, page 225). If the patient appears to be sleeping heavily, continue to monitor for 72 hours.

- Provide supportive treatment plus sedation if agitation and anxiety are severe.
- Monitor the course of withdrawal to prevent suicide.

Substance-induced psychosis has been associated with stimulant intoxication and may persist after drug use has been discontinued. Individuals who have psychotic symptoms and are still intoxicated because of stimulants should be managed in an in-patient setting. Antipsychotic medication may be helpful.

Liaison and advice for discipline and other staff 💾

It is essential to provide information and advice for any officers or other staff who are involved in supervising individuals during and after they are going through a detoxification programme. Wing managers and personal officers may also be very helpful sources of information about the prisoner's behaviour on ordinary location.

Advice that can be given

- Strange and difficult behaviours in people who use illicit drugs are not always caused by the drug use or withdrawal. They must be treated seriously and reported.
- Individuals undergoing and just after withdrawal/detoxification are emotionally vulnerable and at a considerably increased risk of suicide and self-harm.
- Behaviour that can be expected from prisoners withdrawing from drugs includes:
  — a 'crash' into exhaustion/excessive sleep following stimulant use
  — irritable outbursts or aggression following the sudden cessation of treatment for depression or withdrawal from illicit drugs (eg opiates or steroids) and
  — the sensation of 'insects crawling under the skin', hallucinations and delusions: symptoms both of cocaine use and of delirium tremens in alcohol withdrawal. The individual may be unaware of the cause of the symptoms. Severe delirium tremens is an acute medical emergency.
- Methadone can be a legitimate, on-going treatment prescribed for good reasons rather than a mode of feeding a drug habit. Issuing and monitoring methadone needs to be undertaken by experienced staff. If this is not understood and accepted, the staff are likely to resent having to escort patients daily to a central location to receive their maintenance dose of methadone.

Action that may be taken

- Remove dangerous objects and consider the use of suicide-prevention procedures.
- Report the behaviour to health-care. A review of medication or the speed of detoxification may be indicated.
- Use control and restraint as a last, not first, resort where irritability and aggression occurs.
- Use 'talking down' skills.
- Consider delaying adjudications until the withdrawal is complete, so that any improved behaviour can be taken into account.

Referral and throughcare (resettlement)

Management within the establishment

This is multi-disciplinary and may involve CARATS staff, probation officers, chaplains, discipline officers and psychologists in addition to health-care staff.

Refer to the psychiatric services (with expertise in both mental illness and substance misuse) the following patients.

- Those with a psychotic illness and a substance misuse problem for an assessment, including a review of medication, and additional support including relapse-prevention strategies. Use of substances may be related to levels of anti-psychotic medication (eg under-medicated patients may use alcohol or other drugs to drown voices).
- Those in whom anxiety symptoms that emerge during or following detoxification are severe/unmanageable.
- Those with severe or persistent self-harm or severe eating disorders.

Rehabilitation programmes

Prisoners with a mental-health problem and who are taking prescribed anti-depressant or anti-anxiety medication should not be coerced into stopping their medication prematurely in order to access a prison-based rehabilitation programme or to be released on to a community programme. The patient's mental-health needs should be assessed by an appropriately trained clinician and the rehabilitation programme asked to accept the person while still on treatment. Those with ongoing major mental-health problems will require maintenance medication. Referrals should only be made to services that recognise the role of medication in the treatment of both addictive disorders and other mental disorders.[5]

Prerelease

Many patients will leave prison before a full treatment programme can be completed. Where feasible (and with patient agreement), refer them as soon as possible to the local drug-treatment services and/or local community mental-health team/primary care. CARATS workers may be able to assist with this. If either the psychiatric or substance misuse problem appears to predominate, refer initially to that service. Make the rationale clear in the letter/fax. If both types of disorder are of equal significance, then negotiate with both agencies about the preferred initial referral route. It may be that the patient will require support and input from both agencies. Some areas provide services jointly. Some voluntary organisations specialise in clients with multiple disorders, working in conjunction with statutory services, eg Revolving Doors, MACA (see **Managing the interface with the NHS and other agencies**, page 149).

Post-release

It is important to prevent the current high death rate due to opiate overdose on release. Prisoners may allow themselves a 'treat' following their period of abstinence in prison. Advise prisoners about to be released of: the risk of overdose due to loss of tolerance to opiates, safer ways of using drugs (eg smoking) and basic resuscitation procedures. A leaflet about the ways to minimise the risk and to handle overdose, should it occur, is useful. It is on the disk and could be adapted by individual establishments ⌹.

Developing services in your establishment

Many establishments (and NHS services) will not yet have organised their services in a way that facilitates the identification and treatment of comorbid mental disorders in inmates who abuse substances.

The key factors in developing such services are the following.

- **Monitoring of mental state and suicide risk** of patients during and after detoxification and appropriate follow-up. Where patients are reviewed in primary-care clinics, it would be valuable to have mental-health-trained nurses (preferably with both mental-health and substance-misuse expertise). It is particularly important to distinguish between delirium tremens, alcoholic hallucinosis, drug-induced psychosis and a psychotic illness.

- **Specialist help in a psychiatric hospital**, if necessary, for patients undergoing withdrawal and who are at risk of severe delirium tremens, Wernicke–Korsakoff's syndrome or who are thought to have an ongoing psychotic disorder (see **Managing the interface with the NHS and other agencies**, page 149).

- **Education for all staff** about the emotional state of inmates during and after detoxification, in particular the potential for strong, volatile emotions and the increased risk of suicide and self-harm. They should also learn that mental-health problems frequently go along with substance use.

- **Hepatitis B injection programme** for all injecting drug users.

- **Supervised opiate agonist maintenance programmes** or extra-gradual withdrawal programmes for those drug users with complex needs and a long history of opiate dependence.

- **Mental-health liaison nurse** who can liaise between the prison and the NHS mental-health and substance-abuse services to facilitate the appropriate aftercare.

More details about detoxification are provided in Prison Service Order 3550 and Department of Health Guidelines 1999 'Drug Misuse and Dependence: Guidelines on Clinical Management'.

Resources for patients and primary support groups

ADFAM National: 020 7928 8900 (helpline)
(For families and friends of drug users)

Al-Anon Family Groups UK and Eire: 020 7403 0888 (helpline: Monday–Friday, 10 am–10 pm); 0141 2217356
(Support for families and friends of alcoholics whether still drinking or not. Also, **Alateen**, for young people aged 12–20 affected by others' drinking)

Alcoholics Anonymous: 08457 697555 (24-hour helpline)
(Helpline refers to telephone support numbers and self-help groups across the UK for men and women trying to achieve and maintain sobriety

CITA (Council for Involuntary Tranquilliser Addiction): 0151 949 0102
(Monday–Friday, 10 am–1 pm)
Cavendish House, Brighton Road, Waterloo, Liverpool
(Confidential advice and support)

Narcotics Anonymous: 020 7730 0009 (10 am–10 pm)

National Drugs Helpline: 0800 776600 (24-hour freephone)
(Confidential advice including information on local services)

Release Helpline: 020 7603 8654 (helpline: Monday–Friday, 6 pm–10 pm;
Saturday and Sunday, 8 am–midnight; 020 7729 9904 (heroin adviceline)
(Advice, support and information to drug users and their friends and families on
all aspects of drug use and drug-related legal problems)

Resource leaflets:
Harm Minimization Advice

Understanding Dual Diagnosis. General information booklet available for £1.00
from: MIND, 13–19 Broadway, Stratford, London E15 4BQ. Tel: 020 8221 9666;
E-mail: publications@mind.org.uk; URL: http://www.mind.org.uk

*Helping You Cope: A Guide to Starting and Stopping Tranquillisers and Sleeping
Tablets.* Available from: Mental Health Foundation, 20/21 Cornwall Terrace,
London NW1 4QL. Tel: 020 7535 7400; URL: http://www.mentalhealth.org.uk.
See the guideline for relevant disorders for organisations that deal with that
problem

1 Farrell M, Howes S, Taylor C *et al*. Substance misuse and psychiatric comorbidity: an
   overview of the OPCS National Psychiatric Morbidity Survey. *Addictive Behaviours* 1998; 23:
   909–918.
2 Jan Palmer, personal communication. Statistics collected at HMP Holloway from 1996 to
   2000 showed that 45% of new receptions required detoxification, of whom 50% required
   alcohol detox in addition to opiate detox; a further proportion required benzodiazepine
   detox in addition to one or both of opiate and alcohol.
3 Crofts N, Stewart T, Hearne P *et al*. Spread of blood-borne viruses among Australian prison
   entrants. *British Medical Journal* 1995; 310: 285–288.
4 Gawin FH, Khalsa ME, Ellinwood E. Stimulants. In Glanter M, Kleber HD (eds), *Textbook of
   Substance Abuse Treatment*. Washington, DC: American Psychiatric Press, 1994, pp. 111–139.
5 Scott J, Gilvarry E, Farrell M. Managing anxiety and depression in alcohol and drug
   dependence. *Addictive Behaviours* 1998; 23: 919–931.

Management of prisoners with complex presentations and very difficult behaviours

Introduction

Some individuals in prison present both healthcare and discipline staff with particularly difficult challenges. Most of these individuals may have multiple diagnoses of personality disorder, substance misuse and often have mental illness. Self-harm is common. Many are accused of or sentenced for crimes of violence. Prisoners may have a history of poor compliance with treatment, not complying with agreed care plans, a reduced recognition of behavioural boundaries and poor cognitive skills. Some prisoners with personality disorder tend to divide carers into rival groups. Prison Service staff often feel that such individuals are in prison for lack of any better disposal by society and the courts.

Challenging individuals are more likely to be found in special accommodation or in segregation units. There may be confusion about when and in what context they should be accountable for their actions.

Management

- Where the individual has had previous contact with NHS psychiatric services, they should have a care plan and a crisis plan within their Care Programme Approach (CPA) documentation. Contact the CPA Coordinator in the NHS psychiatric service in the first instance. He/she should liaise between the prison and NHS healthcare services.
- Regular multidisciplinary assessments of the health and management of prisoners are essential, with contributions from the wing staff, governor, probation officer, psychologist, nurses, psychiatrist and chaplain. Where the Board of Visitors has been involved in the particulars of an individual prisoner, it should be included in the case conference.
- The assessment should include both subjective and objective measures of symptoms and behaviours, identify any mental disorder and personality disorder, assess the risk and seek to explain the relationship between the disorders and problems in behaviour and management being experienced in the social setting of prison and other possible locations for the prisoner.
- Effective coordination of care is essential. Many of these patients need enhanced care plans as set out in the National Service Framework for Mental Health and protocols of the local mental health Trust. Care plans should be developed covering each of the problem behaviours. Care plans should be:
  — realistic: it should either be possible to put them into action within the prison, or include a planned transfer to hospital
  — multidisciplinary: the NHS multidisciplinary team should be asked for its advice/active involvement; staff from other relevant areas in the prison, eg psychologist, probation officer, chaplain and staff from Residential Units, should be involved
  — humane: responses to presenting problems should be non-punitive; attention should be paid to the dangers of protracted isolation (see **Isolation and mental health**, page 308)

- — evidence-based, wherever possible
- — flexible: it should be possible to respond to changes in the individual such as deterioration or improvement in mental state and
- — regularly reviewed: behaviour can change over time and care plans must be adapted. It is important to keep an open mind. The NHS staff involved in the assessment should be involved in reviews at agreed intervals.

- The location of these patients within a prison needs discussion. The benefits of concentrating or diffusing these individuals, and the risk of disruption to other prisoners, should be assessed. If available, consider transfer to an establishment where there is expertise in managing similar problems, where non-punitive responses like solitary confinement or isolation are unnecessary and where the environment allows the individual to socialise with others and to develop personally.

- When a team becomes divided or tired, an outside second opinion is often helpful.

- On-going and post-incident support for staff is essential. For example, consideration should be given to helping staff to become aware of, review and, if appropriate, develop additional coping mechanisms.

- Non-judgmental critical incident debriefing is useful. It may identify assumptions or management arrangements that are hindering management of individuals. Colleagues from within the NHS and prison management should be involved in these. An outsider can often identify a pattern that has not been seen by those closely involved.

Assessing and managing people at risk of suicide

Introduction

The purpose of this section is to enable healthcare staff to play their part within the overall Prison Service suicide prevention strategy and processes. It should be read alongside the relevant strategies. The role of the primary-care team, within the overall multidisciplinary strategy, is to do the following.

- Identify and assess the seriousness of the risk of suicide in prisoners during reception screening, referred by staff and in surgeries.
- Identify and treat depression and other psychiatric disorders, if present.
- Participate in multidisciplinary care planning and through care planning.
- Advise on and advocate for appropriate locations, support and supervision.
- Provide on-going support to staff and prisoners on normal location.
- Contribute to the establishment's suicide prevention strategy, suicide prevention team and staff training.

Important points about risk assessment

- Main method of assessing risk is to ask the patient about his/her thoughts, intentions and plans.
- Be alert to the presence of specific risk factors (see below).
- In addition, be aware that young offenders tend to be more impulsive than older people.
- It is easy to underestimate the risk associated with difficult, uncooperative individuals. The behaviour of aggressive or sullen prisoners may reflect despair and a failure to cope. They should be viewed as objectively as possible.
- Suicide risk fluctuates over time. It is important to keep assessing the risk.
- Risk assessment is difficult and some individuals who are very determined to kill themselves refuse to admit to suicidal intentions. Therefore, decisions about persons considered to be at risk should be made by multidisciplinary teams not individuals alone. All those in regular contact with the individual should be consulted about how he/she behaves on ordinary location (see **Behaviours that indicate raised suicide risk** below).

Assessment of the risk involves considering four domains

- Individual, eg suicidal intentions, presence of mental disorder, coping skills and resources, social problems (eg with their family), housing, finance. Suicidal behaviour in most people, whether in or outside prison, is a 'last straw' phenomenon, ie it happens in the context of underlying associated low mood and suicidal thinking plus multiple social stresses and problems. It is finally triggered by a 'last straw' event that may not in itself be a major event.
- Environment he/she is in, eg access to means of suicide, being left alone for long periods, lack of access to activity.

- Staff (eg level of supervision and support available).
- Specific, known risk factors (see below).

Asking about suicidal thoughts and feelings

If you are managing an individual who is depressed or who you suspect to be suicidal for other reasons, it is important to talk about suicide. Discussing suicide will not make the person more likely to attempt suicide. It is important to be non-threatening, non-judgmental and empathetic when talking to the patient about his/her thoughts or feelings. Give the person the chance to talk freely and openly. Ask about suicidal ideas, plans and history and the feelings of hopelessness. Examples of questions to ask include the following:

Suicidal ideas[1]

- 'Have you been feeling very low for several days at a time?'
- 'Have you ever thought you wouldn't mind if you didn't wake up in the morning?'
- 'When you feel this way, have you ever had thoughts of killing yourself?'
- 'When did these thoughts occur?'
- 'What did you think you might do to yourself?'
- 'How often do these thoughts occur?'
- 'Have your thoughts ever included harming someone else as well as yourself?'

Suicidal plans

- 'Recently, what specifically have you thought about doing to yourself?'
- 'Have you taken any steps towards doing this?' (eg making a noose/hoarding pills).
- 'Have you thought about when and where you would do this?'
- 'Have you made any plans for your possessions or left any instructions for people for after your death, such as a note or a will?'
- 'Have you thought about the effect your death would have upon your family or friends?'

Generally, risk increases as a person moves from thoughts to intention to making plans. Concrete plans indicate a high risk.

Suicide history

- 'Have you acted on these thoughts in any way in the past? Tell me about that.'

If the individual expresses regret that a previous suicide attempt was not successful, this is an individual at high risk.

Feelings of hopelessness and the strength of protective factors

- 'What has stopped you from acting on your thoughts so far?'
- 'What are your thoughts about staying alive?'
- 'What help could make it easier for you to cope with your problems at the moment?'

If a person replies to this last question with answers like 'Nothing can help. It really doesn't matters what happens to me any more,' this is also an indication of high risk.

Assess for depression, psychosis and other mental disorder

- Persistent low mood with intensifying suicidal thoughts is a significant risk.
- Any psychotic symptoms increase risk. Voices commanding the patient to commit suicide mean a high risk.
- Bipolar disorder is the mental disorder most highly correlated with completed suicide.
- For more information on taking a psychiatric history and assessing a patient's mental state, see the 'Assessment' section of **Managing the interface with the NHS and other agencies** (page 149) for guidelines on relevant disorders, and the Mental State Examination on the disk 💾.

Risk factors and protective factors for suicide

It is important to supplement information about thoughts and feelings with information from other sources, eg prisoner escort record, residence manager.

Prisoner groups at increased risk of suicide[2]

- Those in prison on remand for the first time, those who have returned from court with a sentence longer than expected or those whose status has recently changed, eg from remand to sentenced.
- People with a history of self-harm.
- People with a history of mental disorder (especially depression, psychosis and bipolar disorder).
- People with a history of drug or alcohol abuse.
- Those with chronic or painful physical illness.
- Those convicted of murder, sex or arson offences.
- People with communication difficulties or poor coping skills.
- People with a history of sexual assault or abuse.
- People who are socially isolated either within or outside of prison.

Relationship between suicide and self-harm and substance misuse

- Prisoners undergoing detoxification are especially likely to develop suicidal feelings. Detoxification should be carried out under medical and nursing supervision.
- Look out for prisoners who used cocaine before coming into prison. They are particularly vulnerable to suicidal feelings during withdrawal. Cocaine has a low half-life in the blood stream, does not have a substitute and prisoners often fail to disclose their habit.
- Prisoners emerging from detoxification regimens are at raised risk of depression, anxiety and self-harm. These should not automatically be attributed to the substance abuse. They may be painful feelings or underlying mental disorders that the substance abuse previously masked.

Events that may make self-harm or suicide more likely

Any stressful situation may increase risk. Examples include the following.

- Bullying, intimidation or assault by other prisoners, especially sexual assault.
- All court appearances and outcomes, including appeals.

- Relationship or family problems: children taken into care, social isolation, 'Dear Johns'.
- Bereavement.
- Refusal of parole.
- Disciplinary problems/segregation.
- Home leaves and approaching release.
- Anniversaries — of a death, of the sentence or of the crime.
- Frequent moves within the prison system.
- Identification parades and interviewing about offences.
- Suicide attempts by others in the prison environment or in family members and friends.

Behaviours that may indicate an increased risk

- Withdrawal from the company of others and/or refusal to see visitors.
- Self neglect — not eating or paying attention to washing, hair and clothes.
- Refusal to participate in work, education or association.
- Marked change in mood or behaviour; acting out of character.
- Lack of motivation, eg not planning for home leave/release.
- Tidying up affairs/giving away possessions.

Contact the residential staff for information about these factors.

Protective factors that reduce the likelihood of suicide

- Social support:
  — Confiding relationships (someone trusted to talk to). More is better.
  — Involvement in community or religious organisations.
- Family links:
  — Concern about the impact of suicide on their family.
  — Having children (especially for female prisoners).
- Personal resources:
  — High self-esteem.
  — Good coping skills, especially problem-solving abilities.
  — Spiritual beliefs; a sense of meaning and purpose in life.
- Safe environment:
  — Personal security, eg freedom from bullying.
  — Being with someone. Most suicides take place alone. Shared cells should be used where possible for someone at risk.
  — Lack of access to lethal means of suicide.
- Meaningful occupation:
  — Regular exercise.
  — Opportunities for creative expression.
  — Employment.

Caring for a person who is contemplating suicide or recovering from a suicide attempt

Although any act of self-harm, whether single or repeated, will increase the risk of suicide, you may, after conducting a suicide risk assessment, decide that a patient who has self-harmed is currently at low risk of suicide. For advice on a management plan, see **Assessment and management following an act of self-harm** (page 211).

Where the person is contemplating suicide or recovering from an attempt at suicide, it is important to develop a management plan to help them get safely through the period of distress. Many patients who are vulnerable to attempted suicide are managed on a normal location. Therefore, in the prison context, the care plan needs to be multidisciplinary, with the key elements recorded in the F2052SH (in Scotland, an Act to Care form), though additional clinical points will be recorded on the inmate medical record (IMR) only. Different elements of the management plan will be carried out by different disciplines depending on their skills. Once a plan has been agreed, a key-worker should be nominated to ensure that it is implemented. There should be agreed periodic reviews to ensure that it is meeting the needs of the prisoner. Wherever possible, the individual should be involved in agreeing the care plan. The care plan should aim to reduce the risk of suicide and self-harm in the following areas.

- **In the human environment**: ensure appropriate supervision and support from staff and other prisoners; remove a bully.
- **In the physical environment**, eg by placing in a ligature-free cell; not a strip cell.
- **In the individual**, eg by undertaking clinical assessment, treating the mental disorder, increasing coping skills and resources, helping with social problems.

Suggestions for a management plan include the following:

- Ensure appropriate supervision for the patient. The level of observation required varies according to the individual and should be decided in accordance with individual need and Prison Service procedures (F2052SH in England; an Act to Care form in Scotland). More detail is provided in **Observations of patients at risk** (page 220). Do not leave the individual alone and consider options that allow observations to continue during patrol states and for the individual to have a high level of contact with others. Options include the use of a crisis suite or a gated cell. Shared cells are normally preferable to single cells. Transfer to the health centre may be needed to allow a higher level of observation. There may be occasions on which 24-hour observation and clinical care are essential; these should trigger an urgent assessment by mental-health services.
- Ensure appropriate support for the patient:
  — Consider placing the individual in a shared cell with a listener/buddy or a suitable cell mate.
  — Encourage a supportive network, eg education or chaplain.
  — Encourage use of community resource, eg the Samaritans.
  — Help the individual structure time, eg with work or education or exercise; support the acquisition of appropriate reading materials, provide art materials
  — Promote family contact, eg additional telephone calls and longer visits. The home Probation Service may be able to encourage family to visit (see also 'Voluntary agencies' in **Family support**, page x).
  — If the patient is to return to an ordinary location, give the wing officer a copy of *Ideas for Support Plans* 💾 and agree with him/her which of the options should be implemented.
- Arrange a full clinical assessment and clinical care. Most patients who harm themselves have associated psychiatric problems.[3]
  — **For depression, use a mixture of psychosocial approaches and antidepressants.** The risk of suicide is particularly high during the period following starting antidepressants, as the slowing of thought and movement

may improve before depressed feelings. Close monitoring will be required during this critical period. At first, the patient may only notice side-effects. Explain to them that these are a sign that the medication is beginning to work and they will feel better soon.

— **Single acts of major self-mutilation (eg self-castration) should alert healthcare staff to the possibility of psychotic illness.** Psychotic illness is a very high-risk factor for suicide, irrespective of whether the patient admits to suicidal intent. A psychiatric opinion will be needed. See the guidelines of the relevant disorder for more information.

— **Acts of self-harm** that are not suicidal in intent and where the risk of suicide is assessed as being currently low indicate emotional distress (for advice on management, see page 211).

— **Consider the appropriate location for clinical care**: consider the level of support available to the individual on a normal location. Is the individual a loner or does he/she have friends there? Consider mixed healthcare–normal location options, such as attendance at a day centre (if available) during the day and the normal location at night, or a workshop during the day and a healthcare centre at night.

• Engage in ongoing consultation with colleagues and other staff. Discuss the individual with healthcare colleagues. Especially where the individual is managed on a normal location, the residential manager must also be involved. If the risk of suicide is considered serious, and certainly if higher levels of observation are required, refer to the mental-health services for assessment and a second opinion.

• Build a therapeutic relationship with the patient. It is important to be non-judgmental, non-threatening, empathic and clearly willing to help. Do not make judgements about whether the other person's life is no longer worthwhile.

• Try to delay the individual's suicidal impulses. Try to reach an agreement with the individual about what help can be arranged if they feel increasingly suicidal. Ensure that everyone is clear about their role.

• Neutralise the precipitating problem. Encourage the view that all problems can be solved or their effects ameliorated. Even in prison, the individual has options open to him/her. Help the individual to use/learn the skill of structured problem solving. Liaise with staff from other departments, with the patient's permission, to help neutralise the problem, eg contact the wing or personal officer to deal with bullying or conflict with other inmates.

• Consider contacting/informing the patient's solicitor, especially if the individual is on remand in which case the solicitor may be able to speed representation to the court. Obtain the patient's consent first.

• Consider contacting the patient's family. If possible, arrange for a member of staff to meet with the family of the individual at risk, with his/her consent, to talk with them about the care of their relative.

• Reduce access to the means of committing suicide. Wherever possible, provide a safer physical environment by placing patients in safer, ligature-free cells (not strip cells). Medication should be taken under supervision, not given 'in possession'. Be aware that many types of medication, in addition to psychotropics, may be used to self-harm. Repeat prescriptions should be reviewed at regular intervals. Where this has not been the case, consider a review immediately. Where possible, the individual should be allowed to retain his/her belongings, unless it is clearly unsafe to do so. Consider clothes, mattress and a cigarette lighter.

- Agree frequent, regular and planned appointments with the patient. Review progress and continue problem solving. Work to resolve the underlying problems should continue beyond the point at which the immediate crisis is resolved.
- Brief staff on the Residential Unit before the patient is discharged or returned to the unit. Involve the residential care staff in discharge planning, including ideas for a support plan (these are provided on the disk 💾). Agree a review date and ensure that staff are aware of signs of deterioration which might indicate a need to bring the review date forward.
- Contribute to sentence or prerelease planning. The risk of suicide is particularly high following release. Ensure that information about the history and risk of suicide and self-harm is known to those involved in resettlement and through care planning, and to the community general practitioner and mental-health services (if relevant).
- A checklist for prison officers is provided on the disk 💾.

---

[1] Adapted from Fremouw WJ, de Percqel M, Ellis TE. *Suicide Risk: Assessment and Response Guidelines*. New York: Pergamon, 1990.

[2] 'Caring for the suicidal in custody' is a Prison Service training pack published by HM Prison Service, London 1994; Scottish Prison Service. *Prevention of Suicide Strategy (Act and Care)*. Edinburgh, 1996.

[3] Haw C, Hawton K, Houston K, Townsend E. Psychiatric and personality disorders in deliberate self-harm patients. *British Journal of Psychiatry* 2001; 178: 48–54.

Assessment and management following an act of self-harm — Z91

Understanding self-harm

Self-harm must always be treated seriously. It ranges in severity from mild or superficial effects to permanent physical damage and life-threatening danger. Types of self-harm include cutting, burning, head banging, swallowing objects, self-suffocation, self-choking by ingesting large pieces of cloth, inserting objects into wounds, putting ligatures around the neck, overdosing and other forms of self-poisoning.

Self-harm is a sign of emotional distress and may be associated with mental illness, personality disorder, learning disability (mental retardation) or with none of these. It is a common behaviour in mental health centres in the community and in prisons[1] and presents one of the most difficult dilemmas for healthcare staff, often causing anxiety, frustration or anger, not least because the individual is simultaneously a victim and a perpetrator of harm.

Sometimes it will be clear that an act of self-harm was intended as suicide. However, it is often not easy to categorise the behaviour into suicidal or non-suicidal; motivations may be mixed and (where acts are repeated) suicidal intent may vary over time. Those who self-harm have a 100-fold increase in the risk of suicide in the following year compared with those who do not (about 1% per year as opposed to 0.01% per year). Sometimes, however, the act of self-harm reduces suicidal urges in the short-term by reducing tension. Like depression, drug addiction and being a loner, self-harm is a factor that should alert prison staff to the possible risk of suicide.

Self-harm occurs for a variety of reasons, eg to escape from overwhelming emotions, to release tension, to cause physical pain, which reduces emotional distress, to punish oneself or to show others the emotional pain which cannot be expressed in words.[2] Occasionally, inmates will copy the behaviour of others, having been told by them that cutting helps to defuse emotional pain. Self-harm may sometimes be a symptom of a mental illness (eg the requirement to self-mutilate or jump off a balcony may be part of a psychotic patient's delusion) or it may occur during withdrawal from drugs, particularly amphetamines. Self-harm is only seldom and never exclusively caused by a wish to get attention or for manipulative reasons. It should always be taken as representing an important emotional need.

People who self-injure repeatedly may have some or all of the following factors in their lives.

- **Predisposing**: problems in childhood (physical or sexual abuse,[3] bullying or poor self-esteem), adult experiences of victimisation.
- **Coexisting problems**: eating disorders, alcohol and drug abuse, depression, paranoid ideas, low self-esteem, poor social skills.
- **Precipitating**: recent stresses (coming into prison, rejection by a partner, bullying, the anniversary of a bereavement, cancelled home leave or problems with children). Painful feelings associated with such stresses often become more acute during and after detox, leading to self-harm. The length of time spent in cells may also be a contributing factor in self-harm among young prisoners.[4]

- **Maintaining**: having few friends, being a 'loner', guilt or self-blame, hearing voices, the 'addictive' quality of the self-harm, self-hatred or anger turned inwards.

The great majority of repetitive self-harmers begin the behaviour in their teenage years. It is common to find that people who previously harmed themselves no longer do so by the time they are 40 years old.[5]

Immediate crisis management

- If there is any danger to life, resuscitation should be carried out ensuring that **airways** are clear, **breathing** is taking place, **circulation** is adequate, there is no excessive **bleeding**, there is no immediate risk from **flames**, and **burns** (whether from heat or chemicals) are irrigated with cold water. Death by asphyxiation from a ligature round the neck may take several minutes, allowing time for resuscitation, oxygenation and heart massage, as required. First aid information on **Immediate crisis management** for officers or others who are first on the scene is provided the on the disk 💾.
- Referral to the healthcare centre will usually be necessary even where the physical injury is mild. Severe and life-threatening injury and self-poisoning would normally require attendance at A&E (see **Emergency management of poisoning/overdose**, page 225).
- Whether immediate treatment of the wound takes place in A&E or the prison healthcare centre, it is important to treat the patient with respect and care as someone who is communicating distress and not as someone who is not serious about suicide or who is wasting the time of professionals.
- For infected wounds, the use of antibiotics should be kept to a minimum, with good hygiene and antiseptic dressings instead wherever possible.

Assessment

The aims of the assessment following an act of self-injury are the following:
- To identify the underlying reasons contributing to emotional distress.
- To identify the presence and gauge the seriousness of any suicidal intentions or actions.
- To determine the risk of self-harm in the near future.
- To identify what kind of help is appropriate, both for the current crisis and for the underlying problems, and whether the person will accept this help.

Establish a rapport

- Use first names or call the patient Mr or Miss X, depending on what he/she prefers.
- Explain the purpose of the interview is to understand what happened and to arrange for suitable help for problems that might be causing distress. Gauging the risk of suicide is a part (but not all) of the purpose.
- Aim to be non-threatening, non-judgemental and empathetic. Give the patient the chance to talk freely and openly about their thoughts and feelings.
- Take care not to use language that the patient may find unduly emotive or pejorative (eg why are you threatening suicide?).

Understand the act, or attempted act, of self-injury

- Obtain sequential details about the events that occurred in the 48 hours preceding the act of self-injury.

- Explore circumstances surrounding the act or planned act: the reasons, the method, the degree of planning, the location of the act, the presence of a suicide note, the expected extent of injury, any actions after the attempt, whether drugs were consumed (prescribed or illicit), the likelihood of being stopped in time or revived, the extent of the desire to die, feelings about living.
- Previous acts of self-injury.
- Check F2052SH (an Act to Care form in Scotland) documentation, if any, for notes about the patient's behaviour before, during and after the incident, and on any major life events the patient may recently have experienced.
- Be aware that, in the short-term, the individual's painful feelings/problems may be relieved by the act of self-harm, making it easy to underestimate their habitual state.

Indicators that the act was intended as suicide

The patient:

- expected the act to cause death; a non-lethal dose of drug may have been thought to be lethal
- is disappointed to be still alive
- made concrete plans, eg for their possessions after death, a note to other people
- took precautions not to be found
- planned the act for at least several hours and
- feels hopeless about the future; that things will not get much better.

The expression of regret that the act did not lead to death greatly increases the chance that the person will try to kill themselves again in the near future.

Assess the current thoughts about suicide

It is important to talk about suicide, even where the act of self-injury has been repeated many times and a non-lethal method (eg superficial cutting) was used. Motivations for self-injury vary over time; a risk assessment should be repeated at intervals. Discussing suicide will not make the person more likely to attempt suicide. A full discussion of the act of self-injury will lead naturally to questions about current thoughts about staying alive and whether they perceive any positive factors in their lives. For more information on assessing suicide risk, including sample questions that may be asked, see **Assessing and managing people at risk of suicide** (page 204).

Establish current difficulties

- Nature of problems, their duration, recent changes that triggered the act or led to suicidal thinking.
- Psychological and physical problems: the relationship with a partner and other family members, with workmates, other inmates and friends; alcohol or drug use; physical or sexual abuse; financial or legal difficulties, social isolation, bereavement or other threatened loss.

Assess the associated mental disorders

Most patients who harm themselves have associated psychiatric problems.[6] Look for evidence of major depression, anxiety, psychotic or paranoid symptoms, misuse of alcohol or illicit drugs or withdrawal (especially withdrawal from amphetamines or cocaine), and personality disorder.

See the guidelines for the relevant disorder(s) for more information.

Major depression, bipolar disorder and psychotic illness are high-risk factors for suicide.

Assess the background

- Relevant personal and family history.
- Description of usual personality.
- Obtain information from the wing manager, personal officer or, where possible, a relative.

Identify the usual coping methods

- Coping resources, eg family, friends. Access to appropriate coping resources reduces the risk of self-injury and of suicide. The management plan may focus on increasing the number of appropriate coping resources.
- Is the self-harm itself a method of coping with problems or painful feelings? Especially in cases of repeated self-injury, ask what the self-harm does for the patient.

Work with the individual to devise a list of the most important current problems.

Establish what help is required

- Identify what help is required and what help the patient will accept.
- Consider who else should be involved. Involve the patient's personal officer or other designated member of staff (with patient permission). Consider the chaplain, listeners/buddies, friends, relatives and external organisations.
- Ensure that the agreed help is documented in the care plan (currently F2052SH in England and Wales; an Act to Care form in Scotland), and that an appropriate person supervises the plan.

Management where the suicide risk is high

See **Assessing and managing people at risk of suicide** (page 204).

Management where the suicide risk is currently low

Be aware that the risk of suicide fluctuates. It is important to keep assessing the risk.

When caring for a person who is recovering from an incident of self-harm, it is important to develop a management plan to help the person get safely through the period of distress. In the prison context, the plan needs to be multidisciplinary as many patients who are vulnerable to attempted self-harm are managed on a normal location. Different elements of the management plan will be carried out by different disciplines, depending on their skills. Wherever possible, the individual should be involved in agreeing the care plan. The care plan must be realistic (ie the resources to deliver it must be available).

Treat the associated mental disorders

Most patients who harm themselves have associated psychiatric problems,[7] which may respond to medication. See the relevant guidelines for treatment information.

- Depression (page 47).
- Anxiety (page 33).
- Psychotic or paranoid symptoms (see **Acute psychosis** or **Chronic psychosis**, pages 11 and 36). Single acts of major self-harm (eg self-castration) are often associated with psychotic illness. Psychotic symptoms usually indicate a high suicide risk.
- Use of alcohol or illicit drugs (see **Alcohol misuse** or **Drug misuse**, pages 18 and 55).
- Personality disorder: these general guidelines are applicable whether personality disorder (usually 'borderline' or 'dissocial') is present or not.

Refer to the secondary psychiatric services if the patient develops acute psychiatric symptoms.

Appropriate support

- Try to remain supportive to the patient, listening to the problems they express and avoid any critical or judgmental comments. Wherever possible, try to remain open to their views, seeing the patient as a person with a problem rather than as a 'cutter'.
- Ask about associated problems, eg bullying, bereavement, relationship problems, the difficulties of being in prison, separation from their children. Encourage the use of any available support for dealing with these. Consider supporting the patient in obtaining increased contact with friends and family, eg telephone calls, increased visits. The **Resource directory** (page 316) lists agencies that deal with particular problems.
- Facilitate access to purposeful activity such as exercise, education, work or opportunities to be creative. Advocate for increased time out of the cell for all prisoners, if appropriate.
- Consider referral to classes in developing coping skills, if available. Self-harm is more common among those who fail to develop more appropriate coping strategies.
- Consider use of a care suite. Ensure the patient is not punished for having self-harmed.

Consider reviewing the prescribed medication

Most substances taken by prisoners in overdoses are prescribed medications, often for physical as well as for mental disorders. Repeat prescriptions should be reviewed at regular intervals. Where this has not been the case, consider a review immediately.

Agree a follow-up appointment/plan

To review progress, continue problem solving and assess the extent of the suicidal thinking. Suicide risk fluctuates over time, especially in adolescents.

Brief staff in the Residential Unit before a patient is discharged or returned to the unit

Discuss, with patient permission, the relevant parts of the management plan and agree a review date. The care plan should aim to reduce the risk of suicide and self-harm.

- Location.
- Sharing a cell: young people, in particular, may find being temporarily 'doubled up' with someone else helps, but ensure they are not sharing with a cruel or manipulative individual who may encourage them to self-harm.
- Monitor for the possibility of bullying, threats of violence, problems with debts or other problems.
- Facilitate alternative coping strategies, eg exercise.
- Monitor for a reaction to possibly stressful visits, eg visits from children.
- Be aware of important dates that may trigger self-harm, eg children's birthdays, anniversaries, dates of the index offence.

If the patient is to return to an ordinary location, give wing officer a copy of *Ideas for Support Plans* 💾 and agree with him/her which of the options should be implemented.

If the self-injury is recurrent, in addition the following may be useful.

Advice and support

- Involve mental-health staff. A multidisciplinary approach with a key-worker and a long-term care plan involving the patient is desirable.
- Accept that the self-injury may continue for some time. The aim of treatment is not to stop the behaviour but to understand and support the patient in their distress, to help the patient gain more control of their feelings and to increase self-esteem.
- Make it clear that support is available whether or not they are trying to control the self-harm. Avoid threats and promises.
- Ask what the self-harm does for them — suggest a diary to record their feelings just before harming and discuss possible options for alternative responses (eg punching pillows, taking exercise or a shower, talking to someone). It is most important that the patient provides the ideas for alternative responses. With the patient's permission, involve the residential manager in discussing alternatives and how they may be facilitated.
- Support self-nurturing actions, eg the use of antiseptic.
- Try to see the patient, eg for 15 minutes a week, to talk about feelings: it helps if the patient writes things down before the session. Try to find someone for the patient to confide in, eg a listener, a Samaritan, personal officer, counsellor or friend.
- Where self-injury appears to be related to childhood abuse, see **People who disclose abuse as a child** (page 271) for advice on support and therapy.
- Discuss the possibility of joining a mutual support group, if available.
- Serious, repeated self-harm should result in referral for specialist assessment and advice on day-to-day management.

Medication

The use of medication in the management of patients who self-harm is controversial, except where there is evidence of an associated mental disorder.

- There is some evidence that paroxetine reduces further self-harm in non-depressed patients who self-harm repeatedly.[8]
- Fluoxetine has been associated with a reduction in self-harming in patients with personality disorder in a single controlled study.[9]

Developing in-prison resources

- Discuss with other departments the possibility of developing a course in coping skills. These can be helpful but should not replace reducing the unacceptable sources of stress, such as very long lock-up times.
- Consider the development of a crisis intervention or care suite for use by an individual experiencing an emotional crisis.
- Consider introducing an 'emergency contact card' scheme, whereby patients who have self-harmed are allowed access to immediate telephone or personal support when experiencing an emotional crisis.[10] This may be more effective with patients who have self-harmed for the first time than with those who self-harm repeatedly.
- Develop a library of literature to lend to patients (see **Resources** below).
- It is important to have supervision and training available for staff dealing with self-injury patients, since it can be emotionally draining and can lead to burn-out.
- Consider organising a mutual support group. An experienced, trained facilitator, professionally supervised by a specialist is essential. Other issues to consider in setting up such a group include how confidentiality issues will be handled, the time commitment required from participants, the focus of the group (groups should aim to help participants feel less alone and learn skills for coping with their present feelings), and the provision for support for participants who need it between sessions and after the group ends.

Specialist consultation or referral

The management of severe, long-term self-harm should always be overseen by a psychiatrist.

Referral to forensic psychotherapy services should be considered. Psychological therapies that have shown some effectiveness are the following.

- Structured problem-solving may be useful for associated problems that trigger self-harming behaviour.[11]
- Dialectical behaviour therapy has been shown to reduce the frequency of deliberate self-harm in people with emotionally unstable (borderline) personality disorder, although it is complicated and time-intensive to administer and is not widely available.[12] Consider for aftercare plans or, if available, for those with more than 1 year left of their sentence.
- Cognitive analytic therapy and some psychodynamically informed therapy has shown some effectiveness in self-injury in the context of emotionally unstable personality disorder.[13]

A combination of cognitive and solution-focused therapy may be useful for those patients with history of sexual abuse.[14]

Consider these for aftercare plans or, if available, for those with at least 1 year of their sentence left to run.

If counsellors are contracted to provide particular services (eg bereavement counselling, sexual assault or abuse counselling), arrangements must be made to ensure that they are properly trained and supervised.

Resources for patients and primary support groups

Listener or befriender scheme, chaplain, personal officers (where relationships are good). (Where the individual is considered dangerous, steps should be taken to protect listeners, eg personal alarms).

Samaritans: 08457 909090

National Self Harm Network: 020 7916 5472
c/o Survivors Speak Out, 34 Osnaburgh Street, London NW1 3ND
(Publishes a self-harm sheet and 'crisis card' to take to A&E)

Basement Project: 01873 856524
PO Box 5, Abergavenny NP7 5XW

Bristol Crisis Service for Women: 0117 925 1119 (helpline: Friday and Saturday, 9 pm–12:30 am)
PO Box 654, Bristol BS99 1XH
(Late night national helpline. Also provides information, publications and training about self-injury. Publishes a newsletter, *SHOUT*)

Respond: 0845 606 1503 (helpline: Monday–Friday, 1:30–5 pm)
3rd Floor, 24–32 Stephenson Way, London NW1 2HD
(For people with learning disabilities, who have experienced or perpetrated sexual abuse, their carers and professionals)

Bethlem Royal Hospital Crisis Recovery Unit: 020 8776 4273
Bethlem Royal Hospital, Monks Orchard Road, Beckenham BR3 3BX
(In-patient unit for individuals who repeatedly self-harm. Takes referrals from anywhere in the country)

Survivors of Abuse and Self Harming (SASH)
20 Lackmore Road, Enfield EN1 4PB
(Pen friend network that offers support and friendship on a one-to-one basis)

Disfigurement Guidance Centre: 01337 870 281
PO Box 7, Cupar KY15 4PP
(Supports patients and their families, offers advice on camouflage and natural aid techniques)

MIND leaflets on self-harm and personality disorder. Available from: MIND, 15–19 Broadway, London E15 4BQ. Tel: 020 8519 2122

'What's the Harm?' A Book for Young People Who Self-harm. £3.50. Clear and concise, this book is helpful for young people (and adults) beginning to explore their own self-harm. It is also a helpful resource for workers to use in working with individuals or groups.

The Self-harm Help Book. £5.50. An in-depth resource for people who wish to help themselves or others in their struggles with self-harm or self-injury. It is full of ideas found helpful by people who self-harm

L Arnold. *Hurting Inside: A Book for Young People*. 1988 Basement Project, Abergavenny. £3.50. Aims to help young people tackle difficulties they have as a result of physical, sexual or emotional abuse or neglect. It can also be a helpful starting point for adults looking at their experiences.

All three books are available from: Basement Project, PO Box 5, Abergavenny NP7 5XW. Tel: 01873 856524.

The 'Hurt Yourself Less' Workbook. Available from: the National Self Harm Network, c/o Survivors Speak Out, 34 Osnaburgh Street, London NW1 3ND. Self-help workbook — for people who self-harm to understand their behaviour and find safer alternatives.

[1] Singleton N, Meltzer H, Gatward R *et al. Psychiatric Morbidity among Prisoners in England and Wales.* London: ONS, 1998.

[2] Favazza A. Why patients mutilate themselves. *Hospital and Community Psychiatry* 1989; 40: 137–145.

[3] Livingstone M. A review of the literature on self-injurious behaviour among prisoners. In Towl J (ed.), *Suicide and Self-injury in Prisons.* Leicester: British Psychological Society, 1997.

[4] Pickett P. Unpublished research paper, HMYOI Feltham, quoted in Howard League for Penal Reform. *Scratching the Surface: The Hidden Problem of Self-harm in Prisons.* London: Howard League for Penal Reform, 1999.

[5] Crowe M. Deliberate self harm. In Bhugra D, Munro A (eds), *Troublesome Disguises: Underdiagnosed Psychiatric Syndromes.* Oxford: Blackwell Science, 1997.

[6] Haw C, Hawton K, Houston K, Townsend E. Psychiatric and personality disorders in deliberate self harm patients. *British Journal of Psychiatry* 2001; 178: 48–54.

[7] Morgan HG, Burns-Cox CJ, Pocock H, Pottle S. Deliberate self harm: clinical and socio-economic characteristics of 368 patients. *British Journal of Psychiatry* 1975; 127; 564–574.

[8] Verkes RJ, van der Mast RC, Hengeveld MW *et al.* Reduction by paroxetine of suicidal behaviour in patients with repeated suicide attempts but not major depression. *American Journal of Psychiatry* 1998; 155: 543–547.

[9] Markovitz P, Calabrese J, Schulz SC, Mltzer HY. Fluoxetine in the treatment of borderline and schizotypal personality disorders. *American Journal of Psychiatry* 1991; 148: 1064–1067.

[10] Hawton K, Townsend E, Arensman E *et al.* Psychosocial versus pharmacological treatments for deliberate self harm. *Cochrane Database of Systematic Reviews* 2000; 2: CD001764.

[11] Hawton K, Arensman E, Townsend E *et al.* Deliberate self harm: systematic review of efficacy of psychosocial and pharmacological treatments in preventing repetition. *British Medical Journal* 1998; 317: 441–447.

[12] Linehan MM, Heard HL, Armstrong HE. Interpersonal outcome of cognitive behavioural treatment for chronically suicidal borderline patients. *American Journal of Psychiatry* 1994; 151: 1771–1776.

[13] Bateman A, Fonagy P. Effectiveness of partial hospitalisation in the treatment of borderline personality disorder: a randomised controlled trial. *American Journal of Psychiatry* 1999; 156: 1563–1569.

[14] Dolan Y. *Resolving Sexual Abuse.* New York: WW Norton, 1991.

Observation of patients at risk

Observation is an important skill for all nurses and officers at all times, but in acute phases of mental disorder, some individuals become a risk to themselves or others. The aim is to prevent potentially suicidal, violent or vulnerable individuals from harming themselves or others. Observation is not simply a custodial activity. It is also an opportunity for the nurse or officer to interact in a therapeutic way with the individual on a one-to-one basis.

Definition

Nursing observation can be defined as 'regarding the patient attentively' while minimising the extent to which they feel they are under surveillance. Encouraging communication, listening and conveying to the individual that they are valued and cared for are important components of skilled nursing observation.

Deciding that an individual should be observed

Where possible, decisions about observation should be made jointly by the medical, nursing and residential staff. If a nurse or officer becomes aware that an individual is having suicidal thoughts or difficulty with impulse control, he/she should report to the senior nurse who will decide whether, and at what level, observation needs to be implemented. An F2052SH (or an Act to Care form in Scotland) must be opened and health centre managers must also be made aware so that adequate numbers and grades of staff can be made available for future shifts. The fact that an individual is considered to be at serious risk of suicide should trigger referral to mental-health services for assessment and the results of the assessment recorded in the notes.

Signs that may indicate the need for observation

- History of previous suicide attempts, self-harm or attacks on others.
- Hallucinations, particularly voices suggesting harm to self or others.
- Paranoid ideas where the patient believes that other people pose a threat.
- Thoughts and ideas that the individual has about harming themselves or others.
- Specific plans or intentions to harm themselves or others.
- Past problems with drugs or alcohol.
- Recent loss.
- Poor adherence to medication programmes.

What to observe

- General behaviour, level of cooperation and a willingness to accept help.
- Expression of suicidal ideas or hopelessness.
- Mood and attitude.
- Orientation, ie whether the patient knows where he/she is or what day it is
- Memory (where appropriate).

Make your observations as objective as possible, eg 'he kept saying that he was a complete waste of space' as opposed to 'still depressed'.

Supporting the individual during observations

- Ideally, the observer and individual should know each other and the observer should be familiar with the individual's history, social context and significant events since admission.
- Observer should be aware of the needs assessment and the overall plan of care drawn up by the multidisciplinary team.
- Observation is an opportunity for one-to-one interaction. The observer must show the patient positive regard. If a patient is uncommunicative, the observer can initiate conversation and convey a willingness to listen.
- Some individuals will prefer to be active, or may just want to pass the time. It is important that the observer elicit the individual's preferences, eg in music, television and reading, and attempt to provide these.
- Individual is entitled to information about why they are under observation, how long it will be maintained and what may happen. If possible, information should be provided in written form and translated, if necessary, into the individual's own language. For some individuals, a written contract stating the roles and expectations of staff and the individual might have some therapeutic potential.
- Aims and level of observation should be communicated, with the individual's permission, to the nearest relative and, especially if the individual is on remand, to the individual's solicitor, in order to enable speedy representation to be made to the court.

Responsibility for the observation of individuals

It is impossible to stipulate exactly who should carry out this task, but it is clearly undesirable for someone who does not know the health centre or the individual to be responsible for observing an individual who is suicidal, vulnerable or violent.
   Ideally, the nurse or officer responsible for carrying out observation will:

- know the individual well, including their history, background and specific risk factors
- be familiar with the health centre/unit, health centre/unit policy for emergency procedures and the potential risks in the environment and
- have received formal training in observation and in the management of violence.

It is important to note that the registered nurse remains accountable for the decision to delegate observation to a support worker or student in training and ensuring they are sufficiently knowledgeable and competent to undertake the role.

Four levels of observation

- **Level I: General observation** is the minimum acceptable level of observation for all in-patients. Staff should know the location of all individuals, but not all individuals need to be kept within sight. At least once a shift a nurse or officer should sit down and talk with each individual to assess his/her mental state. This interview should always include an evaluation of the individual's mood and behaviours associated with the risk and should be recorded in the notes (see **Mental State Assessment** on the disk 💾).
- **Level II: Closer, more focused observation** means that the individual should be checked at frequent, irregular intervals (exact times to be specified in the notes). Observation should involve close, supportive interaction with the patient. The patient may find it beneficial to have access to a listener or buddy. Level II

observation should be used sparingly as there is some evidence from the NHS that it may not be effective. If in doubt, move to Level III. Close, focused observation may be considered when the prisoner is potentially, but not immediately, at risk. Individuals with depression but no immediate plans to harm themselves or others, or those who have previously been at risk of harm to self or others but who are in a process of recovery, require intermittent observation. Use a gated cell to ensure that observation can continue during patrol states.

- **Level III: Within eyesight** is required when the patient could, at any time, attempt to harm themselves or others. The patient should be kept within sight at all times, by day and by night, and any tools or instruments that could be used to harm self or others should be removed. It may be necessary to search the patient and their belongings while having due regard for the patient's legal rights. In practice, this level of observation is very difficult to achieve in prison. In some prisons, an observation ward or cameras are available to assist staff in observing prisoners. In addition, access to a listener or buddy should be facilitated if the prisoner would find it helpful. The need for Level III observation should trigger referral to the psychiatric services for assessment and possible transfer to a psychiatric hospital.

- **Level IV: Within arm's length.** Patients at the highest levels of risk of harming themselves or others may need to be nursed in close proximity. On rare occasions, more than one nurse may be necessary. Issues of privacy, dignity and consideration of the gender in allocating staff, and the environmental dangers need to be discussed and incorporated into the care plan. In practice, this level of observation is possible within a prison only within a special-care suite, with special staffing rotas and where the person on Level IV observation is unlocked. Where this is not the case, individuals requiring Level IV observation should be transferred urgently to a psychiatric hospital.

Review of observation

Observation status should be reviewed by the medical officer and the primary nurse or the ward sister/charge nurse and residential manager (if appropriate) at least daily (including weekends). For arm's-length observation (Level IV), there should be three reviews, two during the day and one before the night shift. Decisions to shift the level of observation should always be taken jointly between medical and nursing staff, except in an emergency. Beware of false symptomatic improvement, especially when life crises that are associated with depression remain unresolved.

Recording decisions

All decisions about observation should be recorded by the doctor or nurse in the individual's medical/clinical notes. Records should include the following.
- Current mental state.
- Current assessment of risk.
- Specific level of observation to be implemented.
- Clear directions about therapeutic approach, ie occupation, therapy sessions.
- Timing of the next review.

Detailed records of observation should be kept by the staff responsible for carrying out the observation, including:
- the name of the person responsible and the time that they commenced and concluded their period of observation and

- a detailed record of the patient's behaviour, mental state and attitude to observation.

Ensuring continuity

Observation may involve a number of nurses and/or officers, with care being handed over at hourly intervals. Excellent communication among staff must be maintained by, for example, a group briefing of all staff to be involved in observing an individual at the beginning of each shift, during which the individual's status is reviewed, the potential dangers are enumerated and the attitudes to the process discussed.

Before taking over the individual's care, each nurse should have familiarised themselves with the individual's background and recent clinical notes. If possible, the hand over from one nurse to another should involve the individual. Though difficult, involving the individual can increase their sense of autonomy and encourage the development of trust. The individual has a right to information about their care and about what might happen in the future.

Length of observation time for individual staff

No period of observation by a member of staff should be longer than 2 hours except in very exceptional circumstances. At the end of each observation period, the nurse should have a break from observation of at least half an hour.

Limits to observation

Should a more intensive level than general observation continue for more than 1 week a review by the full clinical team should be triggered.

Auditing observation

Observation is a frequent and significant event in patient care and should be audited at 6-monthly intervals. A minimum data set would include the following:

- Reason for observation.
- Specific level or levels of observation.
- Length of time observed.
- Any untoward incidents.

Training for observation

Observing individuals at risk is a highly skilled activity. Every health centre should ensure that nursing staff (qualified, unqualified, other clinical staff, and bank and agency staff) are appropriately trained. Essential components of adequate training include the following:

- Risk assessment.
- Mental state assessment.
- Management and engagement of patients at risk of harming self and others.
- Factors associated with self-harm/harm to others.
- Indications for observation.
- Levels of observation.
- Attitudes to observation.
- Therapeutic opportunities in observation.

- Roles and responsibilities of the multidisciplinary team in relation to observation.
- Making the environment safe.
- Recording observation.
- Use of reviews and audit.

Observation by discipline staff

A prisoner identified as at risk of attempted suicide or self-harm and placed on a F2052SH or Act to care procedure will more often be located on a normal location on a residential wing than in a healthcare centre. Staff on the wing will be responsible for maintaining observation of those prisoners identified as at risk, unless and until the acuteness of that risk means that the prisoner is best located elsewhere. Healthcare staff will play a key role in liaising with and supporting officers on the wings, eg by sharing information about prisoners and advising on good practice in how to carry out and interpret observations.

References

Standing Nursing and Midwifery Advisory Committee. *Practice Guidance: Safe and Supportive Observation of Patients at Risk*. Mental Health Nursing 'Addressing Acute Concerns'. London: Department of Health, 1999.

Emergency treatment of self-poisoning or overdose

This section is for use by nurses in centres without 24-hour medical presence. Further information can be found in the *BNF* under **Emergency treatment of poisoning**. It contains general information about the management of poisons and specific information about the management of those poisons used most commonly in prisons. These are:

- Acids and alkalis.
- Alcohol.
- Amphetamine and MDMA (ecstasy).
- Antibiotics.
- Aspirin.
- Batteries.
- Benzodiazepines.
- Detergent cleaners.
- γ-Hydroxybutyric acid (GHB).
- Heroin.
- Ibuprofen.
- Mefenamic acid.
- Methadone.
- Opiates (other).
- Paracetamol.
- Steroids.
- Tricyclic antidepressants (TCAs).
- White spirit.

Information about the following poisons is provided on the attached disk ▣. These can be printed and stored.

- ACE inhibitors.
- Acids and alkalis.
- Alcohol.
- Amphetamine and MDMA.
- Antibiotics.
- Anticonvulsants.
- Antidepressants.
- Antihistamines.
- Antipsychotics.
- Aspirin.
- Barbiturates.
- Batteries.
- Benzodiazepines.
- β-Blockers.
- Bleach.
- Body packers.

- Button batteries.
- Calcium channel-blocking drugs.
- Cannabis.
- Cocaine.
- Detergent cleaners.
- Digoxin.
- Disinfectant.
- GHB.
- Heroin.
- Hypnotics, non-barbiturate.
- Ibuprofen and other non-steroidal anti-inflammatory drugs (NSAIDs).
- Khat.
- Lithium.
- LSD.
- Mefenamic acid.
- Opiates.
- Paracetamol.
- Salbutamol.
- Sterilizing tablets.
- Steroids.
- Theophylline.
- Toilet blocks and channel blocks.
- Toiletries.
- White spirit.

General information

Most cases of poisoning will result from deliberate self-harm by adults; occasionally such acts are accidental.

When assessing the patient, remember the following:

- The history from the patient may be unreliable; particularly when asked how much of a substance has been ingested or inhaled.
- The patient may have taken more than one poison.
- Many poisons cause symptoms and signs similar to the symptoms and signs of other diseases or injuries.
- A patient may be poisoned **and** be suffering from the effects of another illness or injury. Ask about other medical conditions and look for cuts and bruises and other signs of injury. In particular, hypoglycaemia and head injury may be confused with poisoning.

The patient may present with the following:

- Vomiting, abdominal pain, diarrhoea.
- Confusion, restlessness, irritability, slurred speech, ataxia, dizziness.
- Drowsiness, unconsciousness.
- Constricted or dilated pupils.
- Muscle tremors, convulsions.
- Breathing difficulties.
- Circulatory problems such as hypotension, tachycardia or bradycardia.
- Raised temperature and sweating.

- Burns and stains on or around mouth or on the skin if a corrosive or irritant liquid has been taken.
- A history or circumstances suggestive of deliberate or accidental poisoning, but conscious and fully orientated. A conscious and well patient may be in the early stages of poisoning and therefore still at risk of toxicity.

More information on clinical presentation of the poisoned patient is given below in an overview of the typical syndromes of poisoning.

Commonly encountered poisoning syndromes.

Syndrome	Possible agents	Vital signs	Mental status	Signs and symptoms
Anticholinergic	atropine, phenothiazines, tricyclic antidepressants	↓BP ↑HR	lethargy to coma	confusion, dilated pupils, dizziness, dry mouth, inability to urinate, flushed skin, convulsions
Extrapyramidal	metoclopramide, phenothiazines, some antipsychotics	↓BP ↑HR ↑ or ↓temperature	lethargy	dystonic movements, abrupt muscle contractions especially of the face and neck, torticollis, tongue protrusion, oculogyric crisis
Hyperthermic	amphetamine, cocaine, ecstasy	↑BP ↑HR ↑temperature ↑RR	fluctuating level of consciousness	rigidity, hyper-reflexia, disseminated intravascular coagulation, rhabdomyolysis, renal failure
Neuroleptic malignant syndrome	antipsychotics	↑BP ↑HR ↑temperature ↑RR	fluctuating level of consciousness	rigidity, hyper-reflexia, disseminated intravascular coagulation, rhabdomyolysis, renal failure
Opioid	codeine, heroin, methadone, morphine	↓BP ↓HR ↓RR ↓temperature	lethargy to coma	slurred speech, ataxia, pinpoint pupils
Sedative	barbiturates, ethanol, hypnotics	↓BP ↓RR ↓temperature	lethargy to coma	slurred speech, ataxia, hyporeflexia
Sympathomimetic	aminophylline, amphetamine, caffeine, cocaine, phencyclidine, theophylline	↑BP ↑HR ↑temperature ↑RR	anxiety, agitation, delirium	dilated pupils, sweating, convulsions
Withdrawal of opiates		↑BP ↑HR	normal	dilated pupils, sweating, nausea, vomiting, hyperactivity, piloerection, rhinorrhea
Withdrawal of sedative hypnotics or ethanol		↑BP ↑HR ↑RR ↑temperature		nausea, dilated pupils, tremor, convulsions, sweating

BP, blood pressure; HR, heart rate; RR, respiratory rate.

227

Resuscitation

- Resuscitate the patient if necessary (Airways, Breathing, Circulation — ABC):
  - **Airway**: if the airway is obstructed, pull the tongue forward, remove the dentures or any other foreign bodies, and oral secretions, hold the jaw forward and insert an oropharyngeal airway, if available. Turn patient semiprone and head-down to reduce the risk of inhaling vomit.
  - **Breathing**: assisted ventilation by mouth-to-mouth or Ambu-bag inflation may be needed.
  - **Circulation**: hypotension is common in severe poisoning with central nervous system (CNS) depressants. If the BP is very low, carry the patient head downwards on a stretcher and nurse in this position in the ambulance.
- Give oxygen via Hudson mask to maintain O_2 saturation > 94%.

Immediate management

- Ingested poison: do not give anything to drink if the patient is drowsy or unconscious or if the breathing is abnormal. Do not induce vomiting. When irritant chemicals have been swallowed, if the patient is fully awake and breathing normally, rinse out the mouth with water. A **small** drink of water can be given (< 200 ml) to dilute the chemical. It is best to avoid giving drinks after ingestion of corrosive chemicals because it may make the patient vomit.
- Chemical in the eye: irrigate immediately with copious amounts of water (preferably sterile) or saline for 15–20 minutes. Solid particles should be removed with cotton wool or forceps. Monitor the pH of the cornea and irrigating fluid with universal indicator paper. Continue until the pH is normal and remains so for 2 hours. Use anaesthetic drops if necessary so that the whole eye can be irrigated including under the upper and lower lids.
- Chemical on the skin: remove contaminated clothing. Irrigate the skin with running water or saline for 15 minutes (30 minutes for alkali exposure). Test the pH of the skin and continue to irrigate until the skin is no longer strongly acidic or alkaline. Neutralising chemicals should not be used. Following thorough irrigation, chemical burns should be treated as thermal burns.

Assess the following signs

- Check the blood glucose and give IV glucose if necessary.
- Respiratory rate, BP, HR, temperature, O_2 saturation, blood sugar.
- Conscious state, monitor the Glasgow Coma Scale (note that the scale is not useful for all agents).
- Gag reflex.
- Pupil size.
- Obtain a full history including the details of poisoning (this should not delay transfer of the patient to A&E).

What substance was taken?	Name of the product, its components and manufacturer. Look for a container if possible. Ask officers or witnesses.
How was it taken?	Swallowed, injected, inhaled, absorbed through the skin.
How much was taken?	Try to work out exactly how much was taken.
When was it taken?	Exact time if possible.
Why was it taken?	Accidental or deliberate.
What else taken?	Overdoses of drugs often involve more than one substance
Previous medical history	A medical condition or medication could put the patient more at risk of toxicity following an overdose. For example, alcohol abuse, or use of carbamazepine or warfarin, put patients into a risk group following paracetamol overdose. When it is not clear what substance has been ingested, a previous medical history may indicate which medicines might have been available to the patient.

Continuing management

- **Airway**: all patients who are at risk of becoming drowsy, are unconscious (Glasgow Coma Scale < 8/15), have an absent gag reflex or are fitting will need airway protection and may need intubation.
- **Fits**: ensure the patient is safe from injury and clear the airway. Most fits stop after 2 minutes. Check the blood glucose and give IV glucose if necessary. For prolonged or recurrent fits not controlled by correcting blood glucose, diazepam can be given, but it may cause cardiorespiratory collapse requiring resuscitation. Refer to a medical officer.
- **Transfer to A&E:**
  — After exposure to a toxic amount.
  — After chemical contamination of the eyes or chemical burns to the skin. In particular, all alkali exposures should be referred to A&E even if they seem insignificant. Urgent referral to an ophthalmologist is essential for alkali contamination of the eye and is probably needed after any chemical contamination of the eye.
- **Contacting a poisons information centre** may be useful to find out whether a substance is considered toxic. Centres are open for consultation by health professionals and emergency services day and night (Tel: 0870 600 6266).
- Preventing absorption with activated charcoal. Activated charcoal binds some poisons in the gut, preventing the toxin from being absorbed. The bound toxin is eliminated rectally. Activated charcoal does not bind the following, and therefore should not be used for:
  — Cyanide.
  — Alcohols, glycols.
  — Metal salts, eg iron salts, lithium salts.
  — Acid, alkali.

Indications:

- Patient is thought to have ingested enough toxin to cause serious poisoning.
- The agent ingested is believed to bind to AC.
- Ingestion was more than 1 hour before.
- Patient is conscious and cooperative.

Contraindications:

- Trivial ingestion.
- Patient has taken an agent that does not bind to an AC.
- Ingestion is more than 1 hour before.
- Drowsy, unconscious patient, whose airway cannot be protected.
- Patient has taken an agent that is corrosive.

Dose: 50 g, given as a drink or via oro- or nasogastric tube.

Substances of low toxicity

- These products are considered non-toxic in **acute** ingestion.
- No clinical features other than oral irritation and gastrointestinal upset are expected.
- No specific treatment is required. In the event of a very large ingestion, or if worrying symptoms occur, contact a poisons information centre.
- All products marked '®' are registered trademarks.

Drugs	Cosmetics	Craft/DIY products	Miscellaneous
• Calamine lotion • Emollients (E45® preparations, petroleum jelly) • Evening primrose oil • Folic acid • Oral contraceptives and hormone replacement (HRT) preparations • Simple linctus BP • Steroid creams • Zinc oxide creams/lotions (eg Sudocrem®)	• Moisturiser cream/lotion • Solid cosmetics (eg. lipstick, make-up)	• Emulsion paint • Plasticine® • PVA (polyvinyl alcohol) glue • Superglue/ cyanoacrylate (risk of mechanical injury) • Wallpaper paste	• Artificial sweeteners • Blu Tack® and similar adhesives • Candles • Felt-tip/ball-point pen ink • House plant food (eg Phostrogen®) • Matches • Mercury thermometers (risk from glass) • Pencil 'leads' (graphite) • Silica gel

Acids and alkalis

- Acids and alkalis affect different areas of the gastrointestinal tract.
- Alkalis damage the mouth, throat and oesophagus more than the stomach.
- Alkalis cause liquefaction burns, therefore they have the potential to cause deep, penetrative injuries.
- Acids mainly affect the stomach. They do not penetrate the tissue as deeply as alkalis. However, severe effects are likely with concentrated solutions. Acids form 'coagulation' burns similar to thermal injuries.

Strong acid	Formic acid, hydrochloric acid, nitric acid, sulphamic acid, sulphuric acid	Likely to cause severe injury
Weak acid	Acetic acid, citric acid	Irritant rather than corrosive unless the solution is concentrated
Weak alkali	Sodium carbonate	Irritant rather than corrosive unless the solution is concentrated
Strong alkali	Sodium metasilicate, sodium hydroxide (caustic soda, lye), calcium hydroxide (slaked lime), calcium oxide (lime, quicklime)	Likely to cause severe injury

Household products that may contain acids or alkalis

Use	Acid or alkali	Examples
Car battery	Acid	Sulphuric acid
Descaler, for a kettle or the bathroom	Acid	Sulphamic acid, citric acid, formic acid
Dishwasher liquid/ powder	Alkali	Sodium metasilicate
Drain cleaner*	Acid/alkali	Sulphuric acid, hydrochloric acid, potassium hydroxide, sodium hydroxide
Oven cleaner	Alkali	Sodium or potassium hydroxide
Paint stripper*	Alkali	Sodium hydroxide
Toilet cleaner*	Acid	Hydrochloric acid or phosphoric acid

*Some products with this function do not contain acid or alkali, so it is essential to find out the trade name and constituents of the product involved

May present with:

- Immediate pain in the mouth, oesophagus and stomach, swelling of lips, vomiting, haematemesis, salivation, mucosal burns, dyspnoea, stridor, dysphagia, shock. Note that the oesophagus may be damaged even when there are no burns to the inside of the mouth.

In severe poisoning:

- Burns to the lining of the mouth, oesophagus and stomach.
- Gastrointestinal haemorrhage and perforation, and upper airway obstruction. Acid ingestion may result in collapse, hypotension, acute renal failure and liver damage.
- Contamination of the eyes: there is the possibility of very serious burns, pain and blepharospasm.

231

- Contamination of the skin: pain, erythema, blistering, ulceration and discoloration of the skin. Alkali burns may be painless initially and appear insignificant, but they may be deep, penetrating burns that become worse over several hours.

Complications:
- Oesophageal stricture and pyloric stenosis can occur after 14–21 days.

Management:
- Ensure the airway is clear.
- For ingestion of household bleach, if the patient is fully awake, breathing normally and able to swallow without difficulty, give small amounts of water to drink.
- After ingestion of industrial bleach, oral fluids should be not be given.
- Never give activated charcoal. Never induce vomiting.
- Patients with Grade 1 burns (erythema, oedema) or more severe symptoms, and all who have ingested alkali, even if they are asymptomatic, should be transferred to A&E for assessment. Intensive care may be required.
- **For skin contamination**: as soon as possible, irrigate with water or saline for 30 minutes. Test the pH of the skin. Continue to irrigate until the skin is no longer strongly acidic or alkaline. Treat as a thermal burn. All alkali exposures should be referred to A&E even if they seem insignificant.
- **For eye contamination,** copious and immediate irrigation is essential, with water, preferably sterile, or saline for at least 15 minutes. Solid particles should be removed with cotton wool or forceps. Monitor the pH of the cornea and irrigating fluid, continue until the pH is normal and remains so for 2 hours. Use anaesthetic drops if necessary so that the whole eye can be irrigated, including under the upper and lower lids. Urgent referral to an ophthalmologist is essential for alkali contamination.

Alcohol

Also called ethyl alcohol, ethanol. In tolerant adults, severe effects are rare. Death is usually as a result of aspiration of vomitus.
May present with:
- Impaired visual acuity, coordination and reaction time, and emotional lability.
- Blood levels < 1.5 g l^{-1}: slurred speech, ataxia, muscular incoordination and diplopia. There may be flushing, tachycardia, sweating and incontinence.

In severe poisoning:
- Blood levels 3–5 g l^{-1}: cold clammy skin, hypothermia, stupor, dilated pupils and drowsiness progressing to coma. Severe hypoglycaemia may lead to convulsions.
- Blood levels > 5 g l^{-1}: deep coma, shock, respiratory depression, respiratory arrest and/or circulatory failure.

Management:
- Observation is recommended for at least 4 hours post-ingestion. Ensure the patient is adequately hydrated and monitor the blood sugar.
- Patients with signs of severe poisoning should be transferred to A&E.
- For hypoglycaemia administer glucose/dextrose IV.
- Convulsions usually respond to the correction of hypoglycaemia and diazepam may be used if required. Ventilation may be needed for respiratory depression.

Amphetamine and MDMA (ecstasy)

MDMA is an amphetamine derivative. It is taken as a tablet or powder enclosed in a capsule. Adverse effects more commonly occur after 'recreational' doses rather than with an overdose.

May present with:

- Onset of symptoms from amphetamine according to the route of exposure.

Drug	Onset (IV)	Onset (oral)	Duration
Amphetamine	within minutes	within 3 hours	4–6 hours
MDMA		within 1 hour	4–6 hours

- Transient nausea, increased muscle tone, muscle pain, trismus (jaw-clenching), dilated pupils, blurred vision, sweating, dry mouth, agitation, anxiety, palpitations, vomiting, abdominal pain and diarrhoea.
- Hypertonia, hyper-reflexia, hyperpyrexia, tachycardia, initial hypertension then hypotension, tachypnoea, and visual hallucinations.
- Effects may be prolonged if a patient has alkaline urine.

In severe poisoning:

- Delirium, coma, convulsions and cardiac dysrrhythmias that may be fatal.
- A hyperthermic syndrome may develop with rigidity, hyper-reflexia and hyperpyrexia (> 39°C) leading to hypotension, rhabdomyolysis, metabolic acidosis, acute renal failure, disseminated intravascular coagulation, hepatocellular necrosis, adult respiratory distress syndrome and cardiovascular collapse.
- Death from intracerebral haemorrhage has also been reported in hyperthermic patients.
- MDMA is also associated with hyponatraemia and cerebral oedema. This can occur in patients who have consumed excessive amounts of water (owing to drug-induced repetitive behaviour). These patients present with mild hypothermia and confusion; they may be unresponsive and staring.

Management:

- Activated charcoal can be given within 1 hour of ingestion to reduce absorption unless the patient is drowsy, fitting or vomiting.
- All patients should be transferred to A&E and observed for at least 6 hours for electrocardiogram (ECG) monitoring and the monitoring of electrolytes balance
- Give diazepam for convulsions. Refer to a medical officer.
- If the rectal temperature > 39°C, instigate cooling measures (fan, sponging, ice packs, cool IV fluids). If this is unsuccessful, the patient will need to be paralysed and ventilated.

Antibiotics

Includes: amoxycillin, erythromycin, flucloxacillin, penicillin. These drugs are essentially non-toxic.

May present with:

- Nausea, vomiting, diarrhoea.

Management:

- No specific treatment is needed.

Aspirin (acetylsalicylic acid)

Includes: salicylate.
Toxic dose:

- Ingestion > 120 mg kg^{-1}.

May present with:

- Nausea, vomiting, epigastric pain, tinnitus, deafness and flushing.
- Hyperventilation, sweating, dehydration, tremor and respiratory alkalosis with metabolic acidosis.

In severe poisoning:

- Confusion, drowsiness, delirium and pyrexia.
- Rarely coma, convulsions, renal failure, pulmonary oedema and cardiovascular collapse.

Management:

- Activated charcoal can be given to reduce absorption unless the patient is drowsy, fitting or vomiting.
- Repeated doses of charcoal may be considered. Consult a medical officer. The patient should be transferred to A&E if > 120 mg kg^{-1} aspirin ingested.
- Measurement of plasma salicylate concentration is important.
- In severe poisoning, haemodialysis is recommended.

Batteries: button batteries

Used in calculators, watches, hearing aids, musical greetings cards, etc.

- There are five main types: mercury, lithium, alkaline–manganese, silver and zinc–air. Most contain alkaline hydroxide solutions whatever their type.
- May cause:
  — electrical burns
  — chemical burns as a result of current-induced alkali production or as a result of leakage of alkaline contents and
  — chemical toxicity.
- On ingestion: in most cases, batteries pass through the gastrointestinal tract without causing harm. There is a risk of serious complications if the battery sticks in the oesophagus or the gut, but this is rare.

May present with:

- Delayed effects: a difficulty in swallowing, vomiting, haematemesis, nausea, burns in the mouth, indicating damage to the oesophagus; vomiting, tarry or bloody stools, abdominal pain, pyrexia indicating damage to the lower gut.

Management:

- Activated charcoal is of no benefit.
- Patient should be transferred to A&E for X-rays to confirm ingestion.
- Urgent removal may be necessary if the battery is leaking or is in the oesophagus
- If the battery is intact and small enough to pass through the gut, the hospital stay is unnecessary if the stools can be monitored and the clinical condition of the patient closely observed. X-rays should be repeated at 24 hours post-ingestion. If the patient develops signs or symptoms, particularly gastroenteritis or discoloured stools, or the battery is passed leaking or in pieces, the patient should return to hospital.

Benzodiazepines

Includes: alprazolam, clonazepam, chlordiazepoxide, diazepam, flunitrazepam, lorazepam, nitrazepam and temazepam.

Susceptibility to benzodiazepines varies widely. Taken alone, benzodiazepines rarely cause severe effects in overdose. However, serious effects may occur if taken with alcohol or other CNS depressants, or by elderly people. Patients who have been taking benzodiazepine sedatives for some time may develop a tolerance and experience less severe effects from overdose.

Toxic dose:

- A toxic dose of benzodiazepines is difficult to assess, as individual susceptibilities vary and concomitant ingestion of a CNS depressant (eg ethanol) may enhance toxicity. There is also the risk of aspiration of vomit in a patient with altered mental status who may not have exceeded the toxic dose. Therefore, the following doses are to be interpreted with care:
  — Alprazolam: 10 mg.
  — Clonazepam: 20 mg.
  — Chlordiazepoxide: 300 mg.
  — Diazepam: 100 mg.
  — Flunitrazepam: 10 mg.
  — Lorazepam: 10 mg.
  — Nitrazepam: 100 mg.
  — Temazepam: 200 mg.

May present with:

- Onset of effects within 30 minutes to 3 hours.
- Drowsiness, slurred speech, ataxia and confusion.

In severe poisoning:

- Unconsciousness is unusual, but if it does occur, it may be associated with hypotension and respiratory depression.

Management:
If a toxic dose has been exceeded:

- Activated charcoal can be given within 1 hour of ingestion to reduce absorption unless the patient is drowsy, fitting or vomiting.
- Patient should be observed for at least 4 hours after ingestion for the monitoring of BP, the pulse and the respiratory rate. Patients with impaired consciousness should be transferred to A&E because of the risk of respiratory depression.
- Flumazenil, a specific benzodiazepine antagonist, is not recommended outside hospital. It can reverse the sedative effects of benzodiazepines, but is not licensed for use in benzodiazepine overdose. It may precipitate convulsions or arrhythmias if other drugs have been ingested, and may precipitate withdrawal syndrome in patients addicted to benzodiazepines.

Detergent cleaners

Domestic general cleaners and domestic washing up liquid are of low toxicity.
May present with:

- Nausea, vomiting, diarrhoea. If the patient vomits foam, there is risk of aspiration, which may cause chemical pneumonitis.

Management:

- No treatment is required unless the patient is coughing and may have aspirated. In such cases, the patient should be referred to hospital.

γ-Hydroxybutyric acid (GHB)

Originally developed as an anaesthetic, GHB was found to have steroidal properties and produced effects similar to ecstasy and LSD. It can be in powder or granular form, often presented in a capsule. It is commonly dissolved in water to produce a clear, colourless liquid that may be injected IV or ingested. In addition to its use as a recreational drug, it is also used by bodybuilders, and as a 'date-rape' drug.

May present with:

- Onset of effects within 15–60 minutes of ingestion or 2–15 minutes after IV injection.
- Nausea, vomiting, diarrhoea.
- Drowsiness, headache, ataxia, dizziness, confusion, agitation, hallucinations (rare), euphoria, amnesia, vertigo.
- Urinary incontinence, tremor, myoclonus, hypotonia, hypothermia, sometimes extrapyramidal symptoms.

In severe poisoning:

- Coma usually lasting 1–2 hours, with dizziness lingering for up to 2 weeks.
- Bradycardia, seizure-like activity, hypotension (rarely hypertension with IV use), Cheyne–Stokes respiration and respiratory depression, which may lead to respiratory arrest.
- Effects usually resolve spontaneously within 2–96 hours; most users feel 'high' for 24–48 hours and then suffer a hung-over state for a further 48–72 hours.

Management:

- Activated charcoal can be given within 1 hour of ingestion to reduce absorption unless the patient is drowsy, fitting or vomiting.
- All patients should be observed for a minimum of 2 hours, monitoring BP, the pulse and the respiration. If patients are symptomatic for more than 2 hours after ingestion, they should be transferred to A&E.

Heroin

Slang terms vary locally, but include horse, 'H', brown sugar, smack, stuff and junk.

Street heroin varies in its chemical and physical appearance depending on the country or region of origin. Most heroin is sold in 'bags' or 'wraps' filled with 200–400 mg powder varying in colour from white to light brown. Heroin may be administered orally, sublingually or rectally, by subcutaneous, IM or IV injection, or by smoking, the snorting of powder or by inhalation of a thick, white smoke by heating it with a flame on silver paper ('chasing the dragon').

May present with:

- Onset of effects within 30 minutes of ingestion or within seconds to minutes after IV injection. The peak effects last for about 10–30 minutes and continue in milder form for 2–4 hours.
- Nausea, vomiting.
- Dry mouth, constricted pupils, drowsiness, confusion, euphoria, a sense of calmness, flushing, sweating and a feeling of warmth.

In severe cases:

- Hypotension, coma, bradycardia, respiratory depression with associated hypoxaemia and pulmonary oedema, cardiac arrhythmias. The pupils may be dilated if hypoxic cerebral damage has occurred.

Management:

- Activated charcoal can be given within 1 hour of ingestion to reduce absorption unless the patient is drowsy, fitting or vomiting.
- Naloxone can be given to reverse the signs of severe poisoning (coma, respiratory depression or convulsions) within a few minutes, but it has a short life and the patient may relapse. Refer to a medical officer.
- All patients who have taken an overdose of opioid analgesics should be transferred to A&E and observed for at least 6 hours. Patients who require naloxone should be observed for 24 hours. ECG monitoring and ventilation may be needed.

Naloxone

Form: ampoule
Strength: 0.4 mg ml^{-1}
Route of administration: IV
Recommended dose adult: 0.4 mg
Duration: can be repeated at intervals of 2–3 minutes to a maximum of 10 mg, only on the medical officer's orders

---

Ibuprofen

Serious poisoning is unusual. Some preparations are sustained release; the onset of toxicity may be delayed and the duration prolonged.

Toxic dose:

- Ingestion > 100 mg kg^{-1}.

May present with:

- Nausea, vomiting, abdominal pain.
- Drowsiness, lethargy, dizziness, headache and tinnitus.
- Tachycardia, hypothermia.

In severe poisoning:

- Hypotension, renal failure.
- Coma, convulsions, apnoea or respiratory depression, cardiorespiratory arrest.

Complications:

- Electrolyte disturbances, metabolic acidosis, hyperventilation resulting in respiratory alkalosis.

Management:

- Activated charcoal can be given within 1 hour of ingestion to reduce absorption unless the patient is drowsy, fitting or vomiting.
- Observe for 4 hours, or 12 hours for a sustained-release preparation. All patients with significant symptoms should be transferred to A&E.
- In drowsy or hyperventilating patients, the pH, electrolytes, blood gases and renal function should be monitored.

Mefenamic acid

Can cause convulsions at doses close to those used in therapy, within 1 hour of ingestion, or delayed for 12 hours or more.
Toxic dose:

- Ingestion > 1500 mg.

May present with:

- Nausea, vomiting, abdominal pain.
- Convulsions.

In severe poisoning:

- Renal failure.
- Cardiac arrest has been reported in patients with convulsions following an overdose with mefenamic acid.

Management:

- Activated charcoal can be given within 1 hour of ingestion to reduce absorption unless the patient is drowsy, fitting or vomiting.
- Diazepam can be given to control fits if they are prolonged. Refer to a medical officer.
- Patients should be transferred to A&E and observed for at least 12 hours, or 24 hours if the patient develops convulsions.
- In drowsy or hyperventilating patients, the pH, electrolytes, blood gases and renal function should be monitored.

Methadone

Toxicity is enhanced if other CNS depressants such as alcohol are ingested as well. Methadone has a long half-life; toxicity may be delayed and the duration prolonged.
Toxic dose:

- Difficult to assess as tolerance and therapeutic doses vary greatly
- Hospital management is recommended if the patient has exceeded their established dose.

May present with:

- Nausea, vomiting.
- Some opioids may cause a rash, itching and flushing.
- Drowsiness, pinpoint pupils.

In severe poisoning:

- Unconsciousness, convulsions, hypotension.
- Respiratory depression, with cyanosis and respiratory arrest. Hypoxia due to respiratory depression is the most frequent cause of death from opioid poisoning
- Methadone has a long half-life; the clinical effects may be prolonged. Naloxone infusion may be required.

Complications:

- Non-cardiogenic pulmonary oedema, cardiovascular collapse, renal failure.

Management:

- Activated charcoal can be given within 1 hour of ingestion to reduce absorption unless the patient is drowsy, fitting or vomiting.

- Naloxone can be given to reverse the signs of severe poisoning (coma, respiratory depression or convulsions) within a few minutes, but it has a short life and the patient may relapse. Refer to a medical officer.
- All patients who have taken an overdose of opioid analgesics should be transferred to A&E and observed for at least 6 hours. Patients who require naloxone should be observed for 24 hours. ECG monitoring and ventilation may be needed.

Naloxone
Form: ampoule Strength: 0.4 mg ml^{-1} Route of administration: IV Recommended dose adult: 0.4 mg Duration: Can be repeated at intervals of 2–3 minutes to a maximum of 10 mg, only on the medical officer's orders

Opiates: codeine, dihydrocodeine, morphine

Toxicity is enhanced if other CNS depressants such as alcohol are ingested as well. Toxic dose:

- A toxic dose of opiate is difficult to assess as individual tolerances vary greatly. Therefore, the following doses are to be interpreted with care:
  — Codeine: 350 mg.
  — Dihydrocodeine: 420 mg.
  — Morphine: 30 mg (patients may be on higher doses in therapy; the clinical effects may occur if established dose is exceeded).

May present with:
- Nausea, vomiting.
- Some opioids may cause a rash, itching and flushing.
- Drowsiness, pinpoint pupils.

In severe poisoning:
- Unconsciousness, convulsions, hypotension.
- Respiratory depression with cyanosis and respiratory arrest. Hypoxia due to respiratory depression is the most frequent cause of death from opioid poisoning.

Complications:
- Non-cardiogenic pulmonary oedema, cardiovascular collapse, renal failure.

Management:
- Activated charcoal can be given within 1 hour of ingestion to reduce absorption unless the patient is drowsy, fitting or vomiting.
- Naloxone can be given to reverse the signs of severe poisoning (coma, respiratory depression or convulsions) within a few minutes but it has a short life and the patient may relapse. Refer to a medical officer.
- All patients who have taken an overdose of opioid analgesics should be transferred to A&E and observed for at least 6 hours. Patients who require naloxone should be observed for 24 hours. ECG monitoring and ventilation may be needed.

Naloxone
Form: ampoule Strength: 0.4 mg ml^{-1} Route of administration: IV Recommended dose adult: 0.4 mg Duration: Can be repeated at intervals of 2–3 minutes to a maximum of 10 mg, only on the medical officer's orders

Paracetamol

Note that preparations may combine paracetamol with opioids, aspirin, metoclopramide or antihistamines.

Toxic dose:

- Ingestion > 150 mg kg^{-1} (up to 12 g maximum) may be hepatotoxic in an adult.
- Individual susceptibility is affected by age, metabolic status and co-ingested medication. There are certain high-risk groups who may be at risk of liver damage at lower plasma paracetamol levels (75 mg kg^{-1}). They include:
  — malnourished/ anorexic/ bulimic patients
  — HIV-positive patients
  — patients with pre-existing liver disease or induced liver enzymes, eg due to chronic alcohol abuse
  — patients taking enzyme-inducing drugs: carbamazepine, phenytoin, barbiturates, primidone, glutethimide or rifampicin
  — patients with cystic fibrosis and
  — patients with some viral infections, eg glandular fever.
- If the ingested dose is not known, determination of serum plasma paracetamol is recommended.
- It is important not to delay in treating a patient with a paracetamol overdose. The efficacy of the antidotes decreases greatly if started more than 8 hours after ingestion.

May present with:

- Initially, sometimes nausea, vomiting, abdominal pain, pallor; rarely, drowsiness and coma.
- Patient may be asymptomatic for up to 24 hours, then develop liver damage.

In severe poisoning:

- Coma and metabolic acidosis, hypoglycaemia, delayed liver damage, which occurs about 3 days after ingestion and may result in death 4–18 days after ingestion. Renal damage can occur in the absence of liver toxicity.

Management:

- Activated charcoal can be given within 1 hour of ingestion to reduce absorption unless the patient is drowsy, fitting or vomiting.
- Patient should be transferred to A&E if:
  — toxic dose has been exceeded
  — there is doubt about the amount ingested
  — patient is in a high-risk category (see above) or
  — the overdose is staggered.

Steroids

Includes: prednisolone, beclomethasone, anabolic steroids and corticosteroids. Low, acute toxicity.

May present with:

- Nausea, vomiting, diarrhoea.

Management:

- No specific treatment is needed for acute overdose.

Tricyclic antidepressants

Includes: amitriptyline, amoxapine, clomipramine, dothiepin, doxepin, imipramine, lofepramine, nortriptyline, protriptyline and trimipramine.

Tricyclic antidepressants are the most commonly prescribed antidepressants in the UK. Although the individual TCAs have differences in side-effects and kinetics, most behave similarly in an acute overdose. Peak plasma levels normally occur within 2–8 hours of a therapeutic dose because of delayed gastric emptying. After an overdose, peak levels may occur even later. Life-threatening signs usually develop within 6 hours of ingestion or not at all. The complications most often associated with a fatal outcome are severe hypotension and cardiac arrhythmias.

Toxic dose:

- Hospital observation is recommended for ingestion > 5 mg kg^{-1}.
- Anticholinergic effects, sedation and hallucinations can occur at doses < 5 mg kg^{-1}.

May present with:

- Dry mouth, dilated pupils, urine retention, hallucinations, jerky movements, drowsiness.
- Metabolic acidosis and hypokalaemia.

In severe poisoning:

- Coma, hypotension, hypothermia, convulsions, respiratory depression, pulmonary oedema, cardiac arrhythmias, cardiac arrest. Arrhythmias may not respond to therapy.
- Lofepramine is less likely to cause cardiac effects.
- Amoxapine is more likely to cause arrhythmias and convulsions.

Management:

- Activated charcoal can be given within 1 hour of ingestion to reduce absorption unless the patient is drowsy, fitting or vomiting.
- Diazepam can be given to control fits if they are prolonged. Refer to a medical officer.
- Because of the potential for serious toxicity, all patients should be transferred to A&E for observation and to monitor their ECG, pH and electrolytes for at least 6 hours post-ingestion.
- In serious poisoning, ventilation and intensive care will be necessary.

White spirit

Also called turpentine substitute and is composed of a mixture of petroleum distillates. Petroleum distillates are the hazardous component of some furniture polishes, window cleaners, shoe polishes, lighter fuels and paint brush cleaners.

They are poorly absorbed from the gut and the main risk following ingestion is aspiration, which may occur during ingestion or if the patient subsequently vomits.
  May present with:

- Nausea and vomiting.
- Respiratory distress with coughing, choking, tachypnoea and dyspnoea.
- After prolonged contact with skin: erythema and irritation.

In severe cases:

- Drowsiness and coma after large amounts.
- Chemical pneumonitis and pulmonary oedema.

Management:

- Do not give anything by mouth if the patient is drowsy or having difficulty in breathing, but if the patient is fully awake and breathing normally, give them water to drink.
- Patients with history of vomiting or coughing should be transferred to A&E for a chest X-ray.
- After spills, contaminated clothing should be removed and the skin washed thoroughly. Emollient should be applied to areas of erythema.

Black and other ethnic minorities — including foreign national prisoners and immigration detainees

Introduction

Healthcare workers in prisons will see many people whose nationality, ethnic group, language, culture or religion is different from their own. These differences affect the way individuals express mental distress, their beliefs about their problems, the treatment they find acceptable and also basic communication with the health worker. Ethnic minorities in prison fall into three main groups.

- British ethnic minorities, eg a Briton of Indian, Chinese or West Indian extraction.
- Foreign national prisoners who are sentenced or held on remand for an offence under criminal law.
- Asylum seekers and other immigration detainees who are detained under the Immigration Act 1971.

This section aims to summarise the main issues affecting the delivery of a good primary mental-health service to these groups and outline possible ways of responding. Some problems (eg experience of racial abuse, discrimination, not speaking English) may be common to all groups. Other problems are specific to only one group. It is intended to be read in conjunction with the guidelines on assessing and managing mental disorders.

All groups

Language

It is impossible to diagnose and manage mental (or physical) ill-health if the patient and clinician do not share a common language. Prisoners who have difficulties with English should have access to an interpreter. Healthcare workers have a duty to ensure that they can provide a health service. The governor will authorise any necessary interpretation or translation facilities.

Language Line is a 24-hour telephone interpreting service covering over 100 languages. A central, part subsidised, contract is held by Prison Service Headquarters (Prisoner Administration Group). The prison race relation's liaison officer will have details. All prisons can access Language Line interpreters, subject to governor authority, by telephoning 020 7713 0090 and quoting their individual identification code. The prison race relation's liaison officer will have a copy of the *Interpreters Directory* and may be able to assist with local sources. The Local Authority, the local Health Authority, and some voluntary and community groups may also offer access to interpreters or translators.

Some people from countries where English is usually spoken may not themselves speak it; eg the language of Irish travellers is Gammon.

Negotiating a shared problem description and management plan with patients from other cultures

Some prisoners come from cultures whose ways of expressing distress and whose views of the causes and appropriate treatments of that distress differ markedly from

243

that of the dominant 'Western' culture. For example, in some cultures, depression may be seen as the result of 'thinking too much' or witchcraft.[1,2] Some mental-health treatments, such as counselling, are based on Western values and are not familiar to people from all cultures. Some ethnic groups do not have a Western diagnostic concept, such as alcoholism, in their vocabulary. There may be an even greater stigma attached to mental illness in some cultures than in Western culture. All this may make communication between the healthcare worker and the patient very difficult. The result may be that the doctor or nurse misunderstands the problem and makes a wrong diagnosis or that the patient refuses to follow the management advice given.

There are too many different races, nationalities and cultures represented in prisons to make it possible to describe here how their citizens typically express and think about mental distress and illness. It is, in any event, very dangerous to make such generalisations. What follows is a step-by-step approach to drawing out the patient's own beliefs about his/her problem. Once this is done, it is possible either to discuss management using the patient's own concepts or (where the belief systems are very different) to negotiate a definition of the problem and a management plan that incorporate both the health worker's and the patient's beliefs.

Wherever possible, obtain general information about the patient's cultural norms from local community groups, the local branch of the Racial Equality Council or a healthcare worker from the same nationality, ethnic group or cultural background.

Step 1: Introductions

- Clarify which is the patient's personal name and which name (if any) is the family name and which name is used as a surname. Clarify how the patient wishes to be addressed. Be aware that naming systems generally reflect cultural and religious backgrounds and may have considerable significance for the individual.
- Explain who you are and the purpose of the interview, ie to identify health problems (in the body and also emotional distress) and seek to provide help. Reassure the patient that the interview is confidential. Explain that the rules of confidentiality apply to any interpreter present.

Step 2: Establish what the problem is

Ask: 'What is the problem?' and 'How can I help you?' If the patient says that there is no problem but you have evidence otherwise, gently press further, eg 'The wing officer tells me that you haven't been talking to anyone or eating for some time. This indicates to me that you may have some distress. How do you feel?'

Step 3: Explore the patient's own beliefs about their problem, its causes and his/her expectations of what might help[3]

Ask:

- 'Can you describe your problem?'
- 'What do you think caused your problem?'
- 'Why do you think it started when it did?'
- 'How severe is it?'
- 'What kind of care do you think you should receive?'
- 'What result do you expect from your care?'

- 'What are the direct problems caused by your problems or illness?'
- 'How satisfied are you with the treatment you have received so far?'

Record the answers to these questions, as far as possible, verbatim.

Step 4: Compare the patient's beliefs about their problems with your own

Explain how these differ; eg the patient may attribute their problems to someone wishing them ill and see the solution as persuading a third party to intervene; you see the problem as an illness and see the solution as transfer to hospital and medication. Check that you have each understood your different perspectives accurately.

Step 5: Seek ways of resolving the differences

The following are examples only.

- If the patient sees their symptoms (eg depressive symptoms) as the result of ill-wishing or sorcery and you are not sure if this is a paranoid delusion or a culturally normal explanation, the patient may agree to your seeking further information or opinions from other people, eg relatives, friends.
- If possible and appropriate, use the patient's words to communicate with him/her, eg 'thinking too much' or 'spiritual problems'.
- If possible and appropriate, agree to incorporate elements of both parties' explanatory models in the management plan. For example, the patient may agree to seek advice and support from a spiritual healer and also to take medication.
- If the patient expects a powerful, immediate and lasting response to antidepressant medication, take particular care to explain that there may be a delayed response and that treatment is likely to continue even when they feel better.

Supporting and encouraging links to family and community

Distress, disorientation and loss may be caused by an inability to maintain cultural identity and some links with family and the community. Where the individual is isolated, it can be very helpful to encourage them to form links with an appropriate community group (see **Resources Directory** page 316). Probation officers, chaplains and race relations liaison officers may help maintain family contacts. You may also be able to advocate for institutional changes, eg the celebration of festivals, allowing the wearing of cultural dress and following their religion, the provision of culturally specific food.

Other cultural issues

Issues to consider include the following.

- Religious or cultural implications of admission of abuse, especially sexual abuse or rape. The family may regard any sexual abuse, however it occurred, as bringing shame upon the family. The chaplain may be able to advise.
- Religious or cultural implications of self-harm. An individual may self-harm and then experience added shame as suicide may not be acceptable in their religion (eg Muslims). The individual may then feel cut off from the support of their faith community. Care may need to be taken in liaising with religious leaders.

- Allowing female patients to see a female doctor or nurse if they wish. Modesty and privacy are crucial to many groups, especially so to women.
- Clothes, hygiene and appearance. Will the patient find health centre clothes immodest? Do they observe the right hand/left hand rule of hygiene?

Experience of racism and discrimination

Being the subject of verbal or physical racist abuse can affect mental health by intimidating the individual and causing anxiety and by leading to self-doubt or dilemmas over cultural identity. This is more likely to happen where members of a particular ethnic group are small in number and lack the support of others. Consider supporting the individual to use the appropriate complaints procedure. Where the experience of racial abuse has resulted in feelings of fear or anger, local Victim Support schemes, available in most areas, may help, though they cannot deal with mental disorders. Racial harassment and abuse are unlawful.

British ethnic minorities

African-Caribbeans

African-Caribbeans are over-represented in the prison population. The research on their mental-health needs is inconclusive. Despite evidence that the prevalence of schizophrenia is similar in different countries,[iv] there are consistent reports that, in the UK, mental illness, particularly schizophrenia, is diagnosed more commonly (three to six times more commonly) in African-Caribbeans compared with whites.[5] It is also well established that African-Caribbeans in the UK are more likely to experience compulsory psychiatric treatment, more likely to be diagnosed as violent and be detained in secure Mental Health Units, less likely to receive diagnosis and treatment at an early stage, and less likely to receive psychotherapy and counselling. The reasons are not clear, though possible explanations include the following.

- African-Caribbeans have a greater biological susceptibility to schizophrenia.
- The stress of social adversity, racism and migration leads to a higher rate of schizophrenia.
- African-Caribbeans do not have a higher rate of schizophrenia but white healthcare staff over-diagnose because of their poor understanding of the cultural background of the patients.

Both in prison and in the community, Caribbean-born people have lower rates of suicide and self-harm compared with the general population.

Asians

Although research in India suggests that the prevalence of mental disorders, including schizophrenia and depression, are similar to those in other countries, Asians in the UK are referred for psychiatric treatment less frequently than whites. Again, the reasons are unclear, but explanations include the following.

- Genuinely low rates of mental disorder.
- Under-diagnosis resulting from a reluctance to approach the health services, language and communication difficulties or poor understanding of cultural differences on the part of white staff.

Community suicide rates are higher for Asian-born women, especially those aged 15–34, than for the general population, while Asian-born men have a lower suicide rate than the average.

What can be done to help?

The guidance outlined under **All groups** above may help to reduce misdiagnosis.

Foreign national prisoners

Who are foreign national prisoners?

Foreign national prisoners are either sentenced or held on remand for an offence under criminal law. As at June 1999:

- 8% of the prison population were foreign nationals
- 3% of white prisoners and 24% of black prisoners were foreign nationals
- 15% of women prisoners and 47% of black female prisoners were foreign nationals
- 75% of female foreign nationals were serving sentences for drug offences, often as 'drug mules'
- foreign national prisoners come from many countries in Europe, the West Indies, Asia, Africa, South and North America, and Australia and New Zealand and
- foreign national prisoners have needs that are distinct from those of British ethnic minorities. Some prisons have a foreign nationals' liaison officer. In most prisons, issues relating to foreign national prisoners are the responsibility of the race relations officer.

What are their mental-health needs?

There have been no studies of the particular mental-health needs of foreign national prisoners. However, in addition to the factors affecting all ethnic minority groups, the following factors all increase the likelihood of mental disorders, particularly depression, developing.

- Isolation: many are imprisoned vast distances from home and contact with family and friends is difficult or impossible. Language difficulties make it harder for them to make friends or seek support in the prison.
- Worry about the fate of their family at home. Women, in particular, may be trying to send money home from prison wages to keep their families. Probation officers may assist in maintaining links with the family at home and any children in care in the UK.
- Long sentences may reduce hope. Drug couriers, in particular, often serve long sentences.
- Shame and concern about what will happen to them when they return home on release. In some countries, being in prison may lead to rejection by the family and the community. In Nigeria, Decree 33 states that any Nigerian found guilty in a foreign country of a drugs offence may face another 5 years' imprisonment on their return.

What can be done to help?

The following ideas have all been implemented in some prisons in England and Wales. Healthcare workers may wish to promote with senior managers and others the adoption of some or all of these measures in their own establishment in order to serve better the mental-health needs of this group.

- Improving interpreting and translating services.
- Increasing the letter allowance in lieu of visits, allowing air mail letters or the provision of a telephone call home for those who have not received a visit in the previous month.

- Making telephone calls easier, eg by installing a phone that receives incoming calls or checking that there are no local restrictions on the purchase of phone cards by foreign national prisoners.
- Allowing foreign national prisoners to avoid using the prison address in order to conceal their whereabouts from their family.
- Encouraging the maintenance of cultural and spiritual identity by, for example, taking newspapers and videos from the foreign nationals' own country, allowing the wearing of cultural dress, ensuring that the prison shop stocks ethnic foods, organising cultural events to coincide with religious festivals, providing religious services in the prisoners' own language.
- Adapting educational provision to suit the needs of foreign national prisoners by, for example, providing courses in English as a second language.
- Allowing and facilitating the use of audio- and videocassettes by foreign national prisoners as a means for them to allay their families' fears about their safety.
- Inviting cultural groups into the prison to provide support for foreign national prisoners (see **Resources Directory** page 316).
- Accommodating some prisoners from the same nationality together.
- Facilitating temporary release on licence in this country.
- Helping prepare foreign national prisoners for release, eg by allowing foreign nationals to earn money and save, and by running a prerelease course.
- Facilitating support and information from the embassy and consular staff where a bilateral agreement between the country and the UK exists. The race relations officer will have a list of countries with which the UK has such an agreement. Care must be taken not to reveal prisoner details to diplomats without prisoner permission, in order to prevent possible reprisals.

Immigration detainees

Asylum seekers: who are they?

An asylum seeker, as defined in the Immigration Act 1971, is someone who is applying for refugee status, ie permission to stay in the UK 'on the ground that if he were required to leave, he would have to go to a country to which he is unwilling to go owing to a well founded fear of being persecuted for reasons of race, religion, nationality, membership of a particular social group or political opinion'. Some asylum applicants are detained under the Immigration Act 1971 while awaiting the outcome of their application or appeal following a refusal. Some are detained when applying for asylum at the port of entry; some have applied for asylum after entry and identification as illegal immigrants; some are awaiting removal. If they have been detained when applying for asylum at the port of entry, the immigration officer who decides that detention is appropriate should give the applicant a written explanation for why they have been detained. However, this does not always happen and decisions are often experienced as arbitrary.[6] There is no time limit on their period of detention. The average length of detention is 68 days, but this includes a span of a few hours to over 2 years. Most detainees are men, but around one-quarter are women. In 1997, the top 12 countries of origin of asylum seekers in the UK were: Afghanistan, China, Colombia, Ecuador, India, Nigeria, Pakistan, Somalia, Sri Lanka, Turkey, the former Soviet Union and the former Yugoslavia.[7]

Immigration detainees are held in dedicated Immigration Service detention centres or in centres run by the Prison Service or in prisons. In June 1999, 54% of detained asylum seekers were held in prison establishments, though there are plans to reduce this number. The detainee population varies but, as of May 2001, there were 1787 people in immigration detention, of whom approximately two-thirds have made application for asylum. Because of the nature of healthcare facilities in immigration centres, people may be transferred from them to prisons, following hunger strikes or unsuccessful suicide attempts or where they are thought to be at exceptional risk of suicide, as some prisons have 24-hour medical facilities.[8]

Who else may be detained under the Immigration Act?

Some immigration detainees are individuals who have not claimed or sought asylum, but have overstayed, absconded or who are subject to deportation action on recommendation of a court, following a criminal conviction and custodial sentence. They may be held pending the outcome of appeals or before removal. Some may have been in the UK for some time and may have community or family ties here.

What are their mental-health needs?

Studies of refugee communities (those whose applications for asylum have been successful) in the UK show a high prevalence of mental-health problems and disorders. There are broadly two levels of problems: most common are problems of adjustment, while a smaller proportion of people experience persistent post-traumatic disorders.[9]

Information about the mental-health needs of detainees is more sparse, but shows the same overall pattern: high levels of psychosocial and spiritual distress, acute stress reactions and sleep disturbance, lower levels of severe depression and severe, persistent post-traumatic stress disorder (PTSD) with psychosis being quite rare.[10,11] Substance abuse appears uncommon in detained asylum seekers, though it has been reported as developing later in the community, particularly among young men. Khat usage in the young Somali population in the community may exacerbate an individual's mental distress and lead in some cases to suicide.

A particular feature of immigration detainees is the widespread nature of suicidal thoughts. These may be either a feature of depression or a rational strategy for dealing with the potential event of deportation, should their application for refugee status fail. It is important that these events are dealt with in accordance with ethical principles governing the right to die (see **Food refusal**, page 292).

Factors (causal and exacerbating) include the following.

- The impact of indeterminate detention. Detention with an unknown time limit is a known causal factor in the development of a range of symptoms of mental disorder, including: sleep disturbances, such as nightmares, insomnia, night-sweats and early morning waking, depression, somatic symptoms such as dyspepsia and constipation, brief reactive psychosis, self-injury and (post-release) problems with control of mood or temper, withdrawal, anxiety, mistrust and forgetfulness.[12] Lack of information about why they were detained and what will happen to them in the future is a source of significant stress.

- The experience of detention (eg cells, uniformed security personnel, seclusion or segregation, body searches) may also reactivate and exacerbate previous trauma. The Medical Foundation for the Care of Victims of Torture reports that where indeterminate detention is suffered by someone who has previously been imprisoned and tortured, it may continue the psychological 'demolition' of the person and cause high stress, despair and anxiety.[13]

- Isolation caused by language difficulties, separation from family and friends and cultural isolation. Poor social support and isolation from the family and the community is a more important predictor of depression in refugees than previous trauma.[14]

- Fear and uncertainty about the future and possible deportation.[15]
- Bereavement: this may include loss of country and cultural values (cultural bereavement) as well as loss of family members and close friends. Bereavement reactions may be aggravated by the difficulty of grieving because of the lack of a body or because they cannot take part in the related religious ceremony that normally plays a part in the grieving process (see **Bereavement**, page 23).
- Previous experience of torture and other traumatic events.
- Shame at being detained. Some detainees will not inform their families in their country of origin as they feel that they will not believe that they have not committed a crime.
- Loss of status. Some asylum seekers are successful, educated, professional people. Adapting to detention, especially in a criminal prison, is stressful.
- A sense of guilt at having survived and escaped when other loved ones did not or are still at risk.
- Shock and anger at how they are treated on arrival in the UK. Problems of anxiety and stress are closely related to feelings of acceptance or otherwise in Britain.[15]

A pattern of initial coping, repeated attempts to seek information about the reason for detention and its likely duration, followed by a 'crash' or collapse into depression has been described in detained asylum seekers.[11]

The key protective factors that reduce the likelihood of developing mental-health problems in refugees and asylum seekers in the community are thought to be:

- contact with family members and/or family reunification
- social support and links with local community groups
- a strong religious or political ideology and
- an active problem-solving style.[16]

Range of health problems that may follow torture

Physical	Psychological
• Persistent back or shoulder pain • Aches and arthritic pain • Convulsions • Inability to walk unaided • Organ damage (eg liver, kidney, lung)	• Nightmares • Hallucinations (eg seeing apparitions of torture) • Panic attacks • Sexual problems • Phobias • Difficulty trusting people • Depressive illness/anxiety

Source: Medical Foundation for the Care of Victims of Torture. *Some Background Information.* London, 1999.

Issues affecting access to health services

- Asylum seekers may fear that consultations will not be confidential. Frequent reassurance may be required. Asylum applicants may fear that the doctor will give information about their physical or mental health to the Home Office and that this will jeopardise their chances of being allowed to stay in the UK. They may refuse health screening for this (or other) reasons.

- Experiences of individual and institutional racism may lead to a breakdown in trust, including a reluctance to trust health professionals.
- Asylum seekers and foreign nationals may have very different experiences and expectations of healthcare. They may not understand the appointments system.

What can be done to help?

All asylum seekers/immigration detainees

- Learn about what has happened in the countries from which the individuals have fled. Use this knowledge both to help establish a relationship and to understand the likely context of their distress.
- Ensure that all asylum seekers in your institution have access to information about their legal rights, legal representation and agencies providing support and assistance to detainees (see **Resources Directory** page 316).
- If you have reason to believe that an asylum seeker has been tortured, contact the Medical Foundation for the Care of Victims of Torture (see **Resources Directory** page 316). Home Office policy is to avoid detaining applicants where there is independent evidence of torture. The Medical Foundation will visit the prison to make such an assessment.
- Advocate for increased opportunities for activity, support to resolve practical problems and help in planning post-release accommodation and support before release. People recently released from detention are mentally vulnerable, especially if released to no accommodation or support.
- Ensure that relevant community groups are invited into the establishment to support asylum seekers (see **Resources Directory** page 316).
- Encourage the individual to be active and use any skills they can to play a role in helping others (eg teaching other detainees, learning English). This may raise self-esteem and help them to cope better.
- Encourage individuals to identify the strengths, resilience, skills and coping mechanisms that they have used in the past. Encourage them to use any of these that are feasible in the current situation.
- Provide a comprehensive health screening, including mental-health screening, suicidal ideation and intent, evidence of torture. Screening should occur with the consent of the asylum seeker after appropriate explanation in his/her language.

Management of acute stress reactions, sleep problems and low-level anxiety/depression

- Encourage the individual to see their experience as a normal reaction to severe stress rather than a sign of being a 'sick' or 'disordered' individual within a normal environment. Indeterminate detention is a current trauma and symptoms of distress are a normal reaction to it. Encourage them to seek support from others who have been through similar experiences.[17] Give them a copy of the leaflet *Stress and Stress Reactions* (see **Resources Directory** page 316) 📁.
- If flashbacks or painful memories are a feature, explain that this is a normal reaction to severe trauma and encourage the individual, if possible, simply to allow these thoughts to pass through his/her head and not to suppress them actively. There is some evidence that it is the suppression of the thoughts that leads to their persistence.

- Do not take somatic complaints such as indigestion at face value. They may have a psychological component (see **Unexplained somatic complaints**, page 94).
- Complementary therapies, if available, may be more culturally acceptable than medication. Shiatsu, massage, aromatherapy and herbal remedies may all be useful.
- Yoga and meditation may also be helpful and acceptable. They are widely used in the East as a means of achieving psychological and spiritual well being. Several organisations run meditation sessions in prisons (see **Resources Directory** page 316).
- See **Adjustment disorder** (page 15) for further advice.

Management of persistent post-traumatic stress disorder (PTSD)

It is important to stress that mental-health problems are not an inevitable consequence of trauma, even of severe torture. It is important to avoid diagnosing natural distress as medical pathology.[18] However, a minority of refugees will require specialised trauma services to deal with the severe, long-term psychological effects of trauma.

While the individual remains in detention, it may be helpful to do the following.

- Refer for a psychiatric assessment. A medical report can be influential in deciding what happens to a detainee.
- Provide the opportunity for individuals to talk through their experiences in their own way. This may include not talking about more extreme experiences. The recognition that certain experiences are 'there' but 'unutterable' can be positive.[19]
- Provide counselling that focuses on helping the individual cope better with their current situation and practical problems. Cognitive-behavioural approaches may be particularly appropriate if they work with the individual's own belief systems and encourage them to develop coping mechanisms.
- Encourage the individual to use existing, traditional forms of solace such as traditional healers and religious leaders.
- Provide information about specialist trauma centres for treatment after release from detention. These may be more effective once the asylum seeker's status has been settled, or at least after release from detention. Until then, the asylum seeker may feel that they remain in a traumatic situation and may be less able to move on to more detailed psychological work on their problems.

Therapy based on the retrieval and working through of memories of trauma should only be done by specialists following a culturally sensitive assessment. There is disagreement about when and for whom such therapy is appropriate. While some individuals may benefit greatly from trauma therapy, for others therapy based on the retrieval and treatment of trauma may interfere with culturally normative ways of coping with past difficulties and cause psychological deterioration.[20]

Treatment for PTSD combining antidepressants and cognitive-behavioural therapy can be effective (see **Post-traumatic stress disorder**, page 82).[21] See **Managing the interface with the NHS and other agencies** (page 149) for information about making referrals and the responsibility for funding.

Resources for patients and primary support groups

Stress and Stress Reactions: Information for Asylum Seekers

Leaflets explaining the normal effects of acute stress are available on the disk in English, Albanian, French, Spanish, Portuguese, Russian, Somali and Lingala (spoken in Zaire), and in hard copy for photocopying at the end of the book in Arabic, Tamil, Turkish and Farsi (spoken in Iraq and Afghanistan). 💾

The local Primary Care Trust (especially in London) may provide a range of specific health-promotion resources such as leaflets, posters and videos.

Many agencies are also listed in the **Resource directory** under **Ethnic minorities and foreign nationals** and **Immigration detainees** (see pages 323 and 326)

1   Patel V, Simunyu E, Gwanzura F. *Kufungisisa* (thinking too much): a Shona idiom for non-psychotic mental illness. *Central African Journal of Medicine* 1995; 41: 209–215.
2   Patel V. Spiritual distress: an indigenous concept of non-psychotic mental disorder in Harare. *Acta Psychiatrica Scandinavica* 1995; 92: 103–107.
3   Adapted from Kleinman, A. *Patients and Healers in the Context of Culture*. Berkeley: University of California Press, 1980.
4   Sartorius N, Jablensky A, Korten A *et al*. Early manifestations and first-contact incidence of schizophrenia in different cultures. *Psychological Medicine* 1986; 16: 909–928.
5   King M, Coker E, Leavey G *et al*. Incidence of psychotic illness in London: comparison of ethnic groups. *British Medical Journal* 1994; 309: 1115–1119.
6   Amnesty International. *Prisoners Without a Voice: Asylum Seekers Detained in the United Kingdom*, 2nd revd edn. London: Amnesty International British Section, 1995.
7   Home Office. *Asylum Statistics 1997*. London: Home Office, 1998.
8   Committee for the Prevention of Torture. *Report to the United Kingdom Carried out by the European Committee for the Prevention of Torture and Inhuman or Degrading Treatment or Punishment (CPT) from 15 to 31 May 1994*. Strasbourg: Council of Europe, 1996.
9   Aldous J, Bardsley M, Daniell R *et al*. *Refugee Health in London: Key Issues for Public Health*. London: Health of Londoners Project, East London & the City Health Authority, 1999.
10 Bracken P, Gorst-Unsworth C. The mental state of detained asylum seekers. *Psychiatric Bulletin* 1991; 15: 657–659.
11 Pourgourides CK, Sashidharan SP, Bracken PJ. *A Second Exile: The Mental Health Implications of Detention of Asylum Seekers in the United Kingdom*. Birmingham: Northern Birmingham Mental Health NHS Trust, 1996.
12 Davis P. Medical problems of detainees: a review of 21 ex-detainees seen in the past 2 years in Johannesburg. In Zwi AB, Saunders LD (eds), *Proceedings of the NAMDA Conference 1985, Towards Health Care for All*. Johannesburg: National Medical and Dental Association, 1985, pp. 12–18, as quoted in Pourgourides *et al.*, *A Second Exile*.
13 Medical Foundation for the Care of Victims of Torture. *A Betrayal of Hope and Trust: Detention in the UK of Survivors of Torture*. London: Medical Foundation, 1994.
14 Gorst-Unsworth C, Golderberg E. Psychological sequelae of torture and organised violence suffered by refugees from Iraq: trauma related factors compared with social factors in exile. *British Journal of Psychiatry* 1998; 172: 90–94.
15 Carey-Wood J, Duke K, Karn V, Marshall T. *The Settlement of Refugees in Britain*. Home Office Research Study No. 141. London: HMSO, 1995.
16 CVS Consultants and Migrant and Refugee Communities Forum. *A Shattered World: The Mental Health Needs of Refugees and Newly Arrived Communities*. London: CVS Consultants, 1999.
17 Manson S. Detention rehabilitation. In Seminar presentation, OASSSA Conference, South Africa, 1996, pp. 67–73, as quoted in Pourgourides *et al.*, *A Second Exile*.

18 Summerfield D. Post traumatic stress and mental health. In Symposium on Refugee Health Issues, Selby Centre, Tottenham, London, 1994.

19 Professor Papadopoulos, Tavistock Clinic Refugee Centre, personal communication, as quoted in CVS Consultants, *A Shattered World*.

20 Migrant and Refugees Community Forum. *Refugees and the Use of Mental Health Services in Kensington and Chelsea*, October 1996, as quoted in CVS Consultants, *A Shattered World*.

21 Sherman J. Effects of psychotherapeutic treatments for PTSD: a meta-analysis of controlled clinical trials. *Journal of Traumatic Stress* 1998; 11: 413–435.

Learning disability — F70

May be known internationally as 'mental retardation'

Presenting complaints

- Difficulties with peers, leading to social isolation.
- Inappropriate sexual behaviour.
- Difficulties in everyday functioning, requiring extra support (eg cleaning, working).
- Moodiness or aggression (may be referred by staff concerned about these).
- Problems with normal social development and establishing an independent life (in adulthood) or difficulties making the transition to adulthood (in adolescence).

Diagnostic features

- Slow or incomplete mental development resulting in:
  — problems with learning and
  — social adjustment problems.
- The range of severity includes:
  — severe learning disability (usually identified before 2 years of age); unable to take care of themselves or organise their lives without help
  — moderate learning disability (usually identified by age 3–5, able to do simple work with support, needs guidance or support in daily activities) and
  — mild disability (usually identified during school years; limited in schoolwork, but able to live alone and work at simple jobs).

People with mild and moderate learning disability show an overall excess of offending behaviour, mainly offences against people (generally aggressive and assaultive behaviour). Sex offences and fire-setting also occur and cause most concern. People with severe disability do not have the capacity to form intent and are not often charged with crime in respect of their antisocial behaviour.

The majority of individuals with learning disability have been detected and assessed well before leaving school. If there is any doubt about diagnosis, obtain intelligence and psychometric tests.

Differential diagnosis

The following may also interfere with performance at work or with education.
- Specific learning difficulties (eg dyslexia).
- Attention deficit disorder.
- Motor disorders (eg cerebral palsy, etc.).
- Sensory problems (eg deafness).

Diagnosis of comorbid conditions

Learning disability is associated with an increased prevalence of many other disorders. For example:
- Schizophrenia, depression and manic depression are twice as common as among the general population.
- Autism is particularly common.

- Because people with learning disability often have brain damage, the rates of epilepsy are high (25% people with learning disability, 50% of those with severe learning disability) and so are the rates of epilepsy-related mental-health problems.
- Hearing impairments (40%).
- Visual impairments (40%).
- Hypothyroidism (people with Down's syndrome).
- Dementia (people with Down's syndrome and those over 50 years of age).

People with learning disabilities are more prone to develop mental-health problems when under stress than others. They usually have fewer experiences of personal success, fewer supportive relationships and are less likely to be regarded by others with respect — all factors that protect against mental ill health.

Diagnosis of mental disorder is often overlooked as people with learning disability are prone to emotional problems, and are often changeable and moody.

Mental disorders may also present in slightly different ways.

- **Schizophrenic people** with a learning disability may not admit to hearing 'voices' and may just behave in a very disturbed, excited and bizarre way.
- **Depressed people** with learning disabilities may not be suicidal but may be very tearful and withdrawn.
- **Manic people** with learning disabilities may simply appear to be play acting or generally being silly.
- **Autism** presents as a combination of:
  — lacking a capacity to socialise with others or having little language or an odd style of speech and
  — a preoccupation or obsession with sameness
  — In prison, these individuals often earn themselves nicknames such as 'Mr Bean' or 'Mr Magoo'
  — Individuals with learning disabilities and autism are very likely to become involved in criminal behaviour.
- **Epilepsy** can affect behaviour in many ways. For example, people with epilepsy may:
  — become irritable, on edge or even aggressive before having a fit and
  — become confused, and this might also lead to aggression
  For a variety of reasons — including the fact that people with learning disability in prison might not comply with medication — these problems are quite common.
- Irritability may be an indication of pain or emotional distress.

Support and advice for the patient

- People with a learning disability frequently underreport illnesses. Arranging regular health screening can be useful actively to seek out treatable sensory disorders, depression, obesity, skin infections, diabetes and other conditions. It is valuable to review care also at times of transition (eg before release or transfer to another prison).
- Encourage the patient to see the same doctor at every appointment, if possible, in order to build trust and reduce problems in communication. Staff who know the patient well are invaluable as informants.
- If the patient becomes depressed, it is helpful to review the social networks and support in addition to other treatment (see **Depression — F32#**, page 47).

Advice and information for prison officers and other staff 💾

- People with learning disability need a structure and daily routine. Left to themselves, they do not have the capacity to organise themselves. Help them form a plan for getting out of bed, doing useful work and having adult education. They may need different sorts of activities to be available during association (eg manual jobs, drawing, simple puzzles, painting by numbers). They will also need help with writing letters to those outside prison.
- Inform the residential officers, teachers and workshop supervisors, as appropriate, of any visual or hearing difficulty the individual has.
- Consider asking one or more reliable prisoners on the Residential Unit who may agree to mentor the individual to help him/her to avoid problems with other inmates.
- Reward effort. Allow the individual to function at the highest level of their ability at education, work and on the unit.
- Watch out for exploitation of the individual by others. People with learning disability like to please others by agreeing with them. They are easily duped by more dominant people and may be 'taxed' (encouraged to 'give' tobacco, food or possessions to others) or be victims of theft. They commonly get into debt without understanding that loans are expected to be repaid and may also engage in criminal behaviour at the direction of others. In prison, a fit, young adult with learning disabilities might be used as a 'hit man' for others. A less assertive adult with learning disabilities can easily become a victim of sexual abuse. If exploitation is identified, consider removing the aggressors or placing them on an antibullying regime. If the aggressors cannot be identified, consider protective relocation of the individual.
- People with learning disability have poor concentration and often do not understand what has been said to them the first time or pick things up as well as others. Be aware that what may seem to be non-compliance with instructions may just mean that they have not understood what is required of them.

Medication

- Learning disabilities may occur with other disorders that require medical treatment (eg seizures, spasticity and psychiatric illness such as depression).
- Unnecessary medication should be avoided, and medication reviewed regularly, as side-effects and idiosyncratic reactions are common. People with learning disabilities underreport side-effects, so consideration should be given to proactive checks (eg blood levels for anticonvulsants).

Referral

For court purposes

A remanded prisoner may need an appropriate adult or an expert in learning disability to represent them or comment on the special circumstances of the case in court. Liaise with the court to ensure that all parties can agree a time schedule for legal processes.

For routine care planning

Most individuals with learning disability who come into prison will already be well known to their general practitioner and local, specialist learning disability team.

Involve these routinely, with the individual's permission, in order to devise and implement an appropriate care plan in the prison.

To obtain assessments and initiate contact with specialist teams

Where the individual does not already have contact with a specialist learning disability service, contact should be established (either with the service in their catchment area or the service local to the prison) and an assessment requested for:
- any individual where autism is suspected (they do not cope well with prison life) and
- all inmates with a learning disability (IQ < 70) when they first come into prison, especially if they also have epilepsy.

To assess recent changes

Consult with the specialist learning disability team.
- Urgently if the individual's behaviour becomes disturbed or odd in the prison.
- Non-urgently following the death of a close relative, as there is increased risk of pathological grief.
- Where there is significant weight change that persists for longer than 1 month to exclude emotional or psychiatric disorder.

Prerelease planning

Arrange follow-up care for all with an IQ < 70, if possible, well before release. Where a young person is below school-leaving age, a transition plan can be requested from the social services for when the young person leaves school, whether or not the child has a statement of special educational need.

Structures to support liaison and referral

Satisfactory liaison with other services is more difficult to achieve on an ad-hoc basis, and for prisons with a local catchment there should be established structures to facilitate liaison and referral. It is recommended that each prison forge links with local learning disability and mental-health services. It may also be possible to develop a nurse-led epilepsy clinic with protocols agreed by the local epilepsy team.

Resources for patients and primary support groups

Down's Syndrome Association: 020 8682 4001

Mencap: 020 7454 0454

Mencap Northern Ireland: 02890 6911351, 0345 636227 (family advisory service)

National Autistic Society: 020 7833 2299, 020 7903 3555 (helpline)

SPOD (Association to Aid the Sexual and Personal Relationships of People with a Disability): 020 7607 8851

Respond: 020 7383 0700
(Services for adults with learning disabilities who have been or may have been sexually abused)

Leaflets:
Learning Disability – information for Prison Officers and other staff 💾

Depression in People with a Learning Disability. Free and available from the Royal College of Psychiatrists. Tel: 020 7235 2351

Learning Disabilities and the Family: The Teenager with a Severe Learning Disability. Available from the Mental Health Foundation. Tel: 020 7535 7400

'Books Beyond Words' is a series of picture books for adolescents and adults who cannot read. They may be used by parents, carers, general practitioners, nurses and staff to help communication about important topics. Titles include: *Feeling Blue* (about depression), *You're On Trial, I Can Get Through It* (the story of a woman who is abused), *Going to the Doctor, Going into Hospital, When Dad Died* and *Making Friends.* Available for £10.00 each from: Royal College of Psychiatrists, 17 Belgrave Square, London SW1X 8PG. Tel: 020 7235 2351 ext. 146

The guideline was based on information provided by Dr Gregory O'Brien, Dr E. Milne, Mr Paul Thornton and Graham English from Northgate and Prodhoe NHS Trust, Morpeth, Northumberland.

Helping victims of sexual assault

Although most victims of sexual assault do not develop a chronic mental disorder, it is associated with mental-health disturbance in a significant minority. Patients who disclose sexual assaults may be referring to either recent or more remote events. The level of distress apparent and the treatment needs differ depending on how recently the assault occurred and whether there is a risk of the assault being repeated.

This guideline focuses on recent assault. For information about the impact of abuse in the past, see **People who disclose that they were abused as children** (page 271).

Three per cent of women and 1% of men report being the victim of forced sexual attention during their prison sentence in England and Wales, though the nature of that forced attention is not known.[1] Rates of past sexual assault are almost certainly higher, with about one in three female prisoners and just under one in 10 male prisoners reporting having suffered some form of sexual abuse at some time in their lives. Rates in refugees, illegal immigrants and those seeking asylum may also be high, as sexual assault is a frequent part of torture. Common reasons for not reporting sexual assaults include: fears of not being believed, feelings of shame and fears of being considered unmanly or homosexual.

Presenting complaints

The patient may seek help for the following.
- Sleep problems.
- Generalised anxiety.
- Self-injury.
- Depressive symptoms.
- Vague but troublesome somatic symptoms.

Clinical features

Short-term effects of recent sexual assault

An acute stress reaction is a normal, understandable reaction to the trauma of sexual assault. In the days or weeks following the assault, the patient may experience the following.
- Feelings of panic, fear of danger, of being alone or a similar event happening again.
- Sleep problems, including getting to sleep, waking in the middle of the night, dreams or nightmares.
- Physical symptoms, such as tense muscles, trembling or shaking, diarrhoea or constipation, nausea, loss of appetite, headaches, sweating or tiredness.
- Preoccupation with the assault and why it happened.
- Being easily startled by loud noises or sudden movements.
- Loss of interest in usual activities.
- Tearfulness or feelings of loss or loneliness.
- Problems with thinking, concentration or remembering things.
- Shock or disbelief, feeling numb, unreal, isolated or detached from other people.

- Guilt and self-blame for having in some way caused or brought on the assault.
- Anger and irritability.

Recovery from serious trauma, such as sexual assault as an adult, occurs in the majority of people. In over half of those assaulted as adults, the most acute symptoms resolved within 4–6 weeks, with other symptoms reducing within 3–4 months.[2]

Long-term effects of sexual assault

In a substantial minority of patients, however, common longer-term effects may include the following.

- Self-injury — in both men and women.
- Alcohol misuse.
- Drug misuse.
- Depression: symptoms include retardation, guilt, feelings of worthlessness, hopelessness or suicidal ideation of a severity or duration that significantly interferes with the individual's functioning.
- Generalised anxiety and phobic anxiety.
- Post-traumatic stress disorder (PTSD): symptoms may include re-experiencing the assault, avoidance and hyperarousal.
- Behavioural disturbance.
- Sexual dysfunction (eg erectile dysfunction, loss of libido).

See the relevant guidelines for advice on the management of these conditions.

Essential information for the patient and the primary support group

- Traumatic or life-threatening events often have psychological effects. For the majority, symptoms will subside with support.
- For those who continue to experience symptoms, effective treatments are available.
- Experiencing psychological symptoms after a sexual assault is a reflection of the severity of the trauma; it is not a sign of weakness and does not mean that the individual has 'gone mad'.
- It is not uncommon for men as well as women to be victims of sexual assault. Most male rapes are committed by heterosexual men against heterosexual men or boys, motivated by the desire to hurt and humiliate rather than by simple sexual gratification.

Confidentiality

Explain to the patient the rules of confidentiality in accordance with medical ethics, prison rules and any guidance from your own profession but, if need be, explain the need to break aspects of confidence to protect young people under 18 who are vulnerable. If a current risk to a child is identified (either the patient or another young person), the overriding principle is to secure the best interests of that child (see **Child protection**, page 276).

Advice and support for the patient and the primary support group

- **Ensure the patient is safe from repeated assault.** If the patient alleges sexual assault while in prison, consider a change of location, the use of antibullying procedure and ways in which the patient can extricate him/herself from risk situations. Liaise as appropriate with wing staff (with patient permission).

- **Check the patient's physical and medical needs** where appropriate. Offer a full physical examination, including investigations for HIV and other sexually transmitted diseases. (Consider tests for gonorrhoea, *Chlamydia*, syphilis, *Trichomonas vaginalis* infection, HIV and hepatitis B. Consider prophylaxis for hepatitis B and chlamydial, gonococcal and trichomonal infections and also HIV — if the perpetrator is known to have HIV or is at high risk for HIV. Exams may be repeated at 2 and 12 weeks after the assault[3]).

- **Support the patient in reporting the assault to the police**, if appropriate. Explore whether the patient wishes to report the assault to the police. A full physical examination carried out by a police surgeon is required if the patient wishes to make a complaint to the police about a current assault. Explain that since the Public Order and Criminal Justice Act 1994, there have been prosecutions and convictions for male rape. Explain that if the crime is reported to the police without avoidable delay, he/she may be eligible for criminal injuries' compensation whether or not the perpetrator is charged or prosecuted. Respect the patient's choices.

- **Listen sympathetically** without judging or pushing for details. Acknowledge the strength and validity of feelings of shame, anger and humiliation. Be aware that some people deal with trauma by not talking about it. Patients may become worse if pushed to talk more about the assault than they are ready to.[4]

- **If you do not have time to listen now**, say that you appreciate the importance of the patient's experience and feelings, and make a definite appointment when you (or another person acceptable to the patient such as nurse, counsellor or chaplain) will be available.

- **Gently challenge distorted beliefs**, eg culpability for the assault. Explain that following a sexual assault, victims frequently blame themselves, feeling that they must have done something to attract the assailant.

- **Encourage appropriate coping methods.** Ask about the methods the patient is using to cope with his/her feelings. Explain that some methods such as substance misuse, self-injury, increased aggression, destructiveness and disobedience are likely to make things worse. Encourage the patient to take care of him/herself by, for example, taking up self-defence or assertiveness training if available.[5] Suggest returning to work, having regular exercise and using opportunities for education or creative expression.

- **Assess the risk of suicide.** Ask a series of questions about suicidal ideas, intent and plans (eg Has the patient often thought of death or dying? Does he/she have a specific suicide plan? Has he/she made serious suicide attempts in the past? Can the patient be sure not to act on suicidal ideas?). Ask about risk of harm to others (see **Assessing and managing people at risk of suicide**, page 204).

- **Assess the risk of violence** to the alleged perpetrator, if appropriate (see 'Assessing the risk of violence' in **Aggression**, page 282).

- **Encourage the use of social support.** Is there a friend, family member, listener or officer in whom the patient can confide? If so, with patient permission, offer information to that person to help them respond appropriately.

Medication

Most acute stress reactions will resolve without the use of medication. If severe anxiety symptoms occur, however, consider using anti-anxiety drugs for up to

3 days. If the patient has severe insomnia, use hypnotic drugs for up to 3 days. Doses should be as low as possible (see *BNF*, Sections 4.1.1 and 4.1.2).

See depression and PTSD for medication for these conditions.

Referral

Referral should be in accordance with recommendations for particular, associated mental disorders. Consider treatment if acute symptoms interfere significantly with everyday functioning and if these are not diminishing 4–8 weeks after the assault.

Treatments for symptoms of PTSD following sexual assault that have shown some effectiveness[N6] include the following.

- Supportive counselling.
- Cognitive-behavioural therapy (brief behavioural intervention programmes, stress inoculation training, exposure therapy and imaginal exposure).
- Psychodynamic psychotherapy.

For general support and where symptoms do not meet the criteria for a mental disorder, consider recommending voluntary/non-statutory counselling. Rape crisis centres may provide a counselling service for women.

Resources for patients and primary support groups

Chaplain, listeners, personal officer

London Rape Crisis Centre: 020 7837 1600 (national crisisline: Monday–Friday, 6 pm–10 pm, weekends, 10 am–10 pm)

Samaritans: 08457 909090
(Support by listening for those feeling lonely, despairing or suicidal. It also has local helplines and branches across the country)

Survivors UK: 020 7613 0808 (Tuesday, 7 pm–10 pm); 07949 994886 (office: Monday–Friday, 9:30 am–5:30 pm); URL: http://www.survivorsuk.co.uk
(Counselling and group support for male victims of sexual assault and abuse. It is available in most parts of the UK)

UK Register of Counsellors: 08704 435232
PO Box 1050, Rugby CV21 2HZ
(Supplies names and addresses of British Association of Counsellors and Psychotherapists [BACP]-accredited counsellors)

Victim Support Supportline: 0845 30 30 900 (Monday–Friday, 9 am–9 pm; weekends, 9 am–7 pm)
(Emotional and practical support for victims of crime, including help with Criminal Injury Compensation Board claims. It provides support to female and male victims of sexual assault. It does not usually offer long-term counselling or deal with severe psychiatric problems beyond the immediate crisis)

Resource leaflet:
Stress and Stress Reactions

[1] Singleton N, Meltzer H, Gatward R, Coid J, Deasy D. *Psychiatric Morbidity among Prisoners.* London: Office for National Statistics, 2000.

[2] Steketee G, Foa EB. Rape victims: post traumatic stress responses and their treatment: a review of the literature. *Journal of Anxiety Disorders* 1987; 1: 69–86.

[3] Greifinger RB, Glaser J. Desmoteric medicine and the public's health. In Puisis M, *Clinical Practice in Correctional Medicine.* St Louis: Mosby, 1998.

[4] Wessely S, Rose S, Bisson J. *Brief Psychological Interventions ('Debriefing') for Treating Immediate Trauma-related Symptoms and Preventing Post Traumatic Stress Disorder.* Oxford: Cochrane Database of Neurotic Disorders, 1997.

[5] Anderson CL. Males as sexual assault victims: multiple levels of trauma. In Gonsiorek JC (ed.), *A Guide to Psychotherapy with Gay and Lesbian Clients.* New York: Harrington Park, 1985.

[6] Most available research focuses on the treatment of post-traumatic stress disorder symptoms in women who have been sexually assaulted. Stress inoculation, supportive counselling and prolonged exposure therapy are all significantly more effective in reducing symptoms of anxiety and depression than waiting list controls at 3 months. Stress inoculation may be particularly helpful where there is persistent fear but not avoidance. Imaginal exposure and eye movement desensitisation and reprocessing (EMDR) are emerging as effective treatments. Psychodynamic therapy is little researched but may be appropriate for a victim of a violent sexual assault that triggers a response to a previous episode of childhood victimisation. Specific behavioural treatments may be helpful for sexual dysfunction: (a) Foa EB, Rothbaum BO, Riggs DS *et al.* Treatment of post traumatic stress disorder in rape victims: a comparison between cognitive behavioural procedures and counselling. *Journal of Consulting and Clinical Psychology* 1991; 59: 715–723; (b) Foa EB, Herst-Ikeda D, Perry KJ. The evaluation of a brief cognitive behavioural programme for the prevention of chronic post traumatic stress disorder in recent assault victims. *Journal of Consulting and Clinical Psychology* 1995; 63: 948–955; (c) Tarrier N, Pilgrim H, Sommerfield C *et al.* A randomized trial of cognitive therapy and imaginal exposure in the treatment of chronic post traumatic stress disorder. *Journal of Consulting and Clinical Psychology* 1999; 67: 13–18; (d) Rothbaum B. A controlled study of eye movement desensitization and reprocessing for post traumatic stress disordered sexual assault victims. *Bulletin of the Meuninger Clinic* 1997; 61: 317–334; (e) Brom D, Kleber RJ, Defares PB. Brief psychotherapy for post traumatic stress disorders. *Journal of Consulting and Clinical Psychology* 1989; 57: 607–612; (f) Becker JV, Skinner LJ. Assessment and treatment of rape related sexual dysfunctions. *Clinical Psychologist* 1983; 36: 102–105.

Women who have experienced domestic violence

Introduction

Domestic violence is a common previous experience of imprisoned women. It includes physical violence, such as beating, hitting, forcibly restraining or rape, and emotional or psychological abuse, such as constant criticism, intimidation or threatening future physical violence. Most women who suffer domestic violence are in danger of further violence[1] and are at increased risk of developing a mental disorder. Children living in the family are also at risk of abuse and resulting physical and mental-health problems. The prevalence of domestic violence is similar among people of all income levels and all ethnic backgrounds.

Although imprisoned women are at least temporarily safe from their abusers, without appropriate interventions and reasonable alternatives many women return to the same setting they left. It is important for prison healthcare workers to know about domestic violence in order to:

- be aware of it as an important factor in the mental health of the women they treat

- be able to give appropriate information and support to patients who disclose that they are in violent relationships and

- consider incorporating domestic violence within any out-patient mental-health programme set-up within the establishment to help abused women.

It would, in any event, be valuable for all healthcare centres in female prison establishments to display information about domestic violence. This might act as a signal to women that they can talk to health workers about this issue. The Home Office leaflet *Breaking the Chain* might be used (see **Resources Directory** page 316). A sample copy is provided on the disk.

Effects of domestic violence on mental health

Domestic violence is frequently persistent. Psychological effects may include the following.

- Loss of confidence.
- Low self-esteem.
- Fear.
- Self blame, shame and guilt.
- Anger — unfocused or directed.
- Decreased concentration.
- Eating and sleeping problems.
- Feeling of hopelessness.
- Social withdrawal.
- Feeling of helplessness and passivity.

The following disorders are more common in women who suffer domestic violence than those who do not.

- Substance misuse (see **Alcohol misuse** and **Drug misuse**, pages 18 and 55).

- **Depression** (see page 47).
- **Anxiety disorders** (see **Generalised anxiety**, **Phobias** and **Panic**, pages 64, 79 and 67).
- **Post-traumatic stress disorder (PTSD)** (see page 82). Symptoms may include re-experiencing assaults, avoidance and hyperarousal.
- **Self-injury** (see page 211).

See the relevant guidelines for advice on the management of these conditions.

Management when a woman discloses domestic violence

Essential information for the patient and the primary support group

- Domestic violence affects all kinds of women; it often continues and becomes more severe with time.
- Domestic violence is illegal; offenders can be prosecuted. Even if the perpetrator is not prosecuted under criminal law, some protection may be possible through civil law, by injunctions and court orders.
- Continuing violence may severely affect your health and that of your children.
- There are ways to remove yourself and your children from danger.
- Living with violence usually has psychological effects. This is normal and is not a sign of weakness or madness. For the majority, symptoms will subside with support when the violence is no longer happening. For those who continue to experience symptoms, effective treatments are available.

Be aware that the patient may be in prison herself because of retaliatory violence against her abuser or because of violence to her own children.

Advice and support for the patient and the primary support group

- Listen sympathetically without judging. Acknowledge the strength and validity of feelings of shame, fear or anger. Explain that victims frequently blame themselves as they may find it hard to understand how a loved one can behave in this way and may assume that they themselves must have done something to provoke the violence. Gently challenge distorted beliefs.
- Emphasise confidentiality and that you will seek the woman's consent before sharing information with other health- or socialcare professionals. However, explain that if it is believed that children are at risk of significant harm, you will need to follow child-protection guidelines (see **Child protection**, page 276).
- Help the woman assess the risk that she and any children face. Assess the physical and psychological risks. The greater the risk, the more need there is for structured help to be offered. Consider together the type of abuse, whether any violence has increased in intensity, frequency and severity, whether children are being harmed, the woman's current fears, and the outcome of any previous recent attempts to get help.
- Explore with the woman the options open to her, the sources of support she may be able to call upon and the risks involved in each option. The safety of the woman and any dependent children is the paramount consideration. Reassure her that her children will not be taken into care simply because she leaves her partner. (Some abusers threaten that this will happen.) Point out that it is not uncommon for women to find it difficult to leave despite continued violence. Women who leave their partners, however, can face an increased risk of assault.[2] Respect her choices:

— If the woman decides to return home, do not criticise her decision. She may not wish to leave her partner, may be worried about financial support and accommodation or may not yet be ready to deal with the situation. Give her information about the help available and help her to plan an escape route in an emergency (money and important documents, such as passport and bank book, should be kept in a safe place).[2,3]

— If the woman does not wish to return home, support her in seeking emergency accommodation (see **Resources** below).

• Provide information about domestic violence helplines and emergency women's shelters (see **Resources** below). Encourage the patient to seek help, preferably before release. The prison or home Probation Service may be helpful, but patient consent must be obtained and extra care taken to ensure that nothing is done that could alert the perpetrator to the fact that the woman has taken this course of action.

• While in prison, encourage and, if possible, facilitate access to opportunities for work, creative expression, spiritual counselling or other means of increasing self-esteem. Assertiveness classes may be helpful.

• Consider, if appropriate, parenting classes that help teach alternatives to violence in child rearing.

Record-keeping

Evidence of domestic violence, including the effects on mental health, may be important in helping an abused woman to obtain protection through an injunction or court order, in opposing an immigration/deportation case and may be used by family courts to assess the possible risks in granting access to children to a violent parent. Although prison healthcare staff are unlikely to see the immediate physical effects of domestic violence, they should:

• document clearly the content of the consultation(s), the nature of abuse and any action taken and

• take additional care to ensure the confidentiality of the medical record.

Medication and referral

See the guidelines for relevant disorders.

Developing services in your establishment

Many local areas have multi-agency domestic violence strategies, including protocols and training programmes. Contact the Primary Care Trust/Local Health Group in the first instance to discuss involvement.

NHS and prison health services in female establishments may wish to consider, in response to the needs assessment exercise, including a clinical component focused on recovery from abuse and trauma within the mental-health programme. Models for such services can be found in the Canadian Federally Sentenced Women's Survivors of Abuse & Trauma Program and in some US prisons (see 'The Correctional Program strategy for federally sentenced women' for further information. URL: http://www.csc-scc.gc.ca).

Where active identification of women suffering domestic violence is considered, evidence suggests that routine questioning is likely to be superior to case-finding approaches.[4] Where a screening programme in which all women are routinely asked about domestic violence is set up, it is important that the following factors are in place.

- An explanation to the women that the same inquiry is being made of all women because domestic violence is widespread and often hidden.
- Use of validated screening questions and tools. Most such tools have been developed in the USA. The Department of Health *Resource Manual*[5] contains a suggested screening questionnaire.
- Protocols for referral to appropriate support services.
- Training for staff in the use of the enquiry tools, interview techniques and responding appropriately.

Resources for patients and primary support groups

Domestic Violence Unit or Community Safety Unit: (contact the local police for details)

Everyman Project: 020 7737 6747 (as a helpline: Tuesday and Thursday, 7:30 pm–10 pm; as an office number: Monday, Wednesday and Friday, 10 am–2 pm) 40 Stockwell Road, Stockwell, London SW9 9ES
(Helpline for anyone concerned about a man's violence. Counselling by appointment for men who want to stop their violent and abusive behaviour)

URL: http://www.womensaid.org.uk
(Provides information, local refuge contact details and sources of help for women experiencing domestic violence)

Kiran — Asian Women's Aid: 020 8558 1986
PO Box 899, London E11 1AA
(Advice, support and refuge accommodation for Asian women experiencing domestic violence. It can provide staff fluent in Urdu, Hindi, Punjabi and Bengali)

Muslim Women's Helpline: 020 8904 8193/8908 6715 (Monday–Friday, 10 am–4 pm); 020 8908 3205 (administration)
(Culturally appropriate emotional support over the telephone for Muslim women. Information and advice on domestic violence, sexual abuse, marital problems and health and bereavement; referrals to other services)

Refuge: 0870 599 5443 (24-hour, 7 days per week helpline); 020 7395 7700/7712 (administration)
(National domestic violence helpline offering counselling, support, and advice for women and children escaping domestic violence. Network of refuges across the UK)

Rights of Women (England, Wales and Northern Ireland): 020 7251 6577 (adviceline); 020 7251 6575 (administration)
52–54 Featherstone Street, London EC1Y 8RT
(Telephone legal advice for women, mainly in the field of family law, also sexual violence, debt, housing and employment. Referrals to other agencies and sympathetic solicitors)

Shelterline: 0808 800 4444 (24 hours)
(Emergency access to refuge services)

Women's Aid Federation England: 08457 023468 (24-hour, 7 days per week helpline); 0117 944 4411 (administration)
PO Box 391, Bristol BS99 7WS
(Helpline for women experiencing physical, emotional or sexual violence in the home. Advice, information and referral)

Victim Support Line: 0845 3030900
PO Box 11431, London SW9 6ZH

Victim Support National Office: 020 7735 9166
Cranmer House, 39 Brixton Road, London SW9 6DZ

Victim Support Northern Ireland: 028 9024 4039
Annsgate House, 70/74 Ann Street, Belfast BT1 4EH

Victim Support Scotland: 0131 668 4486
15/23 Hardwell Close, Edinburgh EH8 9RX

Leaflet:
Domestic Violence: Break the Chain. It is provided on the disk 💾 and is also available from: Home Office Marketing and Communications Group, Room 157, 50 Queen Anne's Gate, London SW1H 9AT. Tel: 0870 241 4680; Fax: 020 7 273 2568; E-mail: homeoffice@prolog.uk.com

Resources for health professionals

Health I. *Domestic Violence: The General Practitioner's Role*. London: Royal College of General Practitioners, 1998

Laurent C. *Domestic Violence: The Role of the Community Nurse*. London: Community Practitioners and Health Visitors Association, 1998

British Medical Association. *Domestic Violence: A Health Care Issue*. London: BMA, 1998

Department of Health. *Domestic Violence: A Resource Manual for Health Care Professionals*. London: Department of Health, 2000. Available free from: Department of Health, PO Box 77, London SE1 6XH. URL: URL: http://www.doh.gov.uk

'Multi-agency guidance for addressing domestic violence'. URL: http://www.homeoffice.gov.uk

'The Correctional Program strategy for federally sentenced women'. URL: http://www.csc-scc.gc.ca

1   Yearnshire S. Analysis of cohort. In Bewley S, Friend J, Mezey G (eds). *Violence Against Women*. London: Royal College of Obstetricians and Gynaecologists, 1997. Reports that on average a woman will be assaulted by her partner or ex-partner 35 times before reporting it to the police.
2   Health I. *Domestic Violence: The General Practitioner's Role*. London: Royal College of General Practitioners, 1998.
3   Laurent C. *Domestic Violence: The Role of the Community Nurse*. London: Community Practitioners and Health Visitors Association, 1998.

[4] Davidson L, King V, Garcia J, Marchant S. What role can the health service plan? In Taylor-Browne J (ed.), *Reducing Domestic Violence: What Works?* London: Home Office Research, Development and Statistics Directorate, 2000.
[5] Department of Health. *Domestic Violence: A Resource Manual for Health Care Professionals.* London: Department of Health, 2000.

Responding to individuals who disclose that they have been abused as children

Many people in prison have been abused, physically, sexually or emotionally, as children. (Figures for sexual abuse range from 5.3% of the general male population,[1] to 15–30% of the general female population, to 42.5% of women detained in special hospitals.[2]) About one in three female prisoners and just under one in 10 male prisoners report having suffered sexual abuse at some time in their lives.[3] The effects can be long-lasting and may manifest in adulthood in disturbed relationships and behaviour, including self-injury.

During consultations for other matters, health workers may find that individuals tell them that they have been abused. The purpose of this section is to enable healthcare workers to respond appropriately and supportively, not to initiate enquiry and not to provide abuse counselling. Counselling/ psychotherapy that helps individuals explore and deal with childhood abuse requires training, a safe and structured environment, and time. Opening issues without the time to deal with them may distress the individual further. If the individual is a young offender who claims that they have been recently abused at home or in their school or children's home, action must be taken to prevent further abuse.

Effects of childhood abuse

Being abused as a child does not automatically condemn a person to a disturbed and disturbing adulthood and it is not itself a mental disorder. However, a proportion of abused children reach adulthood with major emotional problems and dysfunctional personalities. Abuse as a child is associated with the following.

- A sense of helplessness, feelings of vulnerability, a sensitivity to shaming and humiliation, and a difficulty in asking for help.
- Loss of confidence; problems being assertive, difficulties with trust.
- Self-harming behaviour (see **Assessment and management following an act of self-harm**, page 211).
- Aggression and an increased risk of abusing others (some abused children identify with the aggressor).
- Depression, despair and suicidal thoughts (see **Depression**, page 47).
- Substance abuse (see **Alcohol misuse** and **Drug misuse**, pages 18 and 55).
- Relationship difficulties in all areas of life and very disturbed behaviour, consistent with personality disorder (see **Personality disorder**, page 70).
- Eating disorders (see **Eating disorders**, page 60).

The person who is abused sexually may suffer **in addition** from the following.
- Problems with sexual identity.
- Confusion about what sexual behaviours are appropriate.
- Difficulty in describing their experiences. They may experience guilt and self-blame and become very distressed.

See the relevant guideline for advice on managing associated mental disorders.

Action to take initially

- **Listen sympathetically** without judging or asking for details (**unless** there is good reason to believe that another young person is still being abused or is at immediate risk of abuse, in which case ask for more details but refrain from judging).
- **Reduce self-blame.** Explain that some people who have been abused may feel that they are to blame if they did not tell the abuser not to do it or if they did not tell anyone. This is not true. Adults are the powerful ones who are responsible for looking after and protecting children. Children do not have the power to resist overtures and are not to blame for them. Reiterate this whenever blame of self occurs.
- **Explain the rules of confidentiality** in accordance with medical ethics, prison rules and any guidance from your own profession but, if need be, explain the need to break aspects of confidence to protect children who are vulnerable.
- **Ensure that the patient is safe** and does not return to the situation or people where the alleged abuse occurred.
- **Assess the risk of suicide and self-harm.** Ask a series of questions about suicidal ideas, intent and plans (eg has the patient often thought of death or dying? Does the patient have a specific suicide plan? Has he/she made serious suicide attempts in the past? Can the patient be sure not to act on suicidal ideas?). Ask about risk of harm to others (see **Assessing and managing people at risk of suicide**, page 204).
- **Assess the risk of violence** to the perpetrator of abuse, if appropriate (see 'Assessing the risk of violence' in **Aggression**, page 282).
- **Obtain support.** Ensure the individual knows to whom he/she can go for help and support within the institution (eg listener, befriender, chaplain, personal officer) and how to access that support. Explain the sort of support on offer, ie emotional support when the individual is feeling low, help with current practical problems, rather than exploration of the past abuse.
- **Plan activities.** Try to arrange an appropriate plan that offers meaningful activity, study, creativity or work, so time to brood is limited and self-worth may be boosted.

Considering the possible cultural implications

There may be serious cultural or religious problems arising from admitting or being subject to abuse. Examples include:

- The family may regard any abuse, however it occurred, as bringing shame upon the family. Liaison with the family may not be straightforward.
- Because of the shame attached to abuse, the individual may self-harm and then experience added shame if suicide is not acceptable in their religion (eg Muslims). The individual may then feel cut off from the support of their faith community. Care may need to be taken in liaising with religious leaders.

If at all concerned, consult the chaplain. The Local Authority's race relations officer may be helpful. Voluntary agencies that specialise in helping people from particular cultural or religious groups are listed in the **Resource directory** (page 316).

Child protection

Child-protection issues arise:

- if the patient is under 18 years of age and claims that they have been abused at home, school or in a children's home. If they return, they risk being abused again

- if the patient fears that a younger sibling, relative or other child is at risk or is suffering abuse and
- if the patient is an adult, the abuser is still alive and the patient reveals details indicating that a specific child is being abused or is at risk of abuse.

See **Child protection** (page 276).

Arranging therapy, counselling or self-help support

- Explain that many people who have been abused come to terms over time with what has happened to them and regain control of their lives. Contact with others who have had the same experience may be helpful, if this is available (see below). There are several books that can be helpful, eg in enabling the individual to see that their reactions are normal and to feel less alone (see below).
- Be aware that the effects of childhood abuse can be severely disabling with long-lasting effects on the development of the personality, for which the treatment is long-term, specialist psychotherapy. Except where long-term support can be offered to the patient, and especially in the context of remand or a short sentence, appropriate types of help will encourage the patient to focus on the present, and help him/her deal with current problems, for which solutions may be possible, for example:
  — relaxation techniques may be helpful for anxiety
  — self-assertiveness classes may help with self-destructive passivity
  — anger management may help an individual channel their anger constructively and
  — counselling focused on learning coping skills, such as gaining control of intrusive imagery and compartmentalising experiences rather than on the abuse itself, may help reduce immediately disturbing symptoms.
- Treatments for abused adolescents include group work, family therapy and cognitive-behaviour therapy focused on traumatic responses.[4]

If these interventions are not available in prison or the individual is not in the prison long enough to benefit from them, try to ensure that the sentence plan or prerelease plan includes information for the individual about agencies in the community that may provide both support (eg survivors' groups) and long-term therapy.

Developing in-prison resources

- Some individuals will need long-term help either in prison or after release. Consider building into the service agreement with mental-health services' help making appropriate referrals for therapy following release or, where sentences are long, the provision of some long-term psychotherapy in the prison.
- Consider organising a 'Survivors of Abuse' mutual support group, perhaps facilitated by an external counsellor or therapist from a voluntary organisation. For women's prisons, local rape crisis centres (see **Resources Directory** page 316) may have counsellors with special training in working with women who have been sexually abused as children. Issues to consider in setting up such a group include the training of the facilitator, how confidentiality and child-protection issues will be handled, the time commitment required from participants, the focus of the group (groups should aim to help participants regain some sense of control, feel less alone and learn skills for coping with their present feelings) and the provision for support for participants who need it between sessions and after the group ends.
- Develop a library of literature to lend to patients (see **Resources** below).

Resources for patients and primary support groups

Breaking Free: 020 8648 3500 (helpline)
Suite 23–25 Marshall House, 124 Middleton Road, Morden SM4 6RW
(Support and information by telephone and letter primarily for women.
Information and referral service for men and women. Some face-to-face group
support sessions)

Childwatch: 01482 325552 (national helpline: Monday–Friday, 9:30 am–4 pm)
206 Hessle Road, Hull HU3 3BE
(Telephone and face-to-face counselling for adults who have been abused as
children and for their families)

London Rape Crisis Centre: 020 7837 1600 (national helpline: Monday–Friday,
6 pm–10 pm; Saturday and Sunday, 10 am–10 pm)
PO Box 69, London WC1X 9JN
(For women and girls who have been raped or sexually abused, and for their
friends, families and for professionals. Also provides information about local
self-help groups and face-to-face counselling services)

Men as Survivors Helpline (MASH): 0117 9077100 (Thursday, 7–9 pm)
c/o Victim Support, 36 Dean Lane, Bedminster, Bristol BS1 1BS

Reach Out: 020 8905 4501
(For men and women who have suffered abuse as children)

Respond: 020 7383 0700
(Services for adults with learning disabilities who have been, or may have been,
sexually abused)

Survivors UK: 020 7833 3737

Youth Access: 020 8772 9900
(Provides information and advice for young people and the names of counsellors
in local areas)

Videos and books may be available via your Health Authority Health Promotion
Unit or Prism (for addresses, see page 316)

Video:
To a Safer Place. National Film Board of Canada, 1987. 58 minutes. Available
from: Educational Media, 235 Imperial Drive, Rayners Lane, Harrow HA2 7HE.
Tel: 020 8868 1908/1915. Documents the journey of an adult survivor of sexual
abuse. All participants are white. It has a very positive message about recovery
and can be useful in explaining the healing process to adolescents. Suitable for
adults and teenagers

The Survivors' Directory. Manchester: Broadcasting Support Services. Available
from: Broadcasting Support Services, Westminster House, 11 Portland Street,
Manchester M1 3HU. Tel: 0161 455 1212. £9.00. Produces a resource directory to
unfunded groups and individuals

Helen Kennerley. *Overcoming Childhood Trauma: A Self-help Guide Using Cognitive
Behavioural Techniques.* London: Constable & Robinson, 2000. Available from:
MIND, 15–19 Broadway, London E15 4BQ. Tel: 020 8519 2122. Useful for helpers
as well as those who have experienced childhood abuse. Covers all kinds of
abuse, including physical and emotional. Helpful section on building short-term
coping strategies

L Arnold. *Hurting Inside: A Book for Young People*. 1988 Abergavenny Basement Project
Available for £3.50 from: Basement Project, PO Box 5, Abergavenny NP7 5XW. Tel: 01873 856524. Aims to help young people tackle difficulties they have as a result of physical, sexual or emotional abuse or neglect. It can also be a helpful starting point for adults looking at their experiences

O Bain and M Sanders. *Out in the Open: A Guide for Young People Who Have Been Sexually Abused*. London: Virago, 1990. Excellent book for young people

E Gil. *Outgrowing the Pain: A Book for and About Adults Abused as Children*. New York: Dell, 1983. ISBN 0-440-50006-0. For adults and written in an accessible style with cartoons)

M Wilson. *Crossing the Boundaries: Black Women Survive Incest*. London: Virago, 1993. Personal testimony for black female survivors of sexual abuse; detailed resource section

Ellen Bass and Laura Davis. *The Courage to Heal: A Guide for Women Survivors*, revd edn. New York: Harper Perennial, 1992. Offers hope and encouragement to women abused as children

M Lew. *Victims No Longer: Men Recovering from Incest and Other Sexual Child Abuse*. New York: Harper & Row, 1988. Gives both survivors and therapists essential advice for healing

[1]   Coxell AW, King MB, Mezey GC, Gordon D. Lifetime prevalence, characteristics and associated problems of non-consensual sex in men: a cross sectional survey. *British Medical Journal* 1999; 318: 846–850.
[2]   Bland J, Mezey GC, Dolan B. Special women, special needs: a descriptive study of female special hospital patients. *Journal of Forensic Psychiatry* 1999; 10: 34–45.
[3]   Singleton N, Meltzer H, Gatward R, Coid J, Deasy D. *Psychiatric Morbidity among Prisoners*. London: Office for National Statistics, 2000.
[4]   Monck E, Bentovim A, Goodall G *et al*. *Child Sexual Abuse: A Descriptive and Treatment Study*. London: HMSO, 1996. Cognitive-behavioural therapy focused on traumatic responses shows greatest effect.

Child-protection issues

Introduction

Child-protection issues may arise for healthcare staff at any time, but are more likely to do so when dealing with certain situations.

- In Mother and Baby Units (MBU), where the mother's mental state or relationship with the infant is sufficiently disturbed to result in the risk of significant harm to the infant.
- In young offender institutions (YOI), where disclosures of recent or current abuse may be made.
- In adult prisons, where disclosures of past abuse or domestic violence may reveal that a child is currently at risk.
- In any prison holding sex offenders and/or paedophiles, especially if children visit them.
- Participation in risk assessments of individual prisoners to inform decisions on sentence planning or supervision after release.

This section aims to:

- give broad accepted definitions of when child-protection procedures should be invoked
- outline the relevant legal and professional guidance governing breaching confidentiality in order to protect children and
- signpost the child-protection procedures that exist in different types of establishment.

It does not aim to give detailed guidance on how to deal with particular types of situation. Where there is doubt, healthcare staff are advised to contact and discuss the situation with the prison Child Protection Coordinator (CPC), local social services or the designated doctor or nurse in the local Primary Care Trust. (In England and Wales, all Primary Care Trusts must identify a paediatrician or nurse to take a professional lead on the health service contribution to child protection.)

When are child-protection procedures needed?: definitions

The aim of child-protection procedures and the legislation on which they are based is to prevent 'significant harm' occurring to 'children'.

The relevant legislation is the Children Act 1989. While the Act does not apply to regimens for the treatment of under 18 year olds in prison establishments, the Prison Service is required to reflect the standards imposed by the Act through its own delegated legislation and codes of practice. It is important to be aware of what these protocols are. Relevant Prison Service Orders are: Prison Service Order 4950 'Regimes for Under 18 Year Olds' and 'Regimes for Young Women Under 18 Years Old'.

How old is a 'child'?

The Children Act 1989 covers 0–18 years, although the age of consent for sexual activity is 16. Chronological age does not necessarily correspond with the psychological maturity of a young person, nor their ability to recognise and protect themselves against exploitation. Section 31(10) suggests that the child's health and development should be compared with that reasonably expected of a similar child. The United Nations Convention on the Rights of the Child refers to persons below the age of 18 as children. Effectively, all young persons detained in penal establishments should be considered as vulnerable until they have reached the age of 18, even though the age for sexual consent is 16.

What is child abuse?

The Children Act 1989: Section 31(9) covers both actual and likely harm. Harm includes both ill-treatment (including sexual abuse and non-physical ill-treatment like emotional abuse) and the impairment of health or development.

- 'Health' means physical or mental health.
- 'Development' means physical, intellectual, emotional, social or behavioural.
- **Physical abuse** implies a physically harmful action directed against a child, eg any inflicted injury such as bruises, burns, head injuries, fractures, abdominal injuries or poisoning.
- **Sexual abuse** implies the involvement of dependent, developmentally immature children and adolescents in sexual activities they do not fully comprehend and to which they cannot give informed consent, or that violate the social taboos of family roles.

What is 'significant harm'?

- Physical injury needing prompt medical attention that could incur criminal charges under Sections 18, 20 or 47 of the Offences Against the Person Act 1861.
- Sexual abuse includes direct (eg touching) and indirect (eg exposure) sexual acts in which the young person was exploited because the activity was unwanted when it first began and involved differences in age, authority or gender (ie coercion by an older person or one in a position of authority). The young person's degree of physical and personal maturity may be relevant in deciding the seriousness of the abuse.
- Emotional abuse covers actual or likely persistent or severe psychological ill-treatment, eg persistent verbal denigration, humiliation in the absence of any positive interest, concern and action, or intimidation.
- Neglect covers actual or likely persistent or severe neglect or the failure to afford protection to a young person against any kind of foreseeable danger, including a failure to address needs that result in significant impairment of a young person's health or development.

Which children are healthcare workers responsible for protecting?

The requirement to protect children from significant harm extends beyond current patients (eg a young offender), other inmates (eg other young offenders) and beyond children visiting the prison. If you have reason to believe that another child (eg a younger sibling or the patient's own children) are at risk or are suffering significant harm, you have a duty under the Children Act 1989 to take steps to protect them. Consideration should also be given during a prisoner's pregnancy to possible risk of significant harm to her unborn child after it is born. Examples include a pregnant mother who has previously been convicted or suspected of abusing children, or whose children have been removed from her care via a court order because of significant concern about her care of them.

Patient confidentiality and child protection

The guidance accompanying the Children Act 1989 is clear about the obligations of all agencies to report concerns about child protection. In child-protection cases, the overriding principle is to secure the best interests of the child.

Common law

The common law duty of confidence enjoins on healthcare professionals the duty to keep personal information about children and families confidential, except where the individual patient has given consent. However, the law permits disclosure of confidential information necessary to safeguard a child or children in the public interest. The Caldicott principles for disclosure of medical information, which will soon become law, go further and state that the duty of confidence is superseded by the principle of duty of care for the child, making disclosure to safeguard a child an ethical requirement. Where the patient is a child, they are also entitled to confidentiality, provided that, in the case of those under 16, they have the ability to understand the choices and consequences relating to treatment. However, again, where it is believed that the child is being exploited or abused, confidentiality may be breached following discussion with the child.

The guidance of the General Medical Council, the Royal College of Psychiatrists and The United Kingdom Central Council for Nursing, Midwifery and Health Visiting (UKCC) is set out in the section on confidentiality in **Ethical issues** (page 300).

What action should be taken?

Young offenders who allege that they have been abused recently

Recently remanded or sentenced young offenders may claim that they have recently been abused in the establishment, at home, school or in a children's home. They may fear that a younger sibling, relative or other child is at risk or is suffering abuse.

- Ensure that the young person is safe and does not return to the situation or people where the alleged abuse occurred.
- Document what is said and any physical evidence meticulously, with due regard to confidentiality. Do this as soon as possible, and no later than 24 hours after the event. If a court case is considered, the courts will require evidence of the abuse, whether non-accidental injury, sexual or emotional.
- Discuss the situation with the patient and, if he/she or another child is at risk of serious harm, encourage them to report it. If at all possible, offer to help or accompany him/her, even if only to report it to the prison CPC or a social worker.
- Sometimes a patient may be reluctant to report abuse, especially if it has occurred within the family, as they may not want to prosecute the abuser. Reassure them that the priority in child protection is always the protection of any children at risk, not the prosecution of perpetrators. Disclosure need not lead to prosecution if the victim does not want this.
- If consent is refused, discuss the situation with an experienced colleague or, anonymously, with the prison CPC, local social services, the designated doctor or nurse in the local Health Authority or your professional body.

- If the patient continues to refuse consent, if there is reason to believe that serious harm may occur and it is in the best interests of the child, inform the appropriate person and ask that, if possible, the identity of the informant is concealed from the alleged perpetrator.

Advice on responding to an individual who discloses abuse appears in **People who disclose abuse** (page 271). If the young person has been the victim of a very recent sexual assault, **Victims of sexual assault** (page 260) may also be relevant.

Young persons who are themselves abusers

In a YOI or Young Offenders Unit, the abuser may be an inmate, themselves under 18. A complaint against a fellow inmate should be taken seriously, although care has to be taken that this is not a malicious lie to bring trouble upon another inmate. Young people who have been victims of sexual abuse or who have grown up in a culture of domestic violence are more likely to become abusers. Awareness of a young person's history of abuse might make one alert to the possibility that he/she may abuse a weaker young person. If you suspect that a young offender is an abuser of others do the following.

- Consult an experienced colleague — perhaps the healthcare representative on the prison Child Protection Committee.
- Discuss your concerns with the prison CPC.
- If the CPC is not available, the duty governor should be informed as the alleged abuser may need to be relocated within the establishment. The local Social Services' Child Protection Unit may be also helpful.
- An assessment of the needs of the alleged perpetrator and of why he/she is abusing others should be arranged.

Adults talking about past abuse

During the course of treatment, a young person or an adult prisoner may admit to having been abused as a child. Unless there is reason to believe that the original perpetrator is still committing such offences against children, there are no legal child-protection implications. If the young person or adult prisoner wishes to discuss possible prosecution of their former abuser, they will require legal advice. **People who disclose abuse** (see page 271) gives more advice on responding to a disclosure of abuse.

Mother and Baby Units (MBU)

Staff need to be alert to the possibility of babies suffering significant harm. For more details, see **Problems in the mother–baby relationship** and **Postnatal depression** (pages 144 and 134). Each MBU has a child-protection procedure endorsed by the area CPC within which the prison is located. You should ensure that you have access to a copy of this procedure. If harm to the baby is suspected do the following.

- Express care and attention for the mother. Such mothers frequently have unmet emotional needs and/or are immature. If concern for the baby appears to neglect the mother's needs or fears, this could lead to serious resentment of the baby. However, be aware that the child's welfare is paramount.
- Arrange additional practical help with childcare, offered non-judgementally. For example, a nursery nurse assisting the mother to care for the baby may model good care. She would ideally spend considerable periods with both mother and

baby. The health visitor or the MBU governor may trigger a review of the infant's care plan and arrange additional help.

- If possible, involve the mother in making decisions about who should see the baby. However, if she refuses to have the baby examined or given medical treatment or to cooperate in good baby care, so that the baby is at risk, then inform the Liaison Department at the local social services. The principal duty of care is to the baby and this, as a last resort, may override patient confidentiality and the mother's wishes.
- If you become aware of actual harm to the baby, eg a non-accidental injury, activate the prison's child-protection procedure immediately. Involve the mother in this process if possible, but give priority to protecting the baby from the risk of further harm.
- Record all actions and decisions taken clearly. Describe fully the reasons for concern, the agreed plan, and the names and designations of all who are involved in the care plan. Each person must receive a copy of the plan.

Who should be informed?

The principal responsibility for child protection rests with the local Social Services' Child Protection Unit. Additionally, prisons containing an MBU all have a liaison social worker and a written child-protection procedure. YOI have a prison CPC, a prison CPC on which a representative of healthcare sits and a written child-protection procedure. The procedure usually involves the following.

- Referring child-protection issues to the duty governor or the CPC.
- The duty governor making an assessment as soon as possible and certainly within 12 hours in consultation with the prison CPC, and then taking action as necessary. Action taken may include:
  — ensuring that the individual does not return to the place or people where he/she could be harmed again and
  — informing the parents or a guardian and local social services and organising a child-protection conference.
- In other prisons, it may be necessary to report the matter directly to local social services. It is important that all healthcare staff are aware of the name and contact details of the relevant department of local social services.
- Where there is reason to believe that another child in another area is being abused or is at risk of being abused, the appropriate person to inform is the local Social Services' Child Protection Unit where the alleged abuser and child victim live. If it is not local, obtain help from the prison's local social services. The Local Authority, via social services, has a responsibility under Section 47 of the Children Act 1989 to make enquiries where it has reasonable cause to suspect a child is suffering or is likely to suffer from harm.
- Others who may be helpful include: the health visitor, probation staff and the National Society for the Prevention of Cruelty to Children (NSPCC).

Further information

- The prison's child-protection policy (for YOI and prisons with an MBU).
- Any publication or policy of the local area CPC.
- Department of Health. *Protecting and Using Patient Information: Caldicott Report*. London: Department of Health, 1997.
- *Working Together under the Children Act 1989*, 2nd edn London: HMSO, 1999.

- Howard League Report. *Banged Up, Beaten Up, Cutting Up*. London: Howard League, 1995.
- Birchall E, Hallet C. *Working Together in Child Protection*. London: HMSO, 1995.
- Royal College of Psychiatrists. *Good Psychiatric Practice: Confidentiality*. Council Report CR85. London: Royal College of Psychiatrists, 2000.
- General Medical Council. *Confidentiality: Protection and Providing Information*. London: GMC, 2000.
- United Kingdom Central Council for Nursing, Midwifery and Health Visiting. *Guidelines for Professional Practice*. London: UKCC, 1996.

Resources for young people and primary support groups

Childline: 0800 1111 (24-hour freephone helpline)
(For children and young people)

Children 1st: 0131 337 8539
(Offers help and advice on child abuse in Scotland)

Children's Law Centre Northern Ireland: 0808 808 5678 (Monday, Tuesday and Friday, 10 am–4:30 pm; Thursday, 10 am–5 pm)
(Free legal advice and information about children and young people in Northern Ireland)

The Children's Legal Centre: 01206 873820 (Monday–Friday, 10 am–12:30 pm, 2 pm–4:30 pm)
University of Essex, Wivenhoe Park, Colchester CO4 3SQ. E-mail: clc@essex.ac.uk; URL: http://www2.essex.ac.uk/clc
(Free legal advice and information about children and young people)

Family Rights Group: 020 7923 2628; 0800 731 1696 (freephone adviceline: Monday–Friday, 1.30 pm–3.30 pm)
The Print House, 18 Ashwin Street, London E8 3DL. E-mail: office@frg.u-net.com
(Offers advice, advocacy and publications to families whose children are involved with social services)

Kidscape: 020 7730 3300
2 Grosvenor Gardens, London SW1W 0DH
(Provides booklets, leaflets [some free], videos and other materials to help teach children and young people practical strategies for keeping safe, coping with bullying and preventing child abuse)

National Society for the Prevention of Cruelty to Children (NSPCC):
0808 800 5000 (24-hour helpline)
(For children and anyone concerned about child abuse)

Scottish Child Law Centre: 0131 667 6333
(Gives advice about how Scottish law relates to children)

Youth Access: 020 8772 9900
(Provides information on and referrals to agencies around the country providing advice, support and counselling to young people)

See **People who have been abused as children** (page x) for details of resources for this problem

Managing aggression and violence[1]

Effective risk management is particularly important in prison, as some prisoners have major issues in dealing with anger and aggression. Risk management is a part of the health and safety rights and responsibilities of all staff. The health care manager has additional responsibilities under Health and Safety law to make an environmental risk assessment and take action, as appropriate, to reduce risk.

Aggression and violence are not a mental disorder, though people who are aggressive and violent may have one of a number of disorders. This section aims to give advice to help clinicians reduce the risk of violence and aggression and to deal with it if it occurs. The aim is not to 'cure' the individual of being aggressive, but to reduce aggression so that the clinician can address the individual's other health problems safely.

Preparations to be made in advance

Layout of the healthcare centre

- **Avoid excess stimulation.** Noisy waiting rooms, loud music or bright lights can overload an already tense or disturbed individual. Ensure waiting areas are well ventilated.

- **Consider, if possible, a destimulation area**, eg a lounge area with toilet facilities for use by individuals who pose a particular risk.

- **Consider, in the longer term, developing a de-escalation suite** or snoozelen room for use by patients who have become very agitated.

Layout of the interview room

- **Ensure a safe escape route for the patient** (such as an unobstructed exit). A distressed individual would rather escape than fight; aggression levels rise if the individual feels cornered or has trouble finding an exit.

- **Ensure a safe escape route for yourself** (eg be nearest the door). This is important if violence is premeditated or goal-directed, eg an individual is threatening a doctor to try to obtain particular drugs.

- **Ideally then both individual and clinician will have equal access to a safe exit, preferably separate exits.** If this is not possible, then the clinician should be nearest the exit or the room should have an observation panel that allows a clear view from, say, secretary's desk outside.

- **The door should open outwards or swing both ways to prevent possible barricades.**

- **Discreet buzzer to call for help.**

- **Décor and furniture should be as pleasant and relaxing as possible**, eg easy chairs, pastel colours.

- **Other staff members to be clearly visible** or seen to pass the room at frequent intervals.

- **Interview room to have externally locking doors**, so that help cannot be locked out.

- **Scissors, knives or any other unnecessary objects** that can be picked up and thrown should not be kept in the interview room.

Clothing and jewellery

Remove items of clothing that might cause injury if a potentially violent individual catches hold of them, eg earrings, necklaces, neckties, pens or pencils (from pockets), cigarette lighters. Do not wear clothes or shoes that may make a quick exit difficult.

Standard procedures

- **Fear can lead to violence.** Provide information about the symptoms of the illness, any medical procedures, the names and roles of any clinicians who are also present and the role of the health centre.
- **Behave calmly.** Non-verbal stress and anxiety can be difficult to distinguish from anger. To a patient who is confused, hearing voices or lost in distressing thoughts, a highly anxious clinician may be perceived as threatening.
- **Inform patients about anticipated delays.** Offer appropriate resources (eg magazines, drink, bathroom, etc). Simple consideration can help reduce hostility.
- **If delays are anticipated, have a member of staff search the toilet area for objects that might be used as weapons.** Maintain staffing levels to allow patients to be escorted to and from the toilet area.
- **Have a clear policy**, written or reviewed within the last 3 years and known by all in advance, about the prescription and administration of opiates and benzodiazepines.

Assess the risk of violence

Consider the following questions.[2] The more often you answer 'yes', the greater the risk of violence.

- Is the person I am dealing with facing high levels of stress? Consider recent bad news, bereavement, a court date and significant anniversary dates.
- Is the person likely to be drunk or on drugs?
- Does the person have a history of violence?

Before interviewing an individual who is unknown to you, review old notes (if available) or talk to wing staff to look for reports of previous violence (the strongest predictor of violence).

- Does the person have a history of psychiatric illness?
- Does the person suffer from a medical condition that may result in loss of self-control?
- Has the person verbally abused me or others in the past?
- Has the person threatened me or others with violence in the past?
- Has the person attacked me or others in the past?
- Does the person perceive me as a threat to his/her children?
- Does the person think of me as a threat to his/her liberty?
- Does the person have unrealistic expectations of what I can do for him/her?
- Does the person perceive me as wilfully unhelpful?
- Have I felt anxious for my safety with this person before?
- Are other people present who will reward the person for violence?

Visits to wings/units

If visiting a patient in their cell do the following.

- Make staff aware of your presence before entering the cell.
- Acknowledge the patient's territorial rights and respect his/her personal space and possessions. Always ask whether you may enter the cell, sit down, etc. By doing so, you will allow the individual to retain a sense of control and thus will reduce a perceived threat.
- Do not allow yourself to be directed to a seat you are uncomfortable with, eg sitting on the bed.

Recognising potential aggression at an early stage

Signs include the following.

- Any change in behaviour that varies from what is normal for that individual.
- Pale or flushed face.
- Rising voice.
- Focusing/narrowing of gaze.
- Tensing of muscles.
- Increased agitation and disturbance in behaviour, eg pacing.
- Unusual calmness.
- Disturbed communication.

Defuse aggression before it becomes violence (verbal de-escalation)

Adoption of a non-threatening body posture

- Use a calm, open posture (sitting or standing). Place yourself to the patient's side or take up a side-on stance. Reduce eye contact by use of peripheral vision — as direct eye contact can be confronting.
- Allow the individual adequate personal space. The amount varies between individuals, so be aware of signs that the patient feels you are too close or too far away.
- Keep both hands visible with open palms as a calming gesture.
- Do not stand if the individual is sitting or you will appear threatening.
- Do not whisper or talk over the patient. Keep him/her involved in all relevant discussions wherever possible.
- Avoid sudden movements that may startle or be perceived as an attack. Movement towards the individual may be perceived as a threat. Move backwards or sideways if you move at all. Do not turn your back on the individual.
- Avoid audiences — an audience may escalate the situation.

Display an understanding

- Remain calm and patient.
- Speak firmly, slowly and clearly, but with normal tone and intensity — do not raise your voice. Avoid sounding accusatory or punitive.
- Offer support: do not make retaliatory remarks. Reassure the individual that you accept that he/she is angry. If the individual makes a conciliatory gesture, respond accordingly.

- Ask questions: ask how the patient is feeling. Do not say: 'I know how you feel.' Ask what is causing his/her anger. Ask how he/she thinks the situation can be resolved.
- Give time for the individual to think about the situation, to hear the full story. Do not rush the individual.
- Avoid interrupting the individual. If an interruption is necessary, do it quietly and calmly.
- Show that you are willing to help where possible.
- Make an apology if appropriate.
- Do not take the individual's comments personally. Abusive statements may be the only way the individual can express his/her feelings at the time.
- Try to be honest with the individual and do not make promises that you cannot keep.
- If physical contact is made (eg holding your hand or patting you on the back), try and remain calm. Do not pull away or overreact, as this may trigger suspicion.

Provide supportive feedback

Note the individual's non-verbal cues and feed your impression back to him/her. For example:

> You seem a bit agitated. Perhaps you can tell me why you're feeling agitated, then I may be able to help you in some way.

> I can see that you're very upset about something. Tell me what's upsetting you? Tell me what you would like me to do to help you.

This technique is often useful, but occasionally it infuriates the individual further. If this occurs, move on to another technique.

Provide the individual with choice

A choice of alternatives, even if none are what the individual would ideally like, may help him/her feel in control of their situation, and so may alleviate some of their distress. For example, you could say:

> I can see that you're extremely distressed and agitated by the voices you're hearing. I can help you to feel better by giving you your usual tablets. You always tell me that the pills make the voices quieter. You can then go back to the unit. If you don't want me to help you in that way then you can go into a room on the ward. The choice is yours. Tell me what you'd like me to do.

Set limits

Many individuals struggle to avoid becoming aggressive and by setting limits you show that you will not tolerate aggression and that you will help the individual to remain calm. Thus, limits can act to decrease the individual's anxiety about losing control. Limit-setting may be especially effective if you acknowledge the individual's present emotions, so explaining why limits are being set. For example:

> I can see that you're very angry and it's not surprising given your circumstances today. I'd like to help you but I cannot do so if you lose your temper. First of all I'd like you to sit down, then you can tell me how I can help.

> You're obviously very annoyed about something. I can see that you feel like hitting something and I'm a bit scared that you may hit me. I'm going to ask the

prison officer to stand in the room with us. I'd like you to take a seat and then you can tell me what you're annoyed about.

I'd like to help you but I can't do so if you yell at me. Either you stop yelling and talk to me calmly or I'll have to leave you alone until you've calmed down.

Time out

Time out may involve leaving the individual alone in an unlocked room for a few minutes or asking the person to take a break. It should be clear to the individual that the strategy is not a form of punishment. For example, you could say:

Look — this is getting intense (or emotional). Let's take a break for a few minutes. It will help us (or me) to think.

If the situation escalates despite these efforts

Do not try to handle a violent individual on your own. **If he/she claims to have a weapon, GET OUT of the room or building.** If you cannot escape, then do the following.

- Summon assistance. If possible, give the helpers information about the situation to prevent overreactions. (Staff running into a room where a patient is armed may trigger off an assault).
- Stay calm.
- Do not wrestle or argue with the aggressor.
- Adopt a non-threatening stance. Keep your palms open as a gesture of calm. Minimise eye contact with the use of peripheral vision.
- A side-on stance creates a smaller target with the vital organs protected and with better stability.
- Obey the individual's instructions and try not to upset him/her.
- Speak only as much as is needed to keep the individual speaking — rather than acting.
- If the individual calms down a bit, it may be possible to suggest that he/she puts the weapon on the table or in another safe place. Do not attempt to grab the weapon, but play for time until help arrives. Talk empathetically with the individual to continue to defuse the situation. However, do not agree with ludicrous delusions. It may help to say something like: 'I can see you're upset by this belief. Maybe it's true; maybe it's not'.
- Use surrounding objects and furniture as shields if violence occurs.

Use of control and restraint

Physical restraint should only be used when there is no other more appropriate course of action and there are sufficient people for it to be done safely. This is supported by the relevant Prison Service Order (currently PSO 1600, 'Use of Force'). Staff should be trained in the use of restraint and in CPR. Use only the degree of force appropriate to the actual danger or resistance shown by the violent individual. Healthcare staff must attend situations where the use of restraint is planned in any part of the prison. Although their role is to ensure that restraint is applied only when essential and in such a way that the prisoner's health is protected and not to use it themselves, nurses may find it useful to be trained in control and restraint in order to understand better what is happening. Monitor vital signs throughout the time that restraint is applied.

Dos and don'ts of the use of restraint

Do	Don't
Always call for assistance Ask a patient to summon help when appropriate	Do not try to manage on your own
Be aware of the environment and of the whereabouts of your colleagues	Do not put yourself in a position knowingly where you have no immediate exit or that your colleagues are not in a position to respond should you summon assistance
Be aware of the patient's disabilities, old injuries or medical conditions	Do not apply pressure to parts of the body that could restrict breathing, eg stomach and neck
Be aware of medication that the patient is taking and of the possibility that he/she is using illicit drugs	
Protect the patient's airway	
Continue to hold onto the patient once he/she is immobilised	Do not relax the hold the moment struggling stops
Continue to talk to the patient	Do not stop talking to the patient because he/she does not reply
Remember that a patient struggling during restraint may just be trying to get into a position where he/she can breathe	Do not restrain a patient face down for long periods as natural body weight and anxiety can put severe stress on the heart and lungs
Consider the accessories you wear or pens and other items you carry in your pockets as these can cause injury during a struggle	Do not wear jewellery, cufflinks, brooches, watches, rings, etc. of a design that might cause injury during a struggle

For further guidelines on the use of physical restraint, see PSOs 1600, 'Use of force', and 1700; Department of Health and Welsh Office Code of Practice (1990); Mental Health Act 1983; and UKCC 'Managing Aggression' (June 2001).

Where treatment without consent under common law is considered (eg rapid tranquillisation), see **Emergency treatment under common law** (page 168).

Other forms of management of violent patients

Occasionally it may be necessary to use other means to prevent a patient from being violent. Where the patient has a mental illness and either gives permission for treatment to be administered or is not competent to give or withhold consent, then medication is an option. For advice on the use of rapid tranquillisation under common law, see **Emergency treatment under common law** (page 168).

Currently, in prisons in England and Wales, Prison Service guidance allows that where a patient has a medical condition leading to the violent behaviour, a doctor may order the use of 'medical restraint', ie the use of a 'special cell' or of a loose canvas restraint jacket. In addition, for all forms of violent behaviour, as a very last resort, a prison governor may order the use of 'mechanical restraint', ie the use of a body belt with metal cuffs or the use of special accommodation. Where a governor has ordered the use of either mechanical restraint or special accommodation, the role of the doctor is to assess whether there is any medical reason for not using these and, if there is, to order their use to be ended immediately.

In the use of any such form of physical restraint, the following are essential points of principle.

- It should be used as a last resort and for the shortest time possible.
- Steps should be taken to ensure the minimum possible invasion of the individual's dignity, eg audiences should be moved away.
- The individual should be treated in a way likely to calm rather than aggravate their aggression, eg speaking to them calmly and with respect.
- The individual's mental state should be regularly assessed and an opinion urgently sought from a psychiatrist if there is any history or current indication of mental illness, self-destructive behaviour or substance misuse.
- Where the patient has a mental disorder, care and treatment should be planned if necessary and appropriate under common law (see **Emergency treatment under common law**, page 168). Where indicated, steps should be taken to remove them urgently to a hospital where treatment can be given (see **Interface with the NHS and other agencies**, page 149).
- Where the patient has a history of very difficult behaviour, a full, multidisciplinary assessment and care plan should be arranged (see **Management of prisoners with complex presentations and very difficult behaviours**, page 202).

Action to take after a violent outburst

Staff

- Staff members involved will require support and appropriate attention, if required, to meet psychological or physical needs following an incident.
- It is usually helpful for participants to discuss their experiences of the incident. Staff should together talk about what happened, how they felt, what went wrong, what went right and how to handle such situations more effectively in the future. The new information should be shared with staff who were not directly involved in the incident. This kind of review is equally helpful in situations where a violent outburst seemed very likely but which was prevented.
- Some staff may suffer injury (eg orthopaedic strain) during restraint. Encourage staff members to check any potential injuries with the occupational health service.

Patient

A record should be made in the individual's file. In a prominent position inside the file (**NOT** on the front cover) record: 'See (**date**)' and give the date of documentation of violent episode. Then, in the notes on that date, give a detailed record of the violence. Include the grade or severity of the violence, the circumstances in which the violence occurred (eg whether the individual was psychotic or drunk) and whether the violence was provoked.

Offer to discuss the incident with the individual when he/she has recovered. He/she is likely to feel shaken after such an event, especially if restraint or medication were used. If the violent incident was out of character for the individual, he/she may have trouble understanding why it occurred. If the violence was part of a pattern of aggressive behaviour, the individual may be more willing at this point to accept help for his/her violence.

Assess the individual to exclude possible physical and neurological causes for the violence. Arrange a multidisciplinary psychiatric assessment to determine a management plan. Violence is associated with the following.

- Any cause of confusion, either acute (delirium) or chronic (dementia). A thorough medical check-up is advised (see **Delirium** and **Dementia**, pages 41 and 43).
- Acute psychosis.
- Paranoid states.
- Acute organic brain syndromes.
- Head injuries.
- Substance abuse or withdrawal.
- Personality disorders, eg antisocial characteristics or borderline disorder.

Where the violent outburst is part of a pattern of aggressive behaviour that is relatively mild, assertiveness training and anger management training may be helpful.[3] Where problems in controlling anger or aggression have led to the crime the individual has committed, the individual may be eligible for one of the relevant offending behaviour courses (for more details, see **Offending behaviour programmes**, page x).

Medication

The Royal College of Psychiatrists guidelines[4] allow psychotropic medication to be used in patients with **chronic** aggressive behaviours where there is:

- a high level of arousal/anxiety that cannot be reduced by environmental, behavioural or other therapeutic methods or
- a low threshold of stress tolerance that cannot be reduced by environmental, behavioural or other therapeutic methods.

The lowest dose possible should be used. Medication should be part of a comprehensive plan including environmental factors and other therapies. Consult a specialist about prescribing for this indication. For advice on rapid tranquillisation, see **Emergency treatment under common law** (page 168).

If it is suspected that a patient may be violent to others

Potentially violent individuals raise legal, ethical and clinical problems for clinicians. It is generally accepted internationally that a health professional has a duty to protect a person whom a patient threatens to harm by warning that person or contacting the police. UK case law supports this providing the decision about the serious risk is taken on adequate information and the information is disclosed to the appropriate authorities. This includes all potential victims of violence, including domestic violence and including groups of individuals (eg female staff). Where a clinician believes there is a reasonable chance that a patient will seriously harm someone else (eg a family member or prison officer), you should do the following.

Assess the risk of violence

Factors associated with potential violence.

- History of violence (the single strongest predictor).
- Intention to commit violence (most important clinical variable (see below)).

- Male gender.
- Being unemployed.
- Living or growing up in a violent subculture.
- Coming from a violent family.
- Abuse of drugs or alcohol.
- Having weapons available.
- Having victims available.
- History of poor impulse control.
- Factors that weaken self-control (eg psychotic illness, paranoid thinking).

Assess the **strength of motive and intention**. This is the most important predictive clinical variable. If you suspect violence, ask the following questions.

- 'Are you angry with anyone?'
- 'Are you thinking of hurting anyone?'

If 'yes', then ask the following.

- 'Who are you angry with, or thinking of hurting?'
- 'When do you think you might hurt [the person mentioned]?'
- 'Where will you do this?'
- 'How long have you been thinking this way?'
- 'Are you able to control these thoughts about hurting [the person mentioned]?'
- 'Do you think you would be able to stop yourself from hurting [the person mentioned] if you wanted to?'
- For how long do you think you can control your thoughts about hurting [the person mentioned]?'
- 'Have you ever purposely hurt someone in the past?'
- (If 'no') 'How close have you come to hurting someone in the past?'

Be aware of a hierarchy of expressions of intent.

- 'I wish he were dead': thought — lower risk.
- 'I'm going to kill that bastard': intention — higher risk.
- 'I'm going to stick a knife in Joe Bloggs when he comes to my cell': definite plan — highest risk.

If you believe that the individual is likely to commit serious violence against another person, then you have a legal and ethical obligation to both the patient and the potential victims of violence to try to prevent the violence (see **Ethical issues**, page 300).

Discuss your concerns and intended action with the potentially violent individual

Where possible, it is usually best to tell the patient that you are concerned about his/her threats, and that it is your duty to tell the third party about the threats that have been made against him/her. This line of action demonstrates concern for the patient and is less likely to damage the therapeutic clinician–patient relationship than taking no action.

If in doubt, seek urgent consultation with a superior or secondary mental-health services. Telephone consultation is better than none at all.

Keep careful, detailed, written notes (including notes of the results of any consultation).

Protect the third party against violence.

- Inform discipline staff (SIR — Security Incident Report).
- If the patient satisfies the criteria for mental disorder, admit and obtain an urgent transfer to the NHS (see **Liaison and referral to the NHS**, page 149).
- Take appropriate steps to make sure that the person who is the target of the threat is alerted. If he/she is another prisoner or member of the prison staff, inform the duty governor. If the potential target is outside the prison, inform the police. Once the police are informed of such a threat of violence, they too have a duty to warn that person of the risk of violence and, if necessary for the protection of the public and the individual, to discuss the threat with the local multi-agency public protection panel.
- Evidence of child abuse, where you have reason to believe that a child is at current or future risk, should be reported to the appropriate authorities (see **Child protection**, page 276).
- Inform the patient of the action you are taking. Where possible, carry out the warnings in the presence of the patient (eg telephone the duty governor in the presence of the patient). This will ensure that you talk about the patient in a considered way and will reduce the chance of the patient developing paranoid ideas about what has been said in his/her absence. However, if you believe that discussing your intentions with the patient will put you at risk, then you should warn the third party without informing the patient.

Guidance may also be available from your local multi-agency public protection panel.

Policies and training

Policies are needed on the following.

- Management of critical incidents, including debriefing, recording, staff training.
- Risk assessment.
- Staff training.
- Use of restraint.
- Prescription and administration of opiates and benzodiazepines.
- Use of restraint.

[1] Adapted from Andrew G, Jenkins R (eds). *Management of Mental Disorders*, UK edn. Sydney: World Health Organization Collaborating Centre for Mental Health and Substance Abuse, 1999; and The Bethlem and Maudsley NHS Trust, 1994, *Preventing and Managing Violence: Policy and Guidelines for Practice*. Report of Trust Working Party. London: Maudsley.

[2] Adapted from the dangerousness checklist in Breakwell G. *Facing Physical Violence*. London: British Psychological Society, 1989.

[3] Stermac. Anger control treatment for forensic patients. *Journal of Interpersonal Violence* 1986; 1: 446–722.

[4] Royal College of Psychiatrists. *Strategies for the Management of Disturbed and Violent Patients in Psychiatric Units*. Council Report CR41. London, 1995.

Food refusal and mental illness

Complaints of food refusal are common in prison and place a moral strain on all staff involved. Support for staff involved is needed. Categories of food refusal that have been identified[1,2] relate to the following areas.

- Frustration or protest:
  - To draw attention to political or other beliefs.
  - Often determined to pursue the action to the end.
  - Death is not the objective; there is hope that the demands will be met.
  - Not considered to be suicide under English Common Law.
- Bargaining tool:
  - Action is one of a set of negotiations about, for example, prison life.
  - Compromise possible if a 'reasonable offer' is made.
  - If no offer is made, food refusal may eventually be abandoned.
  - Not considered to be suicide under English Common Law.
- Unclear aims/gain attention:
  - Maybe anger: 'I'll die and you'll be sorry'.
  - Typically of short duration.
  - Lack of clear conditions for ending action.
- Suicidal aims:
  - Death is the desired objective.
  - May have already expressed the intention to die but lacks access to other means.
  - Usually associated with mental disorder (eg severe depression), but where it appears not to be, this is the most complex situation legally.
- Medical reasons:
  - Mental illness: most commonly depression, schizophrenia or anorexia nervosa.
  - Physical illness, eg cancers, delirium.

Presentation

Prisoners making protests make sure that staff know about the refusal. Those with a personality disorder, are depressed or psychotic may stay in their cells more and may not come out for association. Those with delusions of persecution may conceal their food refusal. Other prisoners are often the first to know.

Considering the possible alternative explanations

Is the refusal genuine? The individual may be buying food from others and refusing food provided by the prison. Staff may be concerned when a prisoner misses a meal only to find that he/she is eating later. Is the individual being bullied or in debt?

Consider a possible physical illness. Many physical conditions lead to loss of weight and/or loss of appetite, eg cancers, cirrhosis, diabetes, hyperthyroidism, sprue, tuberculosis, tropical infestations.

Consider a physical illness leading to symptoms of mental illness and food refusal.

- Infectious illness, epilepsy, metabolic changes and many other conditions may cause delirium, especially in older patients or those with dementia. Symptoms of delirium may include suspiciousness, confusion and agitation (see **Delirium — F05**, page 41).

- Some medications may produce symptoms of depression (eg β-blockers, other antihypertensives, H_2-blockers, corticosteroids).

Assessment

- How long has the individual been refusing food or liquids?
- Is the individual refusing all food, some food, or food and liquids?
- Does anyone know some of the reasons the individual is refusing food?

Carry out a physical examination if the patient consents.

- Measure and record their current weight. The body fat index must be taken following accurate weight and height measurements.
- General observations: oral hydration, blood pressure (postural drop?), tissue turgor, muscle wasting.
- Routine blood tests: full blood count (FBC), U&E, LFTs (talk to the local hospital chemical pathologist).
- Urine osmolality.

Assess for suicidal intent (see **Suicide assessment and management**, page 204).

Consider an early psychiatric opinion. Even if the individual has a reason for refusing food, it is important to have a psychiatric evaluation before there is doubt about the capacity of the individual to refuse food and/or treatment.

Disorders that may lead to food refusal include the following.

- Psychotic states such as schizophrenia, where persecutory beliefs that the food is poisoned are possible (see **Acute psychosis** and **Chronic psychosis**, pages 11 and 36).
- Depressive illness (see **Depression**, page 47).
- Anorexia nervosa (see **Eating disorders**, page 60).
- Dementia (see **Dementia**, page 43).

Legal context

It is vital to be aware of the relevant legal framework and to operate within it. It will be necessary to consult the relevant Prison Service guidance (DDL (96) 01) and if food refusal persists, to obtain legal advice from the Prison Service and to discuss the situation with the NHS Trust or Primary Care Trust and the Prison Service area manager before the question of loss of capacity arises. The Prison Service headquarters, including the press office, may need to be informed. Legal advice is required in all cases and especially if it is believed that the food refusal is being undertaken as a means of suicide in the absence of mental disorder.

Other Prison Service documents that provide relevant standards and guidance are on *Treatment without Consent, Emergency Treatment, Restraint, Seclusion* and *Transfer of Prisoners to a Treatment Facility*. The Human Rights Act is pertinent.

Common law in England and Wales

Under the common law of England and Wales the provision of nutrition and hydration by artificial means constitutes medical treatment. No adult may be given medical treatment in the absence of their consent unless they lack the capacity to accept or refuse that treatment and it is in the patient's ' best interests' to administer the treatment proposed and the patient has not made a valid advance statement refusing treatment. An adult is presumed to have capacity until it is demonstrated that they do not. Demonstrating this involves an assessment about whether any aspect of the individual's ability to take in and retain treatment information, to believe it and to weigh it in the balance with regard to risks and needs has been sufficiently compromised to render them lacking capacity.

It is possible for capacity to fluctuate. In such cases, it is good practice to establish while the person has capacity their views about any clinical intervention (including compulsory feeding or hydration) that may be necessary during a period of incapacity and to record these views. The person may wish to make an advance refusal of certain types of treatment.

If it is concluded that the individual has capacity, then the staff should respect the decision to refuse food or liquids unless the individual changes their mind or a worsening mental disorder or other condition leads to a loss of capacity. This also applies to the provision of other medical treatment to prolong the individual's life.

If it is concluded that the individual lacks capacity, then it is lawful to treat in the individual's 'best interests', subject to any valid and applicable advance refusal of treatment. Best interests are not confined to best **medical** interests. Other factors that may need to be taken into account include the patient's values and preferences when competent, their quality of life, their spiritual and religious welfare and their own financial interests. Where there is doubt about an individual's capacity or best interests, obtain legal advice (for a more detailed discussion of capacity and consent to treatment, see page 300).

Advance directives

Even where the individual lacks capacity, consideration must be given to any advance directive that the patient may have made. Also known as a 'living will', an advance directive specifies how the individual would like to be treated in the case of future incapacity. Under the common law, it is now clear that an advance refusal of treatment that is valid and applicable to subsequent circumstances in which the patient lacks capacity is **legally binding**. An advance directive may be verbal as well as written. The law concerning advance directives is evolving. Where an advance directive is in existence, it is prudent to obtain legal advice early about its validity and the current law (for more information, see **Consent**, page 168).

Coexisting mental illness: use of the Mental Health Act

A patient may be transferred to a psychiatric hospital for treatment under the Mental Health Act when they are suffering from mental illness of a nature and/or degree that makes it appropriate for them to be detained in a psychiatric hospital for treatment and the need for such treatment is urgent (see **Use of the Mental Health Act**, page 163). Sometimes this will be the case even though the patient retains the capacity to consent to or refuse treatment. Capacity should be assessed separately from the presence or absence of mental illness.

Such transfer may enable the individual to be fed or rehydrated against their will once the individual is in the psychiatric hospital as a medical treatment for mental disorder under the provisions of the Act, if the food refusal is a symptom, consequence or manifestation of the mental disorder. For example, this would be the case if the food refusal was a symptom of severe depression or anorexia nervosa with impaired insight.

In this context, it is important to remember that advance directives may be overridden by the Mental Health Act to the same extent that the competent wishes of a detained patient may be overridden by the Mental Health Act.

Principles of management: all patients

- Assess and record the patient's physical and mental condition daily. Record an assessment of capacity regularly.
- Assess suicidal thoughts regularly and consider a management plan, including the use of current prison self-harm protocols. Suicidal intent, delusional content and energy to attempt suicide may all fluctuate.
- Obtain a psychiatric opinion early. Even where the doctor does not consider mental illness to be likely, an assessment is needed to confirm this formally and to assess capacity (see below).
- Inform the individual of the natural history of food or fluid refusal, including type of deterioration and pain. The Prison Service Dear Doctor Letter (96)1 is helpful. Leave food where the patient can eat it at meal times.
- Discuss with the patient the issues of capacity and refusal. Discuss confidentiality. Help the patient to plan the future. If appropriate, help the patient with any grievances and problems (eg help with writing to relatives, or access to a lawyer). Consider assisted visits for relatives. Provide information in ways that he/she can understand, if necessary in the patient's own language.
- Maintain a caring and professional attitude to the patient, eg address the individual in the manner preferred by them (first name or as Mr/Miss X). Especially where hunger strikes occur in the context of power struggles between staff and a prisoner, it is important for healthcare staff to maintain a degree of independence and not be drawn into seeing the individual simply as a trouble-maker.
- Act early to avoid having to discuss what might happen when the patient may have lost the capacity to determine their own future. Consult early and consult widely. Seek second opinions. The patient's family and lawyer should be contacted in addition to prison and healthcare staff.
- Involve a dietitian from the Local Trust, wherever possible.
- Hold regular multidisciplinary conferences. It is essential that all those involved in care are aware of any advance directive.
- Keep legible contemporaneous records.
- Ensure that support networks are in place for staff, relatives and those close to the patient.

Additional management advice for individuals where mental illness is present

Referral

- Request an early psychiatric opinion to assess both the capacity and mental state. Assessment should be obtained urgently, initially by telephone or fax (see **How to refer urgently**, page 153).
- If the patient requires transfer to a hospital, coordinate the mental-health teams and the medical teams, and agree where the prisoner would be housed. Exceptionally, a transfer to a general hospital for treatment under common law may become necessary.
- Discuss future transfer to a treatment facility with the Home Office Mental Health Unit early.

- If the prisoner has a high-security category, discuss the case with the prison and with Prison Service security managers.
- Maintain a care plan.

Additional advice and support for the patient

- Some patients, often those who are depressed, will take a little food that they particularly like. Pressure to finish what is in front of them is unlikely to help. Encourage drinking fluids, especially those containing vitamins such as fruit juice and milkshakes.
- Patients who have delusional ideas that the food is poisoned may eat packaged food that they open themselves.

Medication

If medication is accepted, doses may need reducing in the presence of liver or kidney impairment. Liver function tests do not correlate well with impairment of drug metabolism. Consult a specialist.

Additional management advice for adults where mental illness is not present

In the majority of cases, there is only partial food refusal. Close monitoring of eating and drinking may lead the patient to refuse more. Often, negotiations will achieve a mutually acceptable agreement without loss of face on either side. Nearly all food refusers start to eat again on their own.

The individual may wish to consider an advance directive about treatment at any time during food refusal. The individual's lawyer or probation officer should be contacted to arrange a visit. The right of access to legal representation is covered by the Human Rights Act.

Referral

Request a psychiatric opinion early to assess capacity, exclude mental illness and establish a working relationship with the psychiatric team. Relationships are maintained, and good medical practice is more likely when a physician is consulted early. The care plan should make clear the legal issues surrounding the refusal to feed and the reasons for not intervening.

Transfer to hospital may include the following.

- Facilitate visits from relatives and friends.
- Enable specialist rehydration and physical care to be given if the individual changes their mind.
- Enable the patient to be made comfortable in their terminal condition.
- Carers should have discussed where the patient wishes to die.
- It is essential to make clear to the general hospital staff (preferably in writing) when arranging transfer the current assessment of the patient's capacity, the purpose of the transfer to hospital and full details of any advance directive the patient has made, if these are known to anyone in the prison.
- Once the prisoner is at the hospital, clinicians there will continue to assess capacity as part of their management of the patient, taking account of any advance directive. In the absence of any such advance directive, at some stage they may decide that the patient no longer has capacity, in which case they may

then decide to administer treatment without the patient's consent if this is in the patient's best interests.

Resources for patients and primary support groups

Agencies that may support individuals in alternative ways of protesting include the following.

Board of Visitors

The Prisoners' Advice Service: 020 7405 8090 (Monday–Friday, 9:30 am–5.30 pm)
(Provides free legal advice and information to prisoners in England and Wales about their rights, the application of prison rules and the conditions of imprisonment)

1   Williams J. Hunger strikes: a prisoner's right or a wicked folly. *Howard Journal* 2001; 40: 285–296.
2   Bennett S. The privacy and procedural due process rights of hunger-striking prisoners. *New York University Law Review* 1983; 58: 1157–1251.

Dirty protests

Why do people make dirty protests?

People may make dirty protests for a variety of reasons.

- They may be making a political or personal protest.
- They become involved in power struggles, seeking a goal such as a transfer to another prison, and they are unprepared to recognise boundaries or authority. This pattern is much more commonly seen in prisoners with a personality disorder. Lack of cognitive and negotiating skills can lead rapidly to a prisoner progressing from normal accommodation to segregation and a dirty protest.
- Mental illness is less common but does occur. Other disorders, such as a brain tumour, are also possibilities. Prisoners may have both mental illness and a personality disorder.

Assessment

Because of the possibility of mental illness and other disorders, a full assessment is essential. Dirty protests should be assumed to be manifestations of health problems until proven otherwise. Dirty protests may also result in infections.

Healthcare staff engaged in assessing and then attempting to meet the healthcare needs of a prisoner on a dirty protest face a very unpleasant task. Facilities should be made available to allow staff to conduct a full assessment. Examinations of a prisoner's health should be held in adequate conditions, in circumstances that allow the prisoner to express him/herself freely and by a healthcare professional who is competent in assessing their mental state. An interview room is required. The prisoner's inmate medical record (IMR) should be to hand (and read) before the examination and the results of the examination entered into it. Observation of the patient alone, without talking to him/her, is never sufficient. Guidance on conducting a mental state assessment can be found on the disk ⌷.

While it is very important that the prisoner's mental state is regularly assessed, the frequency of such assessments and the need for a physical examination should be assessed on clinical grounds. If the healthcare worker has any concerns around the prisoner's mental health and/or if there is any record on the IMR of previous mental-health problems, he/she should arrange for a specialist assessment to be undertaken as soon as possible.

Management

All prisoners

- It may be possible for the protester to protest in another way. The Board of Visitors, chaplain and probation officers are likely to be able to represent the protester to others.
- Health staff should try not to be drawn into conflicts between the protester and prison staff. A neutral stance can be helpful if the protester starts to self-harm and requires medical treatment. A calm, caring, professional attitude may reduce tension on all sides.

- The physical health of the individual should be monitored. This may require specialist input from local NHS Trust staff. Early discussions with outside staff may be more efficient than more urgent discussions later. In offering these health interventions, the individual's capacity to consent or refuse consent should be considered (see **Consent and capacity**, page 168).
- Subject to considerations of confidentiality, the security implications of medical management should be discussed with prison staff.
- Caring for prisoners engaged in dirty protests is unpleasant and challenging for staff. Even where psychiatric staff have confirmed an absence of mental illness, they may be able to provide support to staff who remain in direct contact with the prisoner.

Prisoners with mental illness and/or personality disorder

The key principles of management are set out in **Management of prisoners with complex presentations and very difficult behaviours** (page 202). Multidisciplinary assessments, enhanced care plans and follow-up are likely to be indicated.

Resources for patients and primary support groups

Agencies that may support individuals in alternative ways of protesting include the following.

Board of Visitors

The Prisoners' Advice Service: 020 7405 8090 (Monday–Friday, 9:30 am–5.30 pm)
(Provides free legal advice and information to prisoners in England and Wales about their rights, the application of prison rules and the conditions of imprisonment)

Ethical issues — equivalent care and consent

> **Key ethical principles**
>
> The healthcare of prisoners requires a sound ethical framework. The key principles are the following.
>
> - The quality of care provided should not be dependent upon fluctuating social and political attitudes towards crime and punishment.
> - Loss of liberty must not entail the loss of a right to medical treatment to a proper ethical and clinical standard. Care of an equivalent standard to that available outside prison should be provided (concept of equivalence of care).
> - The concept of equivalence of care rests in turn upon the principle that imprisonment should be used 'as a punishment, not for punishment'.

Equivalent care

Achieving equivalent care for prisoners requires sustained effort and significant cooperation of healthcare professionals working in the community, those working in prison, other prison staff, Primary Care Trusts and Health Authorities, and central government officials. It is generally recognised that the aim of providing equivalent care is not yet achieved, with particularly disturbing problems in some areas with services for prisoners with mental-health problems and with the recruitment and retention of properly trained healthcare staff. In the interim period, clinicians will need to apply ethical guidelines for professional practice in clinical settings falling short of what is expected of a comprehensive psychiatric service.

To work effectively in prisons, healthcare professionals need to consider the needs of a prison and of the wider organisation. The potential tension between 'care' and 'control' is by no means exclusive to forensic settings; however, it is brought into sharper focus there and potential conflicts of interest are to be expected. Professionals need to deal with these as part of their everyday work, but when doing so they must be careful not to allow their ethical standards to be compromised.

Healthcare staff working in prison have a particular responsibility to act as advocates for adequate healthcare for mentally disordered prisoners by drawing the attention of the prison governor and the local Primary Care Trust/Local Health Group to the need to improve services, where there is a need to do so. The situation where healthcare staff have clear evidence that deficiencies in the service put their patients at unacceptable risk is dealt with below.

There is also an ethical obligation on psychiatric services outside the prison to respond promptly to requests for urgent assessment.

Consent to treatment

Requirement to obtain consent

Generally, health professionals cannot legally examine or treat any adult who has not specifically agreed to the examination or treatment. Treatment in this context includes the administration of food or liquids. Consent must be voluntary and must not be obtained by use of unfair pressure. If it is, the consent is invalid. Healthcare interventions carried out without valid consent, even if they are intended to be of benefit, may constitute an assault. Consent is required on every occasion an examination or treatment is offered, except in some emergencies or where the law prescribes otherwise. Consent can be verbal, written or implied by acquiescence. Acquiescence, when a patient does not know what the intervention entails or that there is an option of declining, is not valid consent.

Not everyone may be able to provide valid consent. Conditions that may interfere with the giving of valid consent include intellectual disability, organic brain dysfunction, the effects of drugs, the level of consciousness, mental illness and tiredness. Therefore, before consent is sought, the person must be judged capable of giving it. This is known as 'capacity' or 'competence' to consent to treatment.

Adults who have capacity are entitled to refuse consent to health interventions (other than treatment for mental disorder under the Mental Health Act 1983) even when doing so may result in permanent injury or death provided they fully understand the consequences of their decision.

Does the patient have capacity?

In the UK, an adult (aged 18 or over) is presumed to have capacity to consent to or refuse treatment until proved otherwise.

In determining whether the presumption of capacity can be rebutted in any individual case, the law requires doctors to examine whether the person concerned can follow the decision-making process of 'first, comprehending and retaining the treatment information, second, believing it (which does not necessarily mean accepting it) and third weighing it in the balance to arrive at a choice'.

Thus, to have capacity, the patient must be able to:

- understand what in broad terms is the nature of the treatment and that somebody has said that he/she needs it and why the treatment is being proposed
- understand its principal benefits, risks and alternatives
- understand what will be the consequences of not receiving the proposed treatment and
- retain the information for long enough to make an effective decision.

In determining any individual case, consideration should be given to the nature of the decision to be made. There may be reduced capacity and what matters is whether at that time the person's capacity was reduced below the level needed to make a decision of that particular importance. Mental illness, learning disability or imprudence do not on their own indicate a lack of capacity.

The capacity to give or refuse consent may come and go over time. It needs to be kept under review. Healthcare staff should record in their notes patients' views about consent or refusal of treatment. Consent once given is not final and can be withdrawn at any time, ie a person can change his/her mind.

Capacity in young people (those under 18)

- **A patient who is under 16 is not presumed to be competent to give consent.** They must demonstrate this. The central test is whether the young person has sufficient understanding and intelligence to understand fully the nature, purpose and possible consequences of the proposed intervention.
- **Where a patient under 16 is competent, he/she can give consent to an examination or treatment.** It is not then necessary to seek consent from those with parental responsibility (ie parents or the Local Authority). Prison staff are not

considered to be *in loco parentis*. It is good practice to involve parents, particularly for important or life-changing decisions, unless the young person requests that the matter remains confidential.

- **However, in England, Wales and Northern Ireland, even where a patient under 18 is competent, he/she may not necessarily refuse treatment if those with parental responsibility or a court allow the treatment to be given.** Where a competent young person refuses treatment, the harm caused by violating the choice must be balanced against the harm caused by failure to treat. If the disagreement is about a serious matter, it will often be better for a court to become involved rather than allowing parents automatically to overrule the young person. In Scotland, it is unlikely that the refusal of treatment by a competent young person can be overridden by parents or the courts.

- **Where a patient under 18 lacks capacity, someone with parental responsibility (ie a parent or Local Authority) can consent to treatment on their behalf.** The Children Act 1989 sets out persons who may have parental responsibility. They include the child's parents if married to each other at the time of conception or birth, the child's mother if not so married, the child's legally appointed guardian, a Local Authority designated in a care order in respect of the child, and a Local Authority who holds an emergency protection order in respect of the child. A full list is set out in Section 2(9) of the Children Act 1989 and in the Department of Health *Reference Guide to Consent for Examination or Treatment*. Where there is any doubt about who has parental responsibility, a specific enquiry should be made.

Has the patient received sufficient information?

To give valid consent, the patient needs to understand in broad terms the nature and purpose of the procedure. When seeking consent, the healthcare worker must give the person an account in simple terms of the benefits and risks of the proposed treatment and explain the principal alternatives to it in a manner the patient can understand.

How the information is presented is important. Information should be presented in the following ways.

- In the patient's own language. This is essential where the decision is one of life and death, eg where an Immigration Act 1971 detainee is refusing food. An interpreter may be required.

- In simple and clear language and, if necessary, broken down into chunks to aid understanding.

- In a form that takes account of any disability or impairment of the patient (eg deafness or blindness).

- Where possible, both verbally and in written form.

- At sufficient length for the patient to be able to understand it.

- On several occasions, especially where the decision is ongoing, eg food refusal.

Is the consent given voluntarily?

To be valid, consent must be given voluntarily and freely, without pressure or undue influence being exerted on the patient. In environments (such as prisons and mental hospitals) where there is a potential for treatment offers to be perceived coercively, extra care should be taken to ensure that the patient makes a decision freely. Pointing out the potential benefits of treatment for the patient's health does not constitute coercion, but threats such as withdrawal of any privileges or loss of remission of sentence for refusing consent does. Coercion invalidates consent.

Advance statements (known as 'living wills' or 'advance healthcare directives')

People who understand the implications of their choices can state in advance how they wish to be treated at such a time as they suffer loss of capacity. Such advance statements may either request a particular form of treatment or refuse particular forms of treatment. Where this statement refers to a refusal, it is sometimes known as an advance directive. For example, a patient who is refusing food may give a clear instruction refusing some or all medical procedures should their physical state deteriorate to such an extent that they lack capacity (an advance directive). An advance statement can be written, or it can be a witnessed oral statement or the note of a discussion recorded in the patient's file.

Advance requests for treatment are not legally binding, but advance refusals of treatment are, providing that the patient is an adult (over 18), had capacity and was properly informed when reaching the decision, the statement is clearly applicable to the present circumstances and there is no reason to believe that the patient has changed his/her mind. If doubt exists about what the patient intended, the law supports a presumption in favour of providing clinically appropriate treatment. Any advance statement is superseded by a clear and competent contemporaneous decision by the patient concerned. Where the patient is under 18, advance statements should be taken into account but do not necessarily have the same status as those of adults (see **Does the patient have capacity?** above).

Treatment without consent

Where a patient is suffering from a mental disorder which is leading to behaviour that is an immediate serious danger to self or to others, compulsory treatment is possible under the Mental Health Act 1983 but only in an NHS psychiatric hospital or appropriately registered mental nursing home to which he/she should be immediately transferred (see **Use of the Mental Health Act 1983**, page 149).

Patients in prisons cannot be treated without consent, except in certain very limited circumstances (for information, see **Emergency treatment under common law**, page 168).

Professional guidance on consent

Please note: this section does not provide comprehensive guidance on all issues surrounding consent. Further guidance can be found in:

- British Medical Association. *Report of the Consent Working Party: Incorporating Consent Toolkit*. London, 2001.
- General Medical Council. *Seeking Patients' Consent: The Ethical Considerations*. London, 1998.
- Department of Health. *Reference Guide to Consent for Examination or Treatment*. London, 2001.
- British Medical Association. *Consent, Rights and Choices in Health Care for Children and Young People*. London, 2001.
- British Medical Association. *The Impact of the Human Rights Act 1998 on Medical Decision-making*. London, 2000.
- British Medical Association. *Assessment of Mental Capacity*. London, 1995.

<hr>

Consent to treatment: a summary

- Health professionals cannot legally examine or treat any adult who has not specifically agreed to the examination or treatment. Treatment in this context includes the administration of food or liquids. The consent must be voluntary and must not be obtained by use of unfair pressure.
- Where a patient suffers from a mental disorder which is leading to behaviour that is an immediate serious danger to self or to others, compulsory treatment is possible under the Mental Health Act 1983, but only in an NHS psychiatric hospital or in an appropriately registered mental nursing home to which he/she should be immediately transferred.
- It may be possible to treat a patient under common law if they do not have the 'capacity' to give valid agreement to treatment. It is also required that the treatment is 'in their best interests' and that it is in accordance with a practice accepted at the time by a reasonable body of medical opinion skilled in the particular form of treatment in question.
- To have capacity, the patient must be able to:
  — understand what in broad terms is the nature of the treatment and that somebody has said that he/she needs it and why the treatment is being proposed
  — understand its principal benefits, risks and alternatives
  — understand what will be the consequences of not receiving the proposed treatment and
  — retain the information for long enough to make an effective decision.
- Advance refusals of treatment are legally binding providing that the patient is an adult (over 18), had capacity and was properly informed when reaching the decision, the statement is clearly applicable to the present circumstances and there is no reason to believe that the patient has changed his/her mind.
- Where a patient lacks the capacity to consent to or refuse treatment and there is no valid advance statement, the doctor has a duty of care under common law to provide treatment that is in their best interests.

<hr>

Confidentiality

Importance of confidentiality

Maintaining confidentiality of health information is one of the keystones of the patient–clinician relationship. Patients must be able to trust their healthcare workers not to reveal information inappropriately about their particular conditions or their behaviours (such as a relapse into drug misuse). Some particular groups of inmates (eg asylum-seekers detained under the Immigration Act 1971) may require considerable reassurance before they can trust healthcare staff. Maintaining confidentiality is particularly difficult in a prison. Prisons are closed societies and non-healthcare staff and inmates alike may surmise something about a patient's health simply by observing which professional a prisoner is going to see or which drug he/she is taking. Consequently, healthcare workers need to take extra care to safeguard patient confidentiality and to be seen by their patients to do so.

Importance of sharing information

On the other hand, there are occasions when it is in the best interest of the patient, or it is essential for the safety of others, that information is shared with others. These occasions include the following.

- Giving information and advice to non-healthcare staff (wing manager, personal officers, teachers, workshop supervisors) about the best way to manage and support a particular patient on ordinary location. It will frequently be appropriate for healthcare staff to act as advocates, eg to promote family contact, extra visits or telephone calls, to influence an appropriate location, to support suitable work placements or to acquire appropriate reading or art materials. In some ways, this is analogous to giving information to relatives and carers in the community.

- Participating in the multidisciplinary processes set up to plan the patient's sentence and then resettlement care in prison and back to the community. In some ways, this is analogous to participating in multidisciplinary Care Programme Approach (CPA) meetings in the community. It is essential to share information outside healthcare to facilitate creative solutions such as moves between wings and the healthcare centre, 'respite' stays in the healthcare centre, a mixed location (eg education centre or sheltered work during the day, the healthcare centre at night) and a planned response to a crisis, eg in the case of chronic self-injury in the presence of personality disorder, where several disciplines may be involved.

- Participating in procedures to support the multidisciplinary care of patients thought to be at risk of suicide or self-harm (currently in England and Wales F2052SH, in Scotland the Act to Care). Healthcare staff must provide clear guidance to other staff about the most effective ways of managing risk factors and what signs or symptoms should trigger a request for a further healthcare intervention.

- When the healthcare worker becomes aware that the patient presents a risk of serious harm to some other individual or group of individuals.

- When the healthcare worker becomes aware that a child is at risk of serious harm, including abuse (see **Child protection**, page 276).

Ways of sharing information while maintaining confidentiality

There are several ways to maximise the sharing of information required for multidisciplinary care while maintaining the requirements of confidentiality and the trust of the patient. These include the following.

- **Agreements allowing confidentiality to be held within a designated team.** This is what occurs within general practice teams and within multi-agency mental-health teams (usually consisting of doctors, nurses, social workers, occupational therapists, psychologists and non-professional 'support workers'). Patients are informed at the assessment stage that information about them may be shared on a need-to-know basis with the team and that confidentiality is maintained within the team boundary. Your local 'Caldicott Guardian' may be able to help you draw up a suitable protocol. (All Health Authorities and Primary Care Trusts/Local Health Groups have a Caldicott Guardian — a senior clinician on the Board — who is responsible for agreeing and reviewing protocols governing the disclosure of patient information across organisational boundaries).

- **Asking the patient for permission to share certain information with others.** Emphasise that the purpose is to ensure that the patient is treated as well as

possible on ordinary location and receives appropriate aftercare when he/she is released. Where this is explained sympathetically, many prisoners will agree to appropriate levels of disclosure. Permission is required on every occasion you are planning to disclose significant information. Permission should be written if possible. A copy of a template confidentiality agreement with a patient can be found on the disk 💾.

- **Giving general information about how to treat a group of prisoners.** It is often possible to give residential managers and workshop managers general information about how to manage prisoners with particular problems (eg those who are withdrawn, who hear voices, who have paranoid delusions) without giving confidential details which are on the inmate medical record (IMR) of a particular individual.

- **Providing the prisoner with the opportunity to talk directly with other staff.** The prisoner may be willing to disclose the relevant information to another member of staff (eg counselling, assessment, referral, advice and throughcare services [CARATS] worker, probation officer) themselves. Gaining patient permission to share information may be easier if the patient sees the report that is being shared or is present at the discussion about them.

When confidentiality may be overridden

Where there is a grave risk of serious harm to the individual or to others and the individual refuses consent to disclose information to avert such harm, the duty of confidentiality can be overridden by the duty in the public interest to prevent serious harm. In this case, information relevant to managing that risk should be shared on a need-to-know basis. Unless doing so risks serious harm, the patient should be informed about who has been told what and why.

What constitutes 'serious harm' is not defined in law and may be difficult to judge. Consultation with appropriate colleagues is advised and staff may find the guidance given to assist prison and probation staff assess the risk of serious harm helpful: 'a risk which is life-threatening and/or traumatic and from which recovery, whether physical or psychological, can be expected to be difficult or impossible'.

Professional guidance

The guidance of the most relevant professional bodies on confidentiality is summarised below.

General Medical Council (GMC)

The GMC in its guidance *Confidentiality: Protection and Providing Information* (2000) emphasises the importance of seeking patient consent to disclosure:

> You must obtain express consent where patients may be personally affected by the disclosure.... When seeking express consent you must make sure that patients are given enough information on which to base their decision, the reasons for the disclosure and the likely consequences of the disclosure. You should also explain how much information will be disclosed and to whom it will be given. If the patient withholds consent, or consent cannot be obtained, disclosures may be made only where they can be justified in the public interest, usually where disclosure is essential to protect the patient, or someone else, from risk of death or serious harm. (paragraph 14)

Where third parties are exposed to a risk so serious that it outweighs the patient's privacy interest, you should seek consent to disclosure where practicable. If it is not practicable, you should disclose information promptly to an appropriate person or authority. You should generally inform the patient before disclosing the information.

The GMC has confirmed that its guidance on the disclosure of information that may assist in the prevention or detection of abuse applies both to information about third parties (eg adults who may pose a risk of harm to a child) and about children who may be the subject of abuse).[1]

The Royal College of Psychiatrists

The Royal College of Psychiatrists in *Good Psychiatric Practice: Confidentiality*. Council Report CR85 (2000) suggests that decisions about whether a breach of confidence is justifiable depends on consideration of the following factors.

- Risks of non-disclosure: the probability of consequences and the seriousness of consequences. In general, disclosure should only be considered where there is risk of death or serious harm, including abuse.
- Benefits of disclosure: the likelihood that disclosure will have the desired result.
- Ability to identify a potential victim.
- Risk of disclosure: there may be occasions when the potential harmful effects of disclosure outweigh potential benefits.
- Context and role in which the doctor is working.

United Kingdom Central Council for Nursing, Midwifery and Health Visiting (UKCC)

The UKCC's *Guidelines for Professional Practice* (1996) contains the following advice on providing information.
Disclosure of information occurs:

- with the consent of the patient or client
- without the consent of the patient or client when the disclosure is required by law or by order of a court **and**
- without the consent of the patient or client when the disclosure is considered to be necessary in the public interest.

The public interest means the interests of an individual or groups of individuals or of society as a whole and would, for example, cover matters such as serious crime, child abuse, drug trafficking or other activities which place others at serious risk. (paragraphs 55 and 56)

Confidentiality: a summary
- Maintaining the confidentiality of health information is one of the keystones of the patient–clinician relationship.
- It may be in the best interest of the patient or it is essential for the safety of others that information is shared with others in order to:
  — give advice to residential staff about how best to care for a patient on ordinary location
  — participate in multidisciplinary care planning, eg sentence planning, prerelease planning

---

— participate in prison multidisciplinary processes to prevent suicide and self-harm, and

— prevent serious harm to the patient, to others or to a child.

- Ways to reconcile these two imperatives include the following.

— Forming agreements allowing confidentiality to be held within a designated team

— Asking the patient for permission to share certain information with others

— Giving general information to residential staff about how to care for prisoners with particular problems.

- Where there is a grave risk of serious harm to the individual or to others, and the individual refuses consent to disclose information to avert such harm, the duty of confidentiality can be overridden by the duty in the public interest to prevent the serious harm. In this case, information relevant to managing that risk should be shared on a 'need-to-know' basis. Unless doing so risks serious harm, the patient should be informed about who has been told what and why.

Isolation and mental health

Medical officers are required to visit prisoners held in segregation units or in seclusion to ensure that their mental state does not deteriorate to unacceptable levels and to check for other health issues. The relevant Prison Service Orders, PSO 1700A and 1700B, deal respectively with the maintenance of humane conditions in segregation units and with the management of prisoners who are segregated for any reason — whether for reasons of good order or discipline, in their own interests or protection or because of dirty protests.

Effects of isolation on mental health

There is a high risk that isolation, seclusion and segregation may damage mental health. There is no direct evidence for the precise psychological mechanisms operating in detention in isolated conditions. However, sensory deprivation experiments provide a situation that is analogous in at least some aspects. These experiments have led to dramatic and bizarre effects including anxiety, visual hallucinations and psychotic-type symptoms.[2] Prisoners held in solitary confinement may suffer similar symptoms, reporting loss of memory and impaired concentration.[3] The English Special Units Study, which looked at the treatment of some disruptive and dangerous prisoners, found that a subgroup had spent long periods in segregation and that psychotic symptoms had emerged, unbeknown to the prison staff.[4] Suicide and all types of psychiatric morbidity are common in prisoners held in isolation. Although the most extreme symptoms may often be associated with the most extreme environmental conditions, there is by no means a uniform effect across individuals. Some individuals can tolerate isolation better than others. Some people who have suffered severe and repeated traumas in childhood and their youth may be especially prone to stress-response syndromes.

Prisoners at increased risk of spending time in isolation

Some prisoners are more likely than others to spend extended periods in isolation or segregation. These include people who are mentally ill and/or have other disorders such as emotionally unstable (borderline) personality disorder, antisocial personality disorder and narcissistic personality disorder. They may be isolated because they present a risk to themselves or others, or because they engage in other difficult or dangerous behaviour. They may be isolated while awaiting assessment or transfer to hospital though, in current practice, individuals with personality disorder but lacking evidence of severe mental illness are unlikely to be transferred to an NHS hospital. Individuals who are seen as deliberately provocative or challenging of authority are also likely to spend long periods in isolation.

Until recently, prisoners considered at risk of suicide were sometimes managed in isolation in 'strip cells'. This is now against Prison Service instructions as it was found to be unacceptable and counter-productive (as it may increase suicidal thoughts). Use of crisis suites or shared cells is preferred. Prisoners assessed as being at a current risk of suicide or with a history of self-harm may receive some degree of protection by their placement in a dormitory. Where the risk of harm to (or from) other prisoners makes this impractical, their placement in a safer (ligature-free) cell is an alternative option (see **Assessing and managing people at risk of suicide**, page 204).

Management of prisoners in isolation

Prisoners who are mentally ill

Individuals who are mentally ill within the meaning of the Mental Health Act 1983 and who are held in segregation or seclusion, as that is the only way they can be safely contained, should be transferred immediately (within 24 hours) to a psychiatric hospital. Immediate transfer is often difficult, given variations in the availability of secure psychiatric beds. Nevertheless, it is an important standard (for NHS services to work towards) that such individuals should be accepted by them within 24 hours. A standard of assessment and, if necessary, admission within 24 hours for emergency cases is commonly set in the community and operates in most Scottish prisons. Where paranoid features of the illness mean that the individual refuses the limited access to exercise that is available, transfer is even more urgent (see **Liaison and referral to the NHS** and **Emergency treatment under common law**, pages 149 and 168).

Where the prisoner has any history, or current indication, of mental illness, self-destructive behaviour or substance misuse, an opinion should be sought from a psychiatrist and the appropriateness of relocating the prisoner in the healthcare centre considered. Where any current mental disorder is identified, a treatment plan should be drawn up and implemented.

Prisoners who spend frequent or extended periods in isolation

Prisoners who are not transferred to an outside psychiatric hospital and who are at increased risk of spending frequent or extended periods in segregation or seclusion should be managed as described in **Prisoners with complex presentations and very difficult behaviours** (page 202). Frequent or extended use of segregation, especially but not exclusively transfer from the segregation unit in one prison to that in another in order to provide respite to staff, should trigger a multidisciplinary assessment and the development of appropriate multidisciplinary care plans.

Such prisoners may benefit from admission to specialist units providing humane specialist management approaches such as the 'exceptional risk units' for prisoners with severe personality disorder who are also dangerous (eg at HMP Belmarsh). In whatever environment they are managed in, it is important to bear in mind the factors that characterise a good environment for people with a history of violence and which reduce the chances of violence being repeated. These factors include the following.

- Access to open space.
- Fresh air.
- Privacy, eg, toilet, washing and shower facilities.
- Personal space, including avoidance of overcrowding.
- Control of noise.
- Natural lighting.
- Controls of ambient temperature and ventilation.

See the Royal College of Psychiatrists' *Management of Imminent Violence.*[v]

All prisoners

Medical officers are required to assess the health of prisoners held in segregation.

There are conditions that are required for adequate health assessments. Examinations of a prisoner's health should be held in adequate conditions in circumstances that allow the prisoner to express him/herself freely and by a healthcare professional who is competent in assessing their mental state. An interview room is required. The prisoner's IMR should be to hand before the examination and the results of the examination entered into it.

The appropriate level and frequency of assessment will vary according to the time the prisoner is held in segregation upon the doctor's clinical judgement of the prisoner's state of health and the requirements of Prison Service standards.

- **Prisoners held in segregation for a few hours only pending adjudication.** In these circumstances, the assessment may only be about whether the prisoner is 'fit' for adjudication (eg they are capable of rational thought) and of their risk of suicide. It is also useful to look for signs of depression. Depression may sometimes lead to increased irritability and aggression, and have triggered the incident that led to the use of segregation.
- **Prisoners held for longer periods in segregation.** In these circumstances, a fuller Mental State Examination (MSE) should be conducted, looking in particular for signs of stress-induced psychosis or depression. The doctor's responsibility is to assess the health (including the mental health) of the prisoner and not simply to judge their 'fitness' (eg for punishment).
- **Prisoners with long-term behavioural problems** should be assessed particularly carefully. They are at increased risk of developing stress-induced psychosis and of self-harm.
- It is recommended that prisoners held in isolation are assessed on a daily basis. Should a mental disorder be identified, the prisoner should be managed as described in **Prisoners who are mentally ill** above.

Use of physical restraints

Doctors may sometimes be called upon to give advice about the appropriate use of mechanical restraints, which are more likely to be used in Segregation Units than in other parts of the prison. Currently, in prisons in England and Wales, where a patient has a medical condition leading to the violent behaviour, a doctor may order the use of 'medical restraint', ie the use of a 'special cell' or of a loose canvas restraint jacket. In addition, for all forms of violent behaviour, as a very last resort, a prison governor may order the use of 'mechanical restraint', ie the use of a body belt with metal cuffs or the use of special accommodation. Where a governor has ordered the use of either mechanical restraint or special accommodation, the role of the doctor is to assess whether there is any medical reason for not using these and if there is, to order their use to be ended immediately.

In the use of any form of physical restraint, the following are essential points of principle.

- It should be used as a last resort and for the shortest time possible.
- Steps should be taken to ensure the minimum possible invasion of the individual's dignity, eg audiences should be moved away.
- The individual should be treated in a way likely to calm rather than aggravate their aggression, eg speaking to them calmly and with respect.
- The individual's mental state should be assessed regularly and an urgent opinion sought from a psychiatrist if there is any history or current indication of mental illness, self-destructive behaviour or substance misuse.
- Where the patient has a mental disorder, care and treatment should be planned, if necessary and appropriate, under common law (see **Emergency treatment under common law**, page 168). Where indicated, steps should be taken to remove them urgently to a hospital where treatment can be given (see **Interface with the NHS and other agencies**, page 149).
- Where the patient has a history of very difficult behaviour, a full, multidisciplinary assessment and care plan should be arranged (see **Management of prisoners with complex presentations and very difficult behaviours**, page 202).

The relevant Prison Service instructions contain more detail about the management of prisoners who are segregated or physically restrained. Currently, in England and Wales, they are Prison Service Orders 1600 (Use of Force), 1700A (Management of Segregation Units) and 1700B (The Removal from Association of Prisoners Under Rule 45).

Isolation and mental health: a summary

- There is a high risk that isolation, seclusion and segregation may damage mental health. The English Special Units Study, which looked at the treatment of some disruptive and dangerous prisoners, found that a subgroup had spent long periods in segregation and that psychotic symptoms had emerged, unbeknown to the prison staff.
- Some individuals can tolerate isolation better than others.
- People who are mentally ill and/or have other disorders such as emotionally unstable (borderline) personality disorder, antisocial personality disorder and narcissistic personality disorder are more likely than others to spend extended periods in isolation or segregation.
- Managing people at risk of suicide in 'strip cells' is against Prison Service instructions, as it is unacceptable and counter-productive.
- Prisoners who are mentally ill within the meaning of the Mental Health Act 1983 and who are held in segregation or seclusion because that is the only way they can be safely contained should be transferred immediately (within 24 hours) to a psychiatric hospital. It is an important standard for NHS services to work towards that such patients should be accepted by them within 24 hours.
- Where a prisoner held in segregation has any history or current indication of mental illness, self-destructive behaviour or substance misuse, an opinion should be sought from a psychiatrist and the appropriateness of relocating the prisoner in the healthcare centre considered. Where any current mental disorder is identified, a treatment plan should be drawn up and implemented.

- Frequent or extended use of segregation and, especially but not exclusively, transfer from the segregation unit in one prison to that in another to provide respite to staff, should trigger a multidisciplinary assessment and the development of appropriate multidisciplinary care plans. Such prisoners may benefit from admission to specialist units providing humane management approaches — such as those being developed for prisoners with 'dangerous severe personality disorder'.

- MSEs should be conducted on prisoners held in segregation, looking in particular for signs of stress-induced psychosis or depression. It is recommended that all prisoners held in isolation are assessed on a daily basis.

- Physical restraints should only be used as a last resort and for the shortest time possible. Steps should be taken to ensure the minimum possible invasion of the individual's dignity.

Potential ethical conflicts for staff

Quality of the environment

While work is in progress to improve the environment in prison establishments, for some prisoners the environment will contribute to the development of depression, anxiety and paranoia (eg restricted activity). Indeed, it can be argued that even where everything possible has been done to provide a humane environment, factors intrinsic to imprisonment itself — such as separation from loved ones and friends, the inability to make decisions for oneself, a lack of access to normal ways of coping — can have a negative impact on mental well-being. Healthcare staff have the professional responsibility to decide at what point prison conditions (such as overcrowding and a lack of activity) have deteriorated to such an extent that there is a professional obligation to take constructive action to bring about change.

Different priorities and perspectives

Other issues where conflict may arise involve the different priorities and perspectives of different groups of management and staff. For example, access to prisoners is controlled by lock-up times. Especially at night when staffing levels are at their most tight and escorts hardest to provide, doctors wishing to transfer a patient to A&E may come under pressure to deal with the situation within the prison. Healthcare staff may also request a particular type of location or treatment for a patient, but this may be seen as unfair to other inmates by non-healthcare staff or their managers, with the result that such arrangements may break down.

Resolving ethical conflicts

Staff, whether in the NHS or the Prison Service, have a duty to work to the highest ethical standards and to disclose situations they believe are damaging to standards of care.

If such a situation arises, healthcare staff should make a contemporaneous record in writing detailing the event and must pass on the information as soon as is practically possible. Concerns should be raised through the Prison Service's grievance procedure, which is set out in the Staff Handbook, paragraphs 21.1–21.5. In addition, all staff working in prisons are entitled to raise concerns with the Board of Visitors. Nurses and doctors may also wish to raise concerns with their respective professional organisations. Doctors should follow GMC guidance in relation to concerns about the medical practice of colleagues. All healthcare workers should be aware of the provisions of the Public Interests Disclosure Act 1998.

Potential ethical conflicts for staff: a summary

- Staff, whether in the NHS or the Prison Service, have a duty both to work to the highest ethical standards and to disclose situations they believe are damaging to standards of care.
- Such situations may occur in relation to the quality of the environment in which prisoners are held or as a consequence of the different priorities and perspectives of different groups of management and staff.
- Such concerns can be raised through the Prison Service's grievance procedure, with the Board of Visitors or via professional organisations.

---

1   Department of Health, Home Office and Department of Education and Employment. *Working Together to Safeguard Children*. London, 1999.
2   Brownfield C. *Isolation: Clinical and Experimental Approaches*. New York: Random House, 1965.
3   Crassian S, Friedman N. Effects of sensory deprivation in psychiatric seclusion and solitary confinement. *International Journal of Law and Psychiatry* 1986; 8: 49–65.
4   Coid J. The management of dangerous psychopaths in prison. In Millon T, Simonsen E, Mirket-Smith M, Davis RD (eds), *Psychopathy, Antisocial, Criminal and Violent Behaviour*. New York: Guilford, 1998.
5   Royal College of Psychiatrists' Research Unit. *Management of Imminent Violence: Clinical Practice Guidelines to Support Mental Health Services*. London: Royal College of Psychiatrists, 1998.

Working with voluntary and community organisations

All sections of this guide give information about voluntary, community and self-help organisations that provide support to people with particular problems. These agencies can be a great resource for: patients, augmenting professional help with mutual support, befriending, information, practical advice and (some agencies) specialised professional counselling. Surveys report that some people with mental-health problems, of all severities, find the support of voluntary agencies very useful in helping them to live with their problems, though women are more likely to find this method of support acceptable than men.[1,2] However, the services of most agencies are not currently available within prisons.

Making use of the information about voluntary and community resources

You can use the information provided in this guide in several ways.

- You can give your patients information about relevant agencies so that they can telephone their helplines using their phone cards or write for advice and information.

- You can contact one or more agencies to obtain publications for distribution to your patients.

- You can give information about relevant agencies to someone before release and encourage them to make contact before or after release.

- You can, in collaboration with other staff from other disciplines (eg probation officers, chaplains), build a relationship with one or more agencies to enable them to provide a service that is particularly needed in your establishment.

Which agencies to involve will depend on the type of establishment. For example, the Citizens Advice Bureau exists in most localities and would be a valuable service in most prisons. Those prisons with Mother and Baby Units (MBU) may wish to consider building links with one of the several agencies that provide volunteer support to pregnant and new mothers. Several establishments already provide bereavement counselling or other specialised counselling. Where contracts are developed with agencies to provide professional services such as counselling, it will be essential to assure the quality of the service provided. The British Association for Counselling can provide information here (see **Resource directory**, page 316).

Sources of further advice and information

- Jo Gordon, Prison Service Voluntary Agencies Coordinator, Administration Group, Abell House, John Islip Street, London SW1P 4LH. Tel: 020 7217 6186 (Thursdays and Fridays).

- Prisons Community Links (CLINKS) is a voluntary organisation whose aim is to facilitate links between voluntary agencies and prisons. It can provide advice and support to both parties. It has a database of organisations that work in prisons and it produces a free newsletter, *Get Linked*, for community-based organisations working in prisons. Contact: Clive Martin, Director, CLINKS, Office 4, Central Methodist Centre, St Saviourgate, York YO1 8NQ. Tel: 01904 673970; E-mail: CLINKS@yorks.globalnet.co.uk.

- HM Prison Service and CLINKS. *Good Practice Guide: Prisons and the Voluntary and Community-based Sector*, 2001. Available from: either the Prison Service Voluntary Agencies Coordinator or CLINKS (see above). This is a very useful guide when inviting a voluntary or community agency to help establish a service within a prison. It includes choosing a partner agency, building a relationship, funding issues, communication and evaluation.

- Other staff in the prison, especially the chaplain and also the organiser of the visitor centre and others, may have valuable local links.

- Councils for Voluntary Service, sometimes known as Councils of Voluntary Organisations or, in rural areas, as Rural Community Councils. These are umbrella organisations that provide services to community and voluntary organisations in their area. A meeting with their director will give a great deal of information and advice about which agencies provide the sort of services that you are interested in and whether they are likely to have the capacity to expand their services. Their telephone number may be in the local telephone directory. In case of difficulty, telephone the reference section of the local library or the local Citizens Advice Bureau and ask for the telephone number.

- Volunteer Bureau. Again most areas have a Volunteer Bureau, which may be attached to the Council for Voluntary Service (see above) or independent of it. The Volunteer Bureau is a voluntary organisation whose purpose is to act as a matching agency for individuals wanting to volunteer in their community and agencies looking to involve volunteers in their work. A meeting with the organiser of the Volunteer Bureau to discuss ideas for possible programmes may be very valuable.

[1] Mental Health Foundation. *Strategies for Living: A Report of User-led Research into People's Strategies for Living with Mental Distress*. London: Mental Health Foundation, 2000.
[2] Scottish Health Feedback. *Mental Health and Primary Care: Needs Assessment Research for the Health Education Board for Scotland*. Final Report to the Health Education Board for Scotland, February 1999.

Resource directory

The following self-help, non-statutory and voluntary organisations are national or regional organisations, and the numbers are head-office numbers. Some of the agencies have networks of support groups across the country and they will be able to tell you where your nearest group is. All encourage self-referral. You may wish to adapt this directory to include details of your local groups.

Abuse: sexual, physical and emotional

Breaking Free: 020 8648 3500
Suite 23–25, Marshall House, 124 Middleton Road, Morden SM4 6RW
Support for men and (primarily) women abused as children, their families and professionals working with them. Support and information by telephone and by letter; additional support for women.

Careline: 020 8514 1177 (Monday–Friday, 10 am–4 pm, 7 pm–10 pm); 020 8514 5444 (administration: Monday–Friday, 9 am–4 pm)
Cardinal Heenan Centre, 326 High Road, Ilford IG1 1QP
Telephone counselling service for young people and adults on issues including child abuse, rape and sexual assault, bullying, depression, addiction, and mental health. Can provide counsellors fluent in Hebrew, Gujarati, Punjabi, Urdu, Hindi, French and Greek.

Childline: 0800 1111 (24-hour, 7 days per week freephone)
Royal Mail Building, Studd Street, London N1 0QW. 020 7239 1000 (administration)
Scotland: 18 Albion Street, Glasgow G1 1LH. 0141 552 1123 (administration)
Freepost address for children: Childline, Freepost 111, London N1 0BR
Telephone support and counselling for children and young people in danger and distress.

DABS — Directory and Book Services: 01302 768689
1 Broxholme Lane, Doncaster DN1 2LJ
Information, specialist mail order book service and referral for those abused in childhood, their families and professionals working with them.

Family Matters: 01474 537392 (helpline, 7 days per week: 10 am–12 noon, 2 pm–4 pm, 7 pm–8:30 pm); 01474 536661 (administration: Monday–Friday, 9 am–4:30 pm)
13 Wrotham Road, Gravesend DA11 0PA
Helpline and counselling for young people and adults who have been victims of sexual abuse, and their (non-abusing) family members. Counselling available in Punjabi, Gujerati, Hindi and French

London Rape Crisis Centre: 020 7837 1600 (Crisis line: Monday–Friday, 6 pm–10 pm; weekends, 10 am–10 pm); 020 7916 5466 (administration)
PO Box 69, London WC1X 9NJ
National helpline and (in London and the South East) face-to-face service for women and girls who have been raped or sexually abused; counselling, advice, information and referral.

NSPCC — Child Protection Helpline — England, Wales and Northern Ireland:
0808 800 5000 (24-hour, 7 days per week helpline); 020 7825 2500 (administration)
National Centre, 42 Curtain Road, London EC2A 3NH
Telephone counselling, information and advice for children or anyone else
concerned about a child at risk of abuse.

**Rape and Abuse Line (Scottish Highlands, Orkney, Shetland and Western
Islands):** 080 8800 0123 (7 days per week helpline answered by women:
7 pm–10 pm); 080 8800 0122 (helpline answered by men: Monday and Wednesday,
7 pm–10 pm)
PO Box 10, Dingwall IV15 9HA
Helpline for anyone affected by rape and/or abuse.

Young Abusers Project: 020 7530 6422
The Peckwater Resource Centre, 6 Peckwater Street, London NW5 2TX
Advice, information, counselling and assessment for juvenile sex offenders under
21. Only accepts referrals from professional bodies such as general practitioners,
social services and the Probation Service.

For those with learning difficulties

Respond: 08456 061503 (helpline: Monday–Friday, 1:30 pm–5 pm); 020 7383 0700
(administration)
3rd Floor, 24–32 Stephenson Way, London NW1 2HD
Telephone counselling and advice for people with learning difficulties who have
been sexually abused and/or who have abused others.

Voice UK: 01332 202555 (Monday–Friday, 9 am–5 pm)
The College Business Centre, Uttoxeter New Road, Derby DE22 3WZ
Telephone support and information for those with learning disabilities who have
been victims of abuse, and for their families and carers.

Addictions

Adfam National: 020 7928 8900 (helpline: Monday, Wednesday–Friday,
10 am–5 pm; Tuesday, 10 am–7 pm); 020 7928 8898 (administration)
Waterbridge House, 32–36 Loman Street, London SE1 0EH
Telephone support, counselling and advice for friends and families of drug users.
Information about drugs and referral to support services nationwide. Prisoners'
families support project.

Alcohol Focus Scotland: 0141 5726700
2nd floor, 166 Buchanan Street, Glasgow G1 2LW

Alcoholics Anonymous: 08457 697555 (24-hour helpline); 01904 644026
(administration)
PO Box 1, Stonebow House, Stonebow, York YO1 7NJ
Helpline refers to telephone support numbers and self-help groups across the UK
for men and women trying to achieve and maintain sobriety.

Battle Against Tranquillisers (BAT): 0117 966 3629 (7 days per week helpline: 9 am–8 pm)
PO Box 658, Bristol BS99 1XP
Telephone support to help people on benzodiazepine tranquillisers and/or sleeping pills to withdraw from them as comfortably as possible.

Drinkline: 0800 917 8282 (freephone helpline: Monday and Friday, 9 am–11 pm; weekends, 6 pm–11 pm); 0151 227 4150 (administration)
Healthwise Helplines, 1st floor, Cavern Court, 8 Matthew Street, Liverpool L2 6RE
Advice, information and referral for people with alcohol problems and concerned others.

Families Anonymous (local groups): 020 7498 4680 (7 days per week, 6 pm–11 pm)
UK Office, Unit 37, DRCA, Charlotte Despard Avenue, Battersea, London SW11 5JE
Runs over 60 self-help groups in the UK for families and friends of those with a drug problem.

Gamblers Anonymous: 020 7384 3040 (24-hour, 7 days per week helpline); 01422 250698 (administration)
PO Box 88, London SW10 0EU
Fellowship of men and women who are compulsive gamblers; local self-help groups across the UK with separate meetings for family and friends who are affected by gambling.

Gamcare: 08456 000133 (helpline: Monday–Friday, 10 am–10 pm); 020 7233 8988 (administration)
Suite 1, Catherine House, 25–27 Catherine Place, London SW1E 6DU
Advice, information and counselling for anyone affected by a gambling dependency.

Narcotics Anonymous: 020 7730 0009 (7 days per week helpline: 10 am–10 pm); 020 7251 4007 (administration)
202 City Road, London EC1V 2PH
Advice, information and counselling for addicts wishing to stop using drugs.

Northern Ireland Community Addiction Service (NICAS):
East Belfast: 219 Albertsbridge Road, Belfast BT5 4PU. 028 9073 1602
South Belfast: 40 Elmwood Avenue, Belfast BT9 6AZ. 028 9066 4434
West Belfast: 461 Falls Road, Belfast BT12 6DD. 028 9033 0499
Counselling, advice and information service for people with alcohol, drug or addiction problems. Any of the three offices will serve anyone from across Belfast and Northern Ireland.

Rehabilitation for Addicted Prisoners Trust (RAPT): 020 7582 4677
Riverside House, 27–29 Vauxhall Grove, London SW8 1SY
Provides full-time programmes in prison for inmates with drug and/or alcohol problems.

Release: 020 7603 8654 (out of hours helpline: Monday–Friday, 6 pm–10 pm; weekends, 8 am–12 midnight); 020 7729 9904 (heroin adviceline); 020 7729 5255 (administration)
388 Old Street, London EC1V 9LT
Information and advice, support and counselling for drug users and their families and friends on health, welfare and legal aspects of drug use. Referrals to specialist lawyers and local drug services.

Adoption

After Adoption: helplines: 08456 010168 (North East England) and 0161 839 4930 (Manchester) (Monday, Wednesday and Thursday, 10 am–12 noon, 2 pm–4 pm; Tuesday, 10 am–12 noon, 2 pm–7 pm); 0161 839 4932 (administration); E-mail: aadoption@aol.com
Canterbury House, 12–14 Chapel Street, Manchester M3 7NN
Advice, information, counselling and support, by telephone or in person, for anyone affected by adoption: adoptees, birth and adopted families.

Talk Adoption: 0808 808 1234 (helpline: Monday–Friday, 3 pm–9pm); 0161 819 2345 (administration); confidential E-mail: helpline@talkadoption.org.uk
12–14 Chapel Street, Manchester M3 7NN
Telephone support and information for under 25s who are adoptees, siblings or friends, or for their birth parents.

Anxiety, phobias, panic

No Panic: 01952 590545 (7 days per week helpline: 10 am–10 pm); 0800 7831531 (7 days per week freephone infoline: 10 am–10 pm); 01952 590005 (administration)
93 Brands Farm Way, Randlay, Telford TF3 2JQ
Telephone counselling, advice, information and referrals for people with phobias, obsessive/compulsive disorders and other anxiety disorders.

Obsessive Action: 020 7226 4000 (Tuesday, 10:30 am–3 pm; Wednesday, 11:30 am–5 pm)
Aberdeen Centre, 22–24 Highbury Grove, London N5 2EA
Advice and information for people suffering from obsessive-compulsive disorder, their families, friends and interested professionals.

Stresswatch Scotland: 01563 574144 (helpline: Monday–Friday, 10 am–6 pm); 01563 570886 (administration)
23 Campbell Street, Kilmarnock KA1 4HW
Information, advice and referrals for people affected by stress, anxiety or panic attacks.

Triumph Over Phobia (TOP UK): 01225 330353
PO Box 1831, Bath BA2 4YW
Coordinates a national network of structured self-help groups for people with phobias or obsessive-compulsive disorders.

Asylum seekers

See **Immigration detainees** below.

Attention deficit hyperactivity disorder (ADHD)

Attention Deficit Disorder Information Services (ADDIS): 020 8906 9068
PO Box 340 Edgware, Middlesex HA8 9HL
Extensive catalogue of books and videos on ADHD.

Bereavement

The Compassionate Friends: 0117 953 9639 (helpline: 7 days per week, 9:30 am–10:30 pm); 0117 966 5202 (administration)
53 North Street, Bristol BS3 1EN
Organisation of bereaved parents offering support and friendship to other bereaved parents who have lost a child of any age through any circumstance.

Cruse Bereavement Care: 08701 67 1677; 020 8940 4818 (administration)
Cruse House, 126 Sheen Road, Richmond TW9 1UR
Head office of national network of Cruse bereavement counselling services.
Provides telephone help and referrals to local Cruse branches and other counselling
services and bereavement support groups.

Foundation for the Study of Infant Deaths (FSID): 020 7233 2090 (24-hour
Helpline); 020 7222 8001 (administration)
Artillery House, 11–19 Artillery Row, London SW1P 1RT
Helpline for people bereaved by, or concerned about, cot death. Telephone support,
advice and information.

National Association of Bereavement Services: 020 7709 9090 (helpline:
Monday–Friday, 10 am–4 pm); 020 7709 0505 (administration)
4 Pinchin Street, London E1 1SA
Telephone counselling and referral helpline advising on the most appropriate local
source of support for bereaved people.

Stillbirth and Neonatal Death Society (SANDS): 020 7436 5881 (helpline:
Monday–Wednesday and Friday, 10 am–3 pm); 020 7436 7940 (administration)
28 Portland Place, London W1B 1LY
Supports bereaved parents and families affected by the death of a baby at or soon
after birth. Coordinates a national network of local self-help groups run by and for
bereaved parents.

Sudden Death Support Association: 0118 979 0790
Chapel Green House, Chapel Green, Wokingham RG40 3ER
Telephone support and advice for those bereaved under sudden and tragic
circumstances. The befriending service matches volunteers who have experienced
sudden bereavement with those who have been recently bereaved.

Survivors of Bereavement by Suicide: 08702 413337 (helpline); 01482 610728
(administration)
Centre 88, Saner Street, Hull HU3 2TR
National network of local self-help groups run by and for people bereaved by suicide.
Telephone support and referral to local groups, bereavement pack and literature.

Bipolar disorder

Manic Depression Fellowship
England and Wales: Castle Works, 21 St George's Road, London SE1 6ES.
020 7793 2600
Wales: 1 Palmyra Place, Newport NP20 4EJ. 01633 244244
Scotland: 7 Woodside Crescent, Glasgow G3 7UL. 0141 400 1867
Advice, information and support for people with manic depression and their
families, carers and mental-health professionals. Supports and develops national
networks of self-help groups. Wide range of resources: specialist publications and a
quarterly magazine.

Counselling and psychotherapy

British Association for Behavioural and Cognitive Psychotherapies: 01254 875277
PO Box 9, Accrington BB5 2GD
Produces a directory of accredited cognitive-behavioural practitioners. The list is
free, but please enclose an SAE.

The British Confederation of Psychotherapists: 020 8830 5173
37 Mapesbury Road, London NW2 4HJ
Register of psychotherapists, including psychoanalysts, analytical psychologists, psychoanalytical psychotherapists and child psychotherapists.

British Psychological Society: 0116 2549 568
St Andrew's House, 48 Princess Road East, Leicester LE1 7DR
Produces a directory of chartered clinical psychologists, which is available in most reference libraries.

Careline: 020 8514 1177 (helpline: Monday–Friday, 10 am–4 pm, 7 pm–10 pm); 020 8514 5444 (administration)
Cardinal Heenan Centre, 326 High Road, Ilford IG1 1QP
Telephone counselling service for young people and adults on issues including child abuse, rape and sexual assault, bullying, depression, addiction, and mental health. Can provide counsellors fluent in Hebrew, Gujarati, Punjabi, Urdu, Hindi, French and Greek.

Institute for Counselling and Personal Development Trust: 02890 330996
Interpoint, 20–24 York Street, Belfast BT15 1AQ
Offers counselling and psychotherapy (normally free), courses for helpers, and community training and development courses.

United Kingdom Council for Psychotherapy: 020 7436 3002
Provides information on registered therapists and training organisations.

UK Register of Counsellors: 08704 435232
PO Box 1050, Rugby CV21 2HZ
Supplies the names and addresses of British Association of Counsellors and Psychotherapists (BACP)-accredited counsellors. They are all appropriately trained and qualified, work to codes of ethics and are subject to complaints procedures.

Dementia

Alzheimer's Society: 0845 300336 (helpline: Monday–Friday, 8:30 am–6:30 pm); 020 7306 0606 (administration)
Gordon House, 10 Greencoat Place, London SW1P 1PH
Helpline for people with dementia, carers and professionals. Support, advice and information. Many local support groups nationwide.

Domestic violence

See also the Muslim Women's helpline under **Ethnic minorities and foreign nationals** below.

Kiran — Asian Women's Aid: 020 8558 1986
PO Box 899, London E11 1AA
Advice, support and refuge accommodation for Asian women experiencing domestic violence. It can provide staff fluent in Urdu, Hindi, Punjabi and Bengali.

Domestic Violence Unit or Community Safety Unit
For details, contact your local police station.

Everyman Project: 020 7737 6747 (helpline: Tuesday and Thursday, 7:30 pm–10 pm; it is used as an office number: Monday, Wednesday and Friday, 10 am–2 pm)
40 Stockwell Road, Stockwell, London SW9 9ES
Helpline for anyone concerned about a man's violence. Counselling by appointment for men who want to stop their violent and abusive behaviour.

Refuge: 0870 599 5443 (24-hour, 7 days per week Helpline); 020 7395 7700/7712 (administration)
National domestic violence helpline offering counselling, support, and advice for women and children escaping domestic violence. Network of refuges across the UK.

Rights of Women (England, Wales and Northern Ireland): 020 7251 6577 (adviceline: Tuesday–Thursday, 2 pm–4 pm, 7 pm–9pm; Friday, 12 noon–2 pm); 020 7251 6575 (administration)
52–54 Featherstone Street, London EC1Y 8RT
Telephone legal advice for women, mainly in the field of family law, but also for sexual violence, debt, housing and employment. Referrals to other agencies and sympathetic solicitors.

Women's Aid Federation England: 08457 023468 (24-hour, 7 days per week helpline); 0117 944 4411 (administration)
PO Box 391, Bristol BS99 7WS
Helpline for women experiencing physical, emotional or sexual violence in the home. Advice, information and referral.

Depression

Aware Defeat Depression Ltd (local groups): 02871 260602
22 Great James Street, Derry BT48 7DA
Provides information leaflets, lectures and runs support groups for sufferers and relatives.

Depression Alliance (local groups): 020 7633 0557/0559
35 Westminster Bridge Road, London SE1 7JB
National network of self-help groups. Gives support and information for people suffering from depression and their carers.

Seasonal Affective Disorders Association: 01903 814942
PO Box 989, Steyning BN44 3HG
Advice and information about seasonal affective disorder (SAD). Information pack for members.

Dyslexia

British Dyslexia Association: 0118 966 8271 (helpline: Monday–Friday, 10 am–12:30 pm, 2 pm–4:45 pm); 0118 966 2677 (administration)
98 London Road, Reading RG1 5AU
Information, advice and support for all those concerned with dyslexia. There is a network of local associations and trained befrienders.

Eating disorders

Centre for Eating Disorders (Scotland): 0131 668 3051
3 Sciennes Rd, Edinburgh EH9 1LE
Information, private psychotherapy and self-help manuals.

Eating Disorders Association: 01603 621414 (adult Helpline: Monday–Friday, 9 am–6:30 pm); 01603 765050 (youth helpline: Monday–Friday, 4 pm–6 pm); 01603 619090 (administration)
1st Floor, Wensum House, 103 Prince of Wales Road, Norwich NR1 1DW
Telephone support and advice for people affected by eating disorders. Runs a UK-wide network of support groups, postal and telephone contacts.

Overeaters Anonymous (local groups): 07000 784985 (7 days per week, 9 am–10 pm); 07626 984674 (administration)
PO Box 19, Stretford, Manchester M32 9EB
Network of approximately 150 local self-help groups providing help and support to compulsive overeaters and those with other forms of eating disorder.

Anorexia Bulimia Careline — Northern Ireland: 02890 614440

Ethnic minorities and foreign nationals

Racial issues

Commission for Racial Equality: 020 7828 7022; E-mail: info@cre.gov.uk
Elliot House, 10–12 Allington Street, London SW1E 5EH
Provides support and advice on all racial issues.

Northern Ireland Council for Ethnic Minorities (NICEM): 01232 238645
73 Botanic Avenue, Belfast BT7 4JL.

General advice and support

Akina Mama Wa Africa: 020 7713 5166
334–336 Goswell Road, London EC1V 7LQ
Advice, information and counselling for African women in prison on immigration, domestic violence, health and legal issues.

Confederation of Indian Organisations (UK): 020 7928 9889
5 Westminster Road, London SE1 7XW
Umbrella body for Asian voluntary groups. Publishes a directory of mental-health services for the South Asian communities. Also houses the Greater London Translation Unit for professional translation and interpreting in 15 Indian, Chinese, European, African and Middle Eastern languages.

Female Prisoners Welfare Project, Hibiscus and **Hibisco:** 020 7329 2384
15 Great St Thomas Apostle, Mansion House, London EC4V 2BB
Provides advice and help with family problems, housing, childcare, fostering, adoption, deportation and immigration to women of all nationalities in prison. Liaises with families abroad and provides presentence and circumstance reports. Hibiscus supports Nigerian and Jamaican women. Hibisco supports Latin American and Spanish-speaking women. Has branches in Lagos and Jamaica.

Grupo Amiga: 020 7226 5879
c/o Women in Prison, Aberdeen Studios, 22 Highbury Grove, London N5 2EA
Gives support to Latin American women in British prisons. Its members are all women and all speak either Spanish or Portuguese.

Irish Commission for Prisoners Overseas: 020 72729843
St Mellitus' Church, Tolington Park, London N4 3AG
Provides advice and support to Irish prisoners and their families, regardless of
crime, status or religious belief.

Muslim Women's Helpline: 020 8904 8193 or 8908 6715 (helpline: Monday–Friday,
10 am–4 pm); 020 8908 3205 (administration)
Culturally appropriate emotional support over the telephone for Muslim women.
Information and advice on domestic violence, sexual abuse, marital problems,
health and bereavement; referrals to other services.

Philemon Project: 020 8746 0328
59 Godolphin Road, Shepherds Bush, London W12 SJF
Offers practical assistance, advice and support to offenders, ex-offenders and their
families from African, Caribbean, Asian and other ethnic minorities.

Mental-health support or counselling

Jewish Association for the Mentally Ill (JAMI): 020 8458 2223
16A North End, Golders Green, London N11 7TH
Telephone advice and information, support and counselling for Jewish people with
severe mental-health problems, and for their families and carers.

Latin American Women's Rights Service (LAWRS): 020 7336 0888
52–54 Featherstone Street, London EC1Y
Provides advice and information on immigration, health, domestic violence and
housing to Latin American women in London. Provides counselling to women
suffering depression, postnatal depression, low self-esteem, loss of cultural identity,
anxiety and PTSD.

Miyad — National Jewish Crisis Helpline: 08457 581999 (Sunday–Thursday,
12 noon–12 midnight; Friday, 12 noon–11 pm); 020 8203 6311 (administration)
23 Ravenshurst Avenue, London NW4 4EE
Telephone support for anyone from the Jewish community on issues including
suicidal calls, mental illness and emotional distress.

NAFSIYAT Intercultural Therapy Centre: 020 7263 4130
278 Seven Sisters Road, Finsbury Park, London N4 2HY
Intercultural therapy centre. Short-term therapy for people from black and minority
ethnic communities. Addresses social, cultural and racial experiences. May be able
to assist in providing information about therapists elsewhere in the UK.

Mental-health support: spiritual, religious and cultural care

Chaplains will be the main first port of call here. The following organisations may
also help.

Islamic Cultural Centre: 020 7724 3633
146 Park Road, London NW8 7RG
Appoints and recommends visiting Imams in prisons, ensures that Muslim inmates
can practise their religion and supplies the Quran and Islamic books to prisoners.

The National Federation of Spiritual Healers: 01932 783164; E-mail:
office@nfsh.org.uk; URL: http://www.nfsh.org.uk
Old Manor Farm Studio, Church Street, Sunbury-on-Thames TW16 6RG
The NFSH has more than 6500 members working individually and in centres
throughout the UK.

National Federation of Spiritual Healers (Scotland): 0141 339 8994
c/o 24 Hamilton Park Avenue, Kelvinbridge, Glasgow G12 8DT
Provided signposting for healing across Scotland. Healing centres in Aberdeen,
Inverness and Edinburgh.

Prison Phoenix Trust: 01865 798647
PO Box 328, Oxford OX1 1PJ
Teaches meditation and yoga and supports prisoner practice via a network,
correspondence and a newsletter.

Brahma Kumaris World Spiritual University: 020 8727 3355
Global Co-operation House, 65 Pound Lane, London NW10 2HH
Work in prisons and the community providing a range of programmes on life skills
and personal development, including teaching and supporting meditation

Families, support for

ATD Fourth World: 020 7703 3231
48 Addington Square, London SE5 7LB
Respite stays and artistic workshops for families affected by long-term poverty and
whose children are at risk or in care.

Family Contact Line: 0161 941 4011 (helpline: Monday–Friday, 10 am–10 pm;
Saturday, 10 am–1pm); 0161 941 4522 (family centre in North West England)
30 Church Street, Altrincham WA14 4DW
Telephone support and counselling for people under stress on issues such as marital
and relationship problems, children and family.

Halow (Birmingham): 0121 551 9799
PO Box 7081, Birmingham B18 4AN
Support for partners and families of prisoners; advice on travel, children's rights,
prison visits, etc.

Home Start: 0116 233 9955
2 Salisbury Road, Leicester LE1 7QR
Support, friendship and practical help for families with at least one child under 5
who are experiencing stress or anxiety. Home visits by volunteers.

Newpin:
England: Sutherland House, 35 Sutherland Square, London SE17 3EE. 020 7703 6326
Northern Ireland: Development Office, 8 Windsor Avenue, Lurgan BT67 9BG.
02838 324843
Befriending and support groups for parents of young children who are under stress.
Work focuses on alleviating maternal depression and distress; it also provides
training in parenting skills and family-play programmes.

POPS — Partners of Prisoners and Families Support Group: 0161 277 9066
Suite 4b, Building 1, Wilson Park, Monsall Road, Manchester M40 8WN
Advice, information, support and a range of services for the families, partners and friends of those in prison. Casework support, welfare and accommodation rights advice, and debt counselling.

Prisoners' Families and Friends Service: 0808 808 3444 (helpline: Monday, Tuesday, Thursday and Friday, 10 am–5 pm; Wednesday, 10 am–8 pm);
020 7403 4091/9359 (administration)
20 Trinity Street, London SE1 1DB
Advice and information for friends and relatives of prisoners.

Immigration detainees

Support for convicted prisoners under threat of deportation

Campaign Against Double Punishment: 0161 740 8600 (Monday–Friday, 9.00 am–4.00 pm)
c/o POPS, St Mark's Cheetham, Tetlow Lane, Cheetham, Manchester M8 7HF
Provides advice and support for convicted prisoners under threat of deportation and their families. Campaigns against the use of deportation as a penalty for convicted prisoners.

Greater Manchester Immigration Aid Unit: 0161 740 7722
400 Cheethamhill Road, Manchester M8 9LE
A leaflet entitled *Information and Advice for Convicted Prisoners Under Threat of Deportation'* is available in a number of translations.

Groups that visit people detained under the Immigration Act or help provide bail for their release

Bail for Immigration Detainees (BID): 020 7247 3590
28 Commercial Street, London E1 6LS
Detainees who are held pending an entry decision or upon lodging an appeal can apply for bail to an adjudicator after 7 days' detention. The detainee needs to find two people willing to put up a sum of money as surety. BID helps find such people for detainees without their own contacts.

London Detainee Support Group: 020 7739 9907
74 Great Eastern Street, London EC2A 3JL
Visits and supports asylum seekers in detention in London.

Association of Visitors to Immigration Detainees (AVID): 01962 863 317
53 Western Road, Winchester SO22 5AH
Association of individual visitors and visitors' groups who befriend and support immigration detainees held in prisons, detention centres and police stations.

Detention Advice Service (DAS): 020 7704 8007
244a Upper Street, London N1 1RU
Offers advice, information and support to anyone detained or threatened with detention under Immigration Act powers in the UK. Visits only in the London area.

326

Legal advice to asylum seekers

Asylum Aid: 020 7377 5123
28 Commercial Street, London E1 6LS
Independent organisation providing free advice and support for refugees and asylum seekers in the UK. Helps people present their asylum applications.

Refugee Legal Centre: 020 7378 6242 (adviceline: Monday–Wednesday, Friday–Sunday, 9.30 am–1.00 pm); 020 7827 9090 (administration)
Sussex House, 39–45 Bermondsey Street, London SE1 3XF
Will provide advice and representation at the place of detention, by telephone, on its premises and at appeal hearings.

Immigration Advisory Service: 020 7357 6917
County House, 190 Great Dover Street, London SE1 4YB
Government-funded services providing legal advice, assistance and representation for asylum seekers.

General advice and support to asylum seekers

The Refugee Council: 020 7820 3085 (enquiry line); 020 7820 3000 (administration); URL: http://info@refugeecouncil.demon.co.uk
3 Bondway, London SW8 1SJ
Gives practical help to refugees and asylum seekers. Offers advice, outreach, free leaflets on housing, health, claiming asylum, women, where to get advice, in English, Arabic, French, Somali, Spanish, Turkish and Russian, and some in additional languages. Publishes a nationwide directory of services for asylum seekers and refugees.

Scottish Refugee Council: 0141 333 1850
98 West George Street, Glasgow G2 1PJ
Provides advice, information and legal representation to asylum seekers through out the asylum process.

Welsh Refugee Council: 01222 666 250
Unit 9, Williams Court, Trade Street, Cardiff DF1 5DQ

Refugee Action (North West, East Midlands, South West, South Central):
Birmingham: 0121 693 9989; Derby: 01332 294 202; Leeds: 0113 244 5345; Leicester: 0116 235 8367; Liverpool: 0151 708 7836; London: 020 7654 7700; Manchester: 0161 740 6711
Provides help and advice to asylum seekers through one-stop shops in different UK regions. Also advises to organisations that provide services to asylum seekers.

Help for asylum seekers in tracing family members

British Red Cross: 020 7235 5454
Family Reunion Section, 9 Grosvenor Crescent, London SW1X 7EJ
Helps trace family members separated by conflict and has a message service where communications have broken down due to war or disaster. It also holds a register of all unaccompanied minors arriving in the UK in order that they may be put in

contact with their families. It also provides food parcels, free clothing and blankets for destitute asylum seekers. (Detainees are not eligible for full family reunification arranged via the Home Office, which is only available to those with full refugee status.)

For mental and emotional distress

Medical Foundation for the Care of Victims of Torture: 020 7813 7777
Star House 96–98 Grafton Road, London NW5 3EJ
Works to relieve the difficulties of individuals and their families who have been subjected to torture and other forms of organised violence. Doctors, therapists and caseworkers giving medical care, psychotherapy, social and welfare support and initial help with housing. In addition, it provides medical reports documenting evidence of torture for asylum purposes. Visits to detainees on one-off basis following referral by solicitors.

The Traumatic Stress Clinic: 020 7530 3666
73 Charlotte Street, London W1P 1LB
Offers treatment to refugees experiencing serious trauma reaction; offers advice on the management of traumatic stress.

Refugee Support Centre: 020 7820 3606
47 South Lambeth Road, Vauxhall, London SW8 1RH
London-wide, face-to-face multilingual counselling and psychotherapy for refugees and asylum seekers experiencing emotional or physical distress. Useful for post-release. Helpline for professionals and individuals.

Tavistock Clinic Refugee Services: 020 7435 7111
Child and Family Department, 120 Belsize Lane, London NW3 5BA
Provides consultation to other bodies, such as general practitioner practices, on working with refugees

Learning disability

For agencies that deal with people with learning disabilities and issues of abuse, see **Abuse**.

Down's Syndrome Association
England, Wales and Northern Ireland: 155 Mitcham Road, London SW17 9PG.
020 8682 4001
Scotland: 158–160 Balgreen Road, Edinburgh EH11 3AU. 0131 313 4225
Information, advice, support and counselling for people with Down's syndrome, their families, carers and professionals. Runs networks of local self-help groups.

Mencap
England and Wales: 123 Golden Lane, London EC1Y 0RT. 020 7696 5593/5503
Northern Ireland: Segal House, 4 Annadale Avenue, Belfast BT7 3JH.
028 9069 1351
National network of support, advice and information services for children and adults with learning disabilities and their families. Provides residential, employment, further education, leisure and holiday services.

National Autistic Society (local groups): 0870 600 8585 (helpline: Monday–Wednesday, Friday, 10 am–4 pm; Thursday, 10 am–8 pm); 020 7833 2299 (administration)
393 City Road, London EC1V 1NG
Telephone information for people who are autistic, their carers and families. Literature, national diagnostic and assessment service, supported employment scheme, befrienders and other services.

Mental health and illness: general

MARCH (Mental Aftercare in Registered Care Homes): 0800 783 4621 (7 days per week freephone helpline: 9 am–5 pm); 01698 852771 (administration)
Silverwells House, 1 Old Mill Road, Bothwell, Glasgow G71 8AY
Telephone advice on all aspects of mental healthcare, as well as other services for people who are, or have been, suffering from a mental disorder.

Mental Aftercare Association (MACA): 020 7436 6194
25 Bedford Square, London WC1B 3HW
Range of community-based services for adults with mental-health needs including advocacy, outreach, community support, respite care and supported accommodation.

Mental Health Medication Helpline: 020 7919 2999 (Monday–Friday, excluding Bank Holidays, 11 am–5 pm); URL: http://www.nmhc.co.uk
Run by the UK Psychiatric Pharmacy Group and staffed by experienced mental-health pharmacists, it provides independent advice and information about drugs to patients and carers. The website contains detailed, user-friendly information for service users on psychiatric drugs.

Mental Health Foundation: 020 7535 7400
20–21 Cornwall Terrace, London NW1 4QL
Wide range of publications including a series of free leaflets about mental illness and learning disabilities for the general public.

MIND (local groups): 08457 660 163 (infoline, outside London: Monday–Friday, 9:15 am–4:45 pm); 020 85221728 (infoline, London: Monday–Friday, 9:15 am–4:45 pm); 020 8519 2122 (administration)
Granta House, 15–19 Broadway, Stratford, London E15 4BQ
Runs network of more than 220 local Mind associations. Information, legal advice and referral for users of mental-health services, carers, professionals and the public.

Northern Ireland Association for Mental Health: 028 9032 8474
80 University Street, Belfast BT7 1HE
Provides services in the community for people with mental-health needs. Information and advice on all aspects of mental health including rights, welfare and law.

Revolving Doors: 020 7242 9222
45–49 Leather Lane, London EC1N 7TJ
Helps people with mental-health problems who have come into contact with the criminal justice system to gain better access to health, housing and socialcare. Casework support to the most vulnerable in a number of projects in the South East of England.

329

SANELINE: 08457 678000 (7 days per week Helpline: 12 noon–2 am); 020 7375 1002 (administration)
1st Floor, Cityside House, 40 Adler Street, London E1 1EE
Telephone information and advice on mental health issues, emotional support for mentally ill people and their families and carers, and referral to sources of help and support.

Scottish Association for Mental Health: 0141 568 7000
Cumbrae House, 15 Carlton Court, Glasgow G5 9JP
Telephone information on any aspect of mental health, including benefits and legal issues. Also, a range of residential, training and employment projects and services in the community.

Parents

Family Rights Group: 0800 731 1696 (freephone adviceline: Monday–Friday, 1:30–3:30 pm); 0800 783 0697 (freephone adviceline for Turkish families: Tuesday, 10 am–12 noon); 020 7923 2628 (administration); E-mail: office@frg.u-net.com
The Print House, 18 Ashwin Street, London E8 3DL
Telephone advice and information and advocacy for parents and carers who have children in care or involved with the social services. Publications available in a range of languages.

Gingerbread Information line: 0800 0184318 (1000–16000 weekdays)
England, Wales and Scotland: 16/17 Clerkenwell Close, London SW10 0EU; 020 7488 9300
Northern Ireland: Information and Advice Department, 169 University Street, Belfast BT7 1HR. 02890 234568/231417 (administration)
Information and advice for lone parents on a range of issues. Runs national networks of self-help groups for support of lone parents.

National Council for One-Parent Families: 0800 018 5026 (freephone helpline: Monday–Friday, 9:15 am–5:15 pm); 020 7428 5400 (administration)
255 Kentish Town Road, London NW5 2LX
Information, advice, support and referral for lone parents. Free publications containing information on a range of issues.

The Orminston Children and Families Trust: 01473 724517
333 Felixstowe Road, Ipswich IP3 9BU
Provides support and guidance for parents on the courts, benefits and welfare systems. Organises prerelease courses for parents in prison and a prison parenting course for fathers.

Parentline Plus: 0808 800 2222 (helpline: Monday–Friday, 8 am–10 pm; Saturday, 9.30 am–5 pm; Sunday, 10 am–3 pm); 020 7284 5500 (administration)
520 Highgate Studios, 53–79 Highgate Road, Kentish Town, London NW5 1TL
Support, information and advice to anyone involved in caring for children.

Postnatal and baby problems

Association for Postnatal Illness: 020 7386 0868 (Monday and Friday, 10 am–2 pm; Tuesday and Wednesday, 10 am–5 pm)
145 Dawes Road, Fulham, London SW6 7EB (SAE needed)
Runs a network of volunteers to support sufferers throughout the UK. Leaflets are available.

Meet a Mum Association (MAMA): 020 8768 0123 (helpline: Monday–Friday, 7 pm–10 pm); 01761 433598 (administration)
26 Avenue Road, South Norwood, London SE25 4DX
Telephone information and support for women experiencing postnatal illness. Network of local groups and contacts providing friendship and support for mothers and pregnant women who are isolated and lonely.

The Miscarriage Association: 01924 200799/200795 (administration)
c/o Clayton Hospital, Northgate, Wakefield WF1 3JS
Information and support for people affected by pregnancy loss. Referral to volunteer-support workers and self-help groups across the UK.

National Childbirth Trust (NCT): 020 8992 8637/2616
Alexandra House, Oldham Terrace, Acton, London W3 6NH
Information and support in pregnancy, childbirth and early parenthood. Referral to counsellors and local support groups.

Serene Cry-Sis: 020 7404 5011 (7 days per week Helpline: 8 am–11 pm)
Helpline for parents or carers of excessively crying, sleepless and demanding babies. Support and practical (non-medical) advice.

Relationship problems

Relate: 01788 573241; URL: http://www.relate.org.uk
Herbert Gray College, Little Church Street, Rugby CV21 3AP
Coordinates local Relate centres in England, Wales and Northern Ireland offering counselling for adults with relationship difficulties, whether married or not; occasionally psychosexual counselling and mediation. Payment according to income.

Rapport: 029 2081 1733
PO Box 488, Cardiff CF15 7YY
UK-wide couple counselling service.

Schizophrenia

National Schizophrenia Fellowship: 020 8974 6814 (adviceline: Monday–Friday, 10 am–3 pm)
England and Wales: 28 Castle Street, Kingston upon Thames KT1 1SS. 020 8547 9230
Scotland: Claremont House, 130 East Claremont Street, Edinburgh EH7 4LB. 0131 557 8969
Northern Ireland: 'Wyndhurst', Knockbracken Health Care Park, Saintfield Road, Belfast BT8 8BH. 02890 402323
Telephone advice and information for people with schizophrenia and other severe mental illnesses, their families and carers, on mental health-related issues including benefits, community care and law. Runs a network of over 300 projects across the UK, including supported accommodation, training and daycare.

Self-care for professionals

British Medical Association Stress Counselling Service: 08459 200169
Free, 24-hour, confidential counselling service available to doctors, their families and medical students to discuss personal, emotional and work-related problems.

331

National Counselling Service for Sick Doctors: 01455 255171
Confidential advisory service. Deals with concerns about own health or that of a colleague.

Medical Council on Alcoholism: 020 7487 4445

RCN Counselling Service: 08457 697064 (helpline, RCN members only);
020 7647 3464 (administration)
Counselling in person and by telephone and for members of the Royal College of Nursing only.

Nurseline: 020 7647 3463 (helpline: Monday–Friday, 9 am–1pm, 2 pm–4 pm)
Advice, information and support for nurses and midwives, including those who are students, retired or unemployed. Deals with personal, professional and employment issues. Service provided through the Royal College of Nursing but is for all nurses, whether or not they are members of the College.

The Listening Friends Scheme: 020 7820 3387
The Royal Pharmaceutical Society of Great Britain, 1 Lambeth High Street, London SE1 7JN
Free and confidential advice to pharmacists suffering from stress. Automated answering service asks callers to leave contact details and a convenient time to be called back. Operates independently of the Society.

Self-esteem and creativity

Burnbake Trust: 01202 548139
PO Box 1839, Bournemouth BH9 2ZQ
Motivates and encourages prisoners to create art by visiting prisons to select work for exhibition and sale. Proceeds are returned to the prisoner.

Prison Phoenix Trust: 01865 512521/521522
PO Box 328, Oxford OX2 7HF
Teaches and encourages use of techniques such as meditation and yoga among prisoners through correspondence and a network of teachers.

Prism Project: 01279 777007; E-mail: info@prismproject.org
PO Box 6031, Bishop's Stortford CM23 1PP
Provides prison libraries with a wide range of self-help books and tapes. Can also supply prison health centres with tapes to loan to prisoners on topics such as relaxation, coping with depression and coping with anxiety.

Prison Writing: URL: http://prisonwriting@aol.com
PO Box 478, Sheffield S3 8YX
'Opening up a closed world.' Promotes creative writing among prisoners with the annual publication of a book compilation of their prose and poetry.

Inside Out Trust: 01273 833050
Hilton House, 55–57a High Street, Hurstpierpoint BN6 9TT
Liaises between prisons and charitable or community organisations to foster projects in which inmates make goods and services available to those in need, while gaining knowledge and skills.

Prisoners' Education Trust: 020 88703820
Suite 39, Argyll House, 1a All Saints Passage, London SW18 1EP
Provides funds for adult prisoners wishing to take distance learning courses, and to make available art and craft materials.

Self-harm

Young Minds produce a resource pack on self-harm; see **Young people**.

Basement Project: 01873 856524
PO Box 5, Abergavenny NP7 5XW
Information and literature on self-harm and abuse. Runs groups and workshops for women who have been abused. Coordinates national forum of people who work with self-harm.

Bristol Crisis Service for Women: 0117 925 1119 (helpline: Friday and Saturday, 9 pm–12:30 am)
PO Box 654, Bristol BS99 1XH
Telephone counselling and information for any woman in distress, with particular focus on self-injury. Publications and training on self-injury.

National Self-Harm Network
PO Box 16190, London NW1 3WW
Provides information sheets and training, and campaigns for the understanding of people who self-harm.

Sexual issues

Beaumont Society: 01582 412220 (24-hour, 7 days per week infoline)
27 Old Gloucester Street, London WC1N 3XX
National self-help organisation for transvestites, transsexuals, and their partners and families. Advice and information on issues of cross-dressing and gender dysphoria; social functions.

Brook Central: 08000 185023 (freephone Helpline: Monday–Thursday, 9 am–5 pm; Friday, 9 am–4 pm); 020 7284 6040 (administration)
Head office for a national network of 33 Brook Advisory Centres that offer the under 25s advice, counselling and medical help around contraception, pregnancy, abortion and sexual health.

Gender Trust: 07000 790347 (information line: 8:45 am–4 pm, sometimes open until 10 pm); 01273 234024 (administration)
PO Box 3192, Brighton BN1 3WR
Volunteer-run telephone information, befriending, self-help and specialist referrals services for transsexuals, gender dysphorics or transgenderists.

Mermaids: 07020 935066 (helpline: usually 12 noon–9pm); 01869 248238 (administration)
BM Mermaids, London WC1N 3XX
Volunteer-run information, support and befriending service for children and young people with gender identity problems. Local contacts around the UK.

Out-Side In: 01689 835566
PO Box 119, High Street, Orpington BR6 9ZZ
Befriending pen-pal service for gay and lesbian prisoners.

Sleep problems

Insomnia Helpline: 020 8994 9874 (Monday–Friday, 6 pm–8 pm)

British Snoring and Sleep Apnoea Association: 01249 701010;
E-mail: snoreshop@britishsnoring.demon.co.uk; URL:
http://www.britishsnoring.demon.co.uk
1 Duncroft Close, Reigate RH2 9DE

Narcolepsy Association UK (UKAN): 020 7721 8904;
E-mail: info@narcolepsy.org.uk
Craven House, 1st Floor, 121 Kingsway, London WC2B 6PA

Suicidal feelings

Samaritans: 08457 909090 (24-hour, 7 days per week helpline); 01753 216500
(administration); URL: http://www.samaritans.org.uk
10 The Grove, Slough SL1 1QP
Emotional support by telephone for anyone in a crisis, feeling lonely, despairing or
suicidal. Local branches and helplines throughout the UK.

CALM — Campaign Against Living Miserably: 0800 585858 (freephone 7 days per
week helpline: 5 pm–3 am); 0161 2372720 (administration)
Telephone counselling for men aged 15–24 who are depressed or suicidal.

Trauma (including assault)

For agencies dealing with various types of abuse, see **Abuse: sexual, physical and
emotional**.

ASSIST — Assistance Support and Self-help in Surviving Trauma: 01788 560800
(freephone helpline: Monday–Friday, 10 am–4 pm); 01788 551919 (administration)
The Penthouse, 11–13 Bank Street, Rugby CV21 3PU
Support and counselling by telephone (UK wide) and in person (the Midlands only)
to people experiencing post-traumatic stress disorder (PTSD). Critical incident
debriefing and clinical assessment for PTSD and depression.

Trauma Aftercare Trust (TACT): 0800 1696814 (24-hours, 7 days per week
freephone helpline); 01242 890306 (administration)
Buttfields, 1 The Farthings, Withington GL54 4DF
Telephone information, counselling, some welfare advice and referrals for people
suffering from psychological trauma from any source.

Victim Support Line: 0845 3030900 (Monday–Friday, 9 am–9pm; weekends,
9 am–7 pm)
PO Box 11431, London SW9 6ZH
England & Wales: Cranmer House, 39 Brixton Road, London SW9 6DZ. 020 7735 9166
Scotland: 15/23 Hardwell Close, Edinburgh EH8 9RX. 0131 668 4486
Northern Ireland: Annsgate House, 70–74 Ann Street, Belfast BT1 4EH. 028 9024 4039
National charity that runs 362 local schemes with trained volunteers offering
emotional support, information and practical help to victims and witnesses of crime,
their families and friends.

Welfare: help and support

For agencies dealing with women prisoners' welfare, see **Women's issues**.

Apex Charitable Trust: 0113 2392416
1 Reginald Terrace, Chapletown, Leeds LS7 3FZ
National charity providing advice and support to help (ex-)offenders and prisoners find employment. The range of employment-focused projects and services across the country for (ex-)offenders.

Benefits Enquiry Line for people with disabilities: 0800 882200 (freephone)
Information about Disability Living Allowance, Invalid Care Allowance and other benefits.

Bourne Trust: 020 7582 6699/1313
Lincon House, 1–3 Brixton Road, London SW9 6DE
Formerly the Catholic Social Services for Prisoners. Practical help, advice and support to (ex-)prisoners and families (regardless of religious belief); volunteer prison visits and some professional counselling to prisoners.

HABAP — Housing Advice for Black and Asian Prisoners: 0113 234 1693
Waterloo House, 58 Wellington Street, Leeds LS1 2EE
Culturally sensitive housing advice service to black and Asian staff and prisoners, taking referrals from prisons across the UK.

The Langley House Trust: 01993 774075
PO Box 181, Witney OX8 6WD
Provides accommodation to ex-offenders with a range of care, support and supervision services to help them integrate into the community and to protect the public from their re-offending. Works with prisons, the Probation Service, and both health and social services.

NACRO — National Association for the Care and Rehabilitation of Offenders: 0800 0181259 (freephone adviceline)
England and Wales: 169 Clapham Road, London SW9 0PU. 020 7582 6500

NIACRO — Northern Ireland Association for the Care and Rehabilitation of Offenders: 01232 320157
169 Ormeau Road, Belfast BT7 15Q

SACRO — Safeguarding Communities, Reducing Offending in Scotland: 0131 624 7270
1 Broughton Market, Edinburgh EH3 6NU
NACRO, NIACRO and SACRO promote the care and resettlement of offenders in the community. Advice, information and a range of services for ex-prisoners including housing, resettlement and education and training.

National Association of Citizens Advice Bureaux (NACAB): 020 7833 2181
Myddelton House, 115–123 Pentonville Road, London N1 9LZ
National office for the national network of Citizens Advice Bureaux, which provides free, confidential advice for the general public on a wide range of issues.

National Debtline: 0808 808 4000 (helpline: Monday and Thursday, 10 am–4 pm; Tuesday and Wednesday, 10 am–7 pm; Friday, 10 am–12 noon); 0121 248 3000 (administration)
Birmingham Settlement, 318 Summer Lane, Birmingham B19 3RL
Helpline offering information and advice on debt.

New Bridge: 020 7976 0779
27a Medway Street, London SW1P 2BD
Provides support and guidance to prisoners and ex-prisoners on employment and family issues, and a befriending service through letters and visits. Publishes prisoners' quarterly national newspaper, which is available in prisons.

Prince's Trust: 0800 842842 (freephone)
Helps offenders and ex-offenders aged 14–30 with various personal programmes, including help in starting a business. Provides loans and bursaries.

Prison Fellowship (England and Wales): 01621 843232
PO Box 945, Maldon CM9 4EW
Christian ministry running a volunteer-based national network of local groups to offer spiritual and practical support for prisoners, ex-prisoners and their families. Sends Christmas presents to prisoners' children, regardless of their country of origin. (Also aims to promote Biblical standards of justice within the criminal justice system.)

Prisoners' Advice Service: 020 7405 8090
Unit 305 Hatton Square, 16/16a Baldwins Gardens, London EC1N 7RJ
Takes up prisoners' complaints about prison treatment and resolves disputes via internal adjudications.

Resource Information Service: 020 7494 2408
The Basement, 38 Great Pulteney Street, London W1R 3DE
Publishes information on resources available to homeless people and other disadvantaged groups. Publications include *London Hostels Directory*, *Telephone Helplines Directory*, *Homeless Pages* and the *UK Advice Finder*.

Shelter Helpline: 0808 800 4444 (24-hours, 7 days per week)
General advice and help on housing problems.

Women's issues

For agencies dealing with domestic violence, see **Domestic violence**. For agencies dealing with ethnic minority women, see **Ethnic minorities and foreign nationals**.

Women in Prison: 020 7226 5879
3b Aberdeen Studios, 22 Highbury Grove, London N5 2EA
Information and support to female prisoners; visiting caseworkers provide advice on after-release accommodation, mental-health projects, drug and alcohol rehab projects, education and training.

Female Prisoners Welfare Project, Hibiscus and **Hibisco:** 020 7357 6543
18 Borough High Street, London Bridge, London SE1 9QG
Provides advice and help with family problems, housing, childcare, fostering, adoption, deportation and immigration to women of all nationalities in prison.

Liaises with families abroad and provides presentence and circumstance reports. Hibiscus supports Nigerian and Jamaican women. Hibisco supports Latin American and Spanish-speaking women. Has branches in Lagos and Jamaica.

Rights of Women (England, Wales and Northern Ireland): 020 7251 6577 (adviceline: Tuesday–Thursday, 2 pm–4 pm, 7 pm–9pm; Friday, 12 noon–2 pm); 020 7251 6575 (administration)
52–54 Featherstone Street, London EC1Y 8RT
Telephone legal advice for women, mainly in the field of family law, also advice on sexual violence, debt, housing and employment. Referrals to other agencies and sympathetic solicitors.

Women Prisoners Resource Centre: 020 8968 3121
1a Canalside House, 383 Ladbrook Grove, London W10 5AA
Advice and information service for women in prison. Part of the National Association for the Care and Rehabilitation of Offenders (NACRO): also runs housing, employment, training and other services for women ex-prisoners.

Young people

For agencies dealing with young people and abuse, see **Abuse**. For agencies that deal with adoption, see **Adoption**. For agencies dealing with young people and self-harm, see **Self-harm**.

Childline: 0800 1111 (24-hour, 7 days per week freephone); 020 7239 1000 (administration)
Royal Mail Building, Studd Street, London N1 0QW
Freepost address for children: Childline, Freepost 111, London N1 0BR
Telephone support and counselling for children and young people under 18 in danger and distress.

Get Connected: 0800 096 0096 (7 days per week freephone helpline: 3 pm–11 pm); 020 8260 7373 (administration)
PO Box 21082, London N1 9WW
Telephone support on any issue for vulnerable young people and children, including runaways and homeless people.

National Youth Advocacy Service: 0800 616101 (freephone helpline: Monday–Friday, 3:30 pm–9:30 pm; weekends, 2 pm–8 pm); 0151 342 7852 (administration)
1 Downham Road South, Heswall CH60 5RG
Information, advice and advocacy for children and young people under 25 via a network of advocates and in-house solicitors.

Who Cares? Linkline: 0500 564570 (helpline: Monday, Wednesday and Thursday, 3:30 pm–6 pm); 020 7251 3117 (administration)
Kemp House, 152–160 City Road, London EC1V 2NP
Telephone information and support for young people who are or have been in care, and carers.

Young Minds Trust: 0800 182138 (freephone parent information service);
020 7336 8445 (administration)
102–108 Clerkenwell Road, London EC1M 5SA
The parent information service provides information and advice for anyone
concerned about the mental health of a child. Produces a range of leaflets for
parents and young people

Youth Access: 020 8772 9900
2 Taylors Yard, 67 Alderbrook Road, London SW12 8AD
National umbrella for youth information, advice, counselling and personal support
agencies (YIACs); gives information on and referrals to appropriate local YIACs,
including youth counselling services that help with self-injury.

Further reading and websites

Further copies of this book can be obtained from: The Prison Health Task Force (prison staff) Tel: 01788 834215 or RSM Press Tel: 020 7290 2900

Clinical

General

Andrew G, Jenkins R (eds), *Management of Mental Disorders*, UK edition. Sydney: World Health Organization Collaborating Centre for Mental Health and Substance Abuse, 1999.
Excellent, accessible textbook for use by general practitioners and generalist mental-health clinicians working in community settings. Covers core management skills, medication, affective disorders, anxiety and somatoform disorders, schizophrenic disorders, personality problems, sexual dysfunction and sleep disorders. Note that it is not available via bookshops or via the Internet. Available from: Management of Mental Disorders, PO Box 55, Aldershot GU12 4FP. Credit card payments: Tel: 01252 322252; Fax: 01252 322315.

British Medical Journal 'ABC of Mental Health' series:

Gerada C, Ashworth M. Addiction and dependence I: Illicit drugs. *British Medical Journal* 1997; 315: 297-300.
Review of drug misuse, dependence and management. Includes a table of benzodiazepines in equivalent doses of diazepam and a table of opioids in equivalent doses of methadone.

Ashworth M, Gerada C. Addiction and dependence II: Alcohol. *British Medical Journal* 1997; 315: 358-360.

Hale AS. Anxiety. *British Medical Journal* 1997; 314: 1886-1889.

Marlowe M, Sugarman P. Disorders of personality. *British Medical Journal* 1997; 315: 176-179.

Davies T. Mental health assessment. *British Medical Journal* 1997; 314: 1536-1539.

Atakan Z, Davies T. Mental health emergencies. *British Medical Journal* 1997; 314: 1740-1742.
Review of the causes of mental-health emergencies, safety and risks, rapid tranquillisation and aftercare.

Dein S. Mental health in a multiethnic society. *British Medical Journal* 1997; 315: 473-476.
Review of the cultural beliefs and practices of a patient, the errors doctors can make and mental health in ethnic cultures.

Watson JP, Davies T. Psychosexual problems. *British Medical Journal* 1997; 315: 239-242.

Pathare SR, Paton C. Psychotropic drug treatment. *British Medical Journal* 1997; 315: 661-664.
Reviews factors affecting the choice of antidepressants, antipsychotics, anti-anxiety medications and anticholinergics. Also covers patient concordance.

Turner T. Schizophrenia. *British Medical Journal* 1997; 315: 108-111.

Armstrong E. *Mental Health Issues in Primary Care: A Practical Guide*. Basingstoke: Macmillan, 1995.
Written for generalist nurses in primary care by a health visitor and mental-health educator. Discusses the treatments available and strategies for prevention of depression, anxiety and schizophrenia.

Medication

Taylor D, McConnel D, Abel K, Kerwin R. *The Bethlem and Maudsley NHS Trust Prescribing Guidelines*. London: Martin Dunitz, 2001. Available from: ITPS Ltd, ISBN 1-853-17963-9. £15.00. Tel: 01264 332424.
Provides detailed, annually updated information on prescribing psychotropic drugs. There are helpful charts and flow-charts.

Bazire, S. *Psychotropic Drug Directory 2000 (The Professionals' Pocket Handbook & Aide-Mémoire)*. Quay, 2000. Salisbury. ISBN 1-85642-180-5.
Compact, up-to-date information on psychiatric drugs. Contains community-orientated information.

Psychological therapies

Padesky C, Greenberger D. *Clinicians Guide to Mind Over Mood*. New York: Guilford, 1995.
Guide to cognitive therapy. It supports clinicians in acting as guides to patients using the companion volume.

Mind Over Mood: A Cognitive Treatment Manual for Clients.
Suitable for use by primary-care counsellors or others with appropriate training.

Daines B, Gask L, Usherwood T. *Medical and Psychiatric Issues for Counsellors*. London: Sage, 1997.

Self Injury

Crowe M. Deliberate self-harm. In Bhugra D, Munro A (eds), *Troublesome Disguises: Underdiagnosed Psychiatric Syndromes*. Oxford: Blackwell, 1997.
Useful overview of the literature plus a description of the treatment methods used at the South London and Maudsley NHS Trusts 'Crisis Recovery Unit' — the leading NHS treatment centre for people who self-harm repeatedly.

Ashworth Hospital Authority and MIND. *Self-injury: A Resource Pack*. Liverpool and London, 1996.
Available from: Ashworth Hospital, Parkbourn Maghull, Liverpool L31 1HW. Tel: 0151 473 0303; Fax: 0151 526 6603.
Information pack that covers personal accounts, the competencies required by healthcare staff and treatment guidelines.

Hawton K, Cowen P. *Dilemma and Difficulties in the Management of Psychiatric Patients*. Oxford: Oxford University Press, 1990.
Self-injury and other challenging behaviour analysed from a medical management perspective. Interesting and easy to access.

Suicide

Department of Mental Health and WHO. *Preventing Suicide: A Resource for Prison Officers*. London and Geneva, 2000.
Available from: www.who.int/mental_health/topic_suicide/
Advice for prison officers, produced as part of the WHO world-wide initiative for the prevention of suicide.

Substance misuse

Department of Health, The Scottish Office, Welsh Office and Department of Health and Social Services, Northern Ireland. *Drug Misuse and Dependence: Guidelines on Clinical Management*. London: HMSO, 1999.

Service development

Department of Health. *Treatment Choice in Psychological Therapies and Counselling: Evidence Based Clinical Practice Guideline*. London, Department of Health, 2001.
Developed by the British Psychological Society Centre for Outcomes Research and Effectiveness, the book makes recommendations relating to the treatment of depression, including suicidal behaviour, anxiety, panic disorder, social anxiety and phobias, post-traumatic disorders, eating disorders, obsessive-compulsive disorders, personality disorders, repetitive self-harm, chronic pain and chronic fatigue where there is an emotional element.

Department of Health and Prison Service. *Nursing in Prisons*. London, 2000.

Mental Health Foundation. *Knowing Our Own Minds: A Survey of How People in Emotional Distress Take Control of Their Lives*. London, 1997.
Valuable summary of what people with mental-health problems find useful; many simple, cost-effective options.

Clinical Advisory Group. *Depression*. London: Department of Health, 2000.
Evidence-based standards for services of depression, a review of the state of current services and recommendations for improving services. It focuses largely on primary care.

Counselling in Primary Care. *Guide to Setting Up and Running a Managed Primary-care Counselling Service.* Available from: Counselling in Primary Care, 95 Hewarts Lane, Bognor Regis PO21 3DJ. Tel: 01243 268322.

Internet resources

Centre for Evidence-Based Mental Health
The centre has established a website with extracts from the journal *Evidence-based Mental Health*, which includes a useful evidence-based mental-health toolkit. It is a gateway to many other related sites through its links.
URL: http://www.cebmh.com/

The Cochrane Collaboration
URL: http://www.update-software.com/ccweb.default.htm

NHS Centre for Reviews and Dissemination
URL: http://www.york.ac.uk/inst.crd.welcome.htm

Health Evidence Bulletins Wales
URL: http://www.uwcm/Ib/pep

Institute of Psychiatry, King's College, London
URL: http://www.iop.kcl.ac.uk/main
The Institute's library website page has links to other resources.

Mental Health Foundation
URL: http://www.mentalhealth.org.uk

PriMHE (Primary Care Mental Health Education)
URL: http://www.primhe.org
Information and links specific to primary-care mental health.

UK Psychiatric Pharmacy Group
URL: http://www.ukppg.co.uk
Useful resources section, including 'Bespoke', an individualised patient information system.

WHO Health in Prisons Project
URL: http://www.hipp-europe.org
Health (in its broadest sense) in prisons in Europe.

Joint Prison Service and Department of Health site on prison health
URL: www.hmprisonservice.gov.uk/prisonhealth/index.htm

Prison Service England and Wales website — health page
URL: http://www.hmprisonservice.gov.uk/life

Prison Service Northern Ireland
URL: www.niprisonservice.gov.uk

Scottish Prison Service
URL: www.sps.gov.uk

Training resources

Training courses may be organised locally via university Departments of General Practice, Psychiatry or Nursing, Strategic Health Authorities or Primary Care Trusts, often utilising locally available skills. The following provides courses or training packs on a national or regional basis.

Training courses for prison staff

Prison Service mental-health training

A prison health-training manager started work in May 2001 to develop bespoke induction programmes and training for all prison healthcare staff, including healthcare officers, nurses, doctors and healthcare managers. Courses in mental health are an early priority, including a course for prison officers and non-healthcare staff. Work also includes the introduction of national occupational standards for prison nursing, the roll out of an NVQ in custodial healthcare for healthcare officers, the development of a modified system for assessing registered nurses against the occupational standards, and the further development and introduction of clinical appraisal models.

Contact: Marc Harrison, Curriculum Development Manager, Prison Service Training College, Newbold Revel, Rugby CV23 0TH. Tel: 01788 834048.

Prison Service suicide and self-harm prevention and management training

Core, multidisciplinary training in the prevention of suicide and self-harm is available from the establishment's training section. Further training, relevant to the needs of staff working in particular parts of the prison, will be developed from 2001 to 2003.

Contact: Lisa Jasper, Training Manager, Safer Custody Group, Abell House, John Islip Street, London SW1 4LH. Tel: 020 7217 2132.

John Moores University training, Liverpool

A certificate in Therapeutic Skills for generic prison officers in the North West is available. There are four modules: Experiential Learning and Reflection; Interpersonal Skills; Personal Stress and Anxiety Management; and Mental Health and Illness. Officers undertaking the course need to travel to the university for regular days spent in the classroom.

Contact: Deb Knott or Christina Lyons, Programme Leaders, School of Health and Human Sciences, Liverpool John Moores University.

Resources for use by trainers of prison staff

- *Understanding and Working with Women in Custody*, 2nd edn (2001).
- *The Nature of Adolescence: Working with Young People in Custody*, 2nd edn (1997).

Developed by the Trust for Study of Adolescence (TSA) in cooperation with the Prison Service, both packs cover normal adolescent development. *Understanding and Working with Women in Custody* also looks at mental-health issues and, in particular, provides a very helpful introduction to the issue of repetitive self-harm. The second edition relates to adult women as well as adolescents. Aimed at all types of prison staff, it provides useful background understanding. It does not address specific treatment issues. Packs are available for £110.45 from: Publishing Department, Trust for Study of Adolescence Ltd, 23 New Road, Brighton BN1 1WZ. Tel: 01273 693311; Fax: 01273 679907; E-mail: tsa@pavilion.co.uk; or Woman's Policy Unit, HM Prison Service, Abell House, John Islip Street, London SW1P 4LH.

Training courses for primary healthcare staff (non-prison specific)

The **Sainsbury Centre for Mental Health** is a mental-health charity that provides a mental-health-training consultancy. Courses are developed to meet the needs of the organisation requesting them. It has extensive experience in primary-care mental-health training, particularly in relation to patients with severe mental illness and in the commissioning of services. It is not experienced in working in prisons. Contact: Dr Alan Cohen, Primary Care Lead, Sainsbury Centre for Mental Health, 134–138 Borough High Street, London SE1 1LB. Tel: 020 7403 8790.

The National Depression Care Training Centre provides a range of short (1- or 2-day) courses primarily for general nurses working in primary care, but also for general practitioners and multidisciplinary groups, on caring for people with depression in primary care, and giving an introduction to mental illness, schizophrenia and anxiety management. It also runs a 3-day Trainers' Course for clinicians who already have some existing training skills. Contact: Elizabeth Armstrong or Martin Davies, National Depression Care Training Centre, University College, Northampton, Thornby 1, Park Campus, Boughton Green Road, Northampton NN2 7AL. Tel: 01604 735 500 ext. 2640; Fax: 01604 712 425.

Courses for pharmacists in mental-health issues are available from the following institutions.

- Aston University, supported by the UK Psychiatric Pharmacists Group. It provides a Postgraduate Certificate, Diploma and MSc in Psychiatric Pharmacy and a Diploma by distance learning. Contact: Penny Delaney, Course Administrator, Aston Pharmacy School, Aston University, Aston Triangle, Birmingham B4 7ET. Tel: 0121 359 3611; E-mail: P.J.Delaney@aston.ac.uk.
- De Montford University provides a Certificate in Psychiatric Therapeutics and a Postgraduate Diploma in Psychiatric Pharmacy, both either part-time or by distance learning. Contact: Dr DM Collet, School of Pharmacy, De Montford University, The Gateway, Leicester LE1 9BH. Tel: 0116 257 7275; E-mail: SASCPD@dmu.ac.uk.
- Centres for Pharmacy Postgraduate Education (England, Scotland and Wales) all provide short workshops and distance-learning modules.

The Counselling in Primary Care Trust keeps information about additional training for counsellors in issues particular to work in general practice, including a Degree programme. Contact: Dr Graham Curtis-Jenkins, Counselling in Primary Care Trust, Majestic House, High Street, Staines TW18 4DG.

PriMHE (Primary Care Mental Health Education) is an initiative to bring together health professionals active in primary mental healthcare to provide a nationally coordinated programme of mental-health education. There are discussion forums for teachers, researchers and Primary Care Trust/Local Health Group mental-health leads. Co-chairs are Dr André Tylee and Dr Chris Manning. PriMHE does not itself provide training. Contact: PriMHE Secretariat, 29 Park Road, Hampton Wick KT1 4AS. Tel: 020 8891 6593; E-mail: PriMHE@compuserve.com; URL: http://www.Primhe.org

Northern and Yorkshire NHS Region 'Teach the Teachers' Course. This is a modular course for clinicians wishing to teach mental-health skills to primary-care teams in their local areas. Contact: Dr Tim Thornton, Mental Health Education Fellow, Strayside Education Centre, Harrogate Health Care, Harrogate District Hospital, Lancaster Park Road, Harrogate HG2 7SX. Tel: 01423 885959.

42nd Street is a voluntary organisation that works with young people with mental-health problems in Manchester. It has undertaken research into self-harm from the young person's perspective and provides courses from that perspective on working with young people who self-harm. Courses are provided on request for organisations in the North West of England. The organisation has some links with HMP Manchester. Contact: Sarah Dimmelow or Keith Green, 42nd Street, 2nd Floor, Swan Buildings, 20 Swan Street, Manchester M4 5JW. Tel: 0161 832 0169.

Bristol Crisis Service for Women provides training workshops, talks and seminars on working with people who self-injure. The training is customised to the needs of the organisation requesting it. Training is focused on the patient perspective. It also produces a modular training pack for professionals who work with people who self-injure. Contact: Hilary Lindsay (Coordinator), Bristol Crisis Services for Women, PO Box 654, Bristol BS99 1XH. Tel: 0117 925 1119.

Resources for use by trainers of primary-care staff (non-prison specific)

Video-based training packages for use in skills-based training (watching the skills demonstrated on the video followed by practising them in role-play) have been produced by the Department of Psychiatry, University of Manchester. Topics include: Counselling Depression in Primary Care; Depression in Primary Care — Part 1: Recognition in General Practice, Part 2: How to Plan and Assess Treatment; Problem-based Interviewing in General Practice; The Diagnosis of Schizophrenia; Interviewing Skills for Family Doctors; Relaxation; Managing Somatic Presentation of Emotional Distress; Helping People at Risk of Suicide or Self-harm; Depression and Suicidal Behaviour in Adolescents; and Cognitive Behaviour Therapy for Adolescents. Most tapes cost £58.75 and can be ordered from: Nick Jordan, Video Producer, University of Manchester, Department of Psychiatry, Withington Hospital, West Didsbury, Manchester M20 8LR. Tel: 0161 291 4359; Fax: 0161 445 9263; E-mail: Nick.Jordan@man.ac.uk; online catalogue: URL: www.man.ac.uk/psych

Multimedia CD-ROM-based training packages are produced by the University of Leeds, Divisions of Psychiatry and Behavioural Studies. Aimed at a broad audience including general practitioners and psychiatrists-in-training, they are designed to teach the diagnosis, assessment and management of the patient's mental state. Topics include: Anxiety Disorders; Affective Disorders; Schizophrenia and Paranoid Disorders; and Disorders in the Elderly. There are also two CD-ROMS designed to be used as self-help materials by patients: Overcoming Depression and Overcoming Bulimia. Contact: Stephen Taylor-Parker, UoL Innovations Ltd, 175 Woodhouse Lane, Leeds LS2 3AR. Tel: 0113 233 3444.

Audio tapes for patients on coping with depression, coping with anxiety, relaxation, tranquilliser addiction and coping with pain; and for primary-care professionals. *The Depression Skills Pack* (three audio cassettes and a book on the recognition, assessment and management of depression in primary care) are available from: Wendy Lloyd Audio Productions Ltd, 30 Guffitts Rake Meols, Wirral L47 7AD. Tel: 0151 632 0662.

344

Learning resource packs for use by health professionals and others on *Understanding Depression in People with Learning Disabilities*, *Understanding Grief in People with Learning Disabilities* and *Mental Health and Learning Disabilities* are available from: Pavilion Publishing Ltd, 8 St George's Place, Brighton BN1 4ZZ. Tel: 01273 623 222. £125, £125 and £195, respectively (plus VAT and p&p).

Other resources are available from MIND, the Mental Health Foundation and the Samaritans. For example, the Mental Health Foundation sells a training pack: *Working With People Who Self-Injure*. £70 (plus £7 p&p). Tel: 020 7535 7400. MIND provides in-house training on mental-health awareness and other mental-health issues. These training courses are generally aimed at a broad audience, including clinicians, but are not specifically produced for primary care. For catalogues, contact: MIND Conference and Training Unit, Granta House, 15–19 Broadway, London E15 4BQ; and Mental Health Foundation, 20/21 Cornwall Terrace, London NW1 4QL.

Definitions

Mental health and illness

Mental health. The term includes both emotional and psychological well-being — being able to take pleasure in life, to form and sustain relationships with others, and to cope with the ups and downs of life.

Mental ill-health or **mental-health problem** are general terms covering a huge range of conditions and difficulties, from mild-or-moderate anxiety or depression to serious and debilitating conditions such as schizophrenia. One definition states that 'whenever a person's abnormal thoughts, feelings or sensory impressions cause him/her objective or subjective harm which is more than transitory, a mental illness may be said to be present'.[1] Terms used to describe different levels of mental ill-health are often used imprecisely and interchangeably, but the following definitions[2] may help.

- **Mental disorders** are any clinically significant mental or behavioural disorder, including alcohol and drug dependence and personality disorders.

- **Mental illness** is a clinically significant mental disorder other than 'behavioural' disorders such as alcohol or drug misuse and personality disorder. The term mainly refers to schizophrenia and 'affective' disorders (including depression and bipolar, or manic-depressive, disorder).

- **Severe mental illness** is a mental illness of sufficient severity that will usually require contact with the mental-health services rather than just with primary healthcare.

- **Neuroses** are conditions such as anxiety, obsessive-compulsive disorders and phobias.

- **Affective disorders** are conditions where mood is disturbed, such as depression.

- **Psychoses** are more serious disorders such as schizophrenia or mania in which insight and contact with reality are lost (for more details, including a description of 'substance-induced psychosis', see **Nursing a patient with a severe, psychotic illness**, page 173).

- **Personality disorders** are characterised by a long-lasting, inflexible and limited range of attitudes and behaviours that are expressed in a wide variety of settings and that deviate markedly from the expectations of the person's culture and cause distress to the person and others.

For a description of the characteristic features of each disorder, see **Specific mental disorders** (page 11).

Psychological therapies

Anxiety management comprises a varying mixture of behavioural strategies often taught in a group setting to people with anxiety problems. The strategies commonly include education about the nature of anxiety (eg fight or flight response), recognising hyperventilation, a slow breathing technique, relaxation training and graded exposure. Stress management, assertiveness training and structured problem-solving may also be included depending upon the training and background of the therapist and the needs of the clients.

Behaviour therapy is a structured therapy originally derived from learning theory that seeks to solve problems and relieve symptoms by changing behaviour and the environmental factors which control behaviour. **Graded exposure** to feared situations is one of the commonest behavioural treatment methods and is used in a range of anxiety disorders. **Social skills training** is a form of behaviour therapy in which patients are taught skills in social and interpersonal relationships.

Cognitive therapy is based on the idea that how you think largely determines the way you feel. It teaches the individual to recognise and challenge upsetting thoughts. Learning to challenge negative or fear-inducing thoughts helps people think more realistically and feel better. Patients are given homework assignments. Cognitive therapy is more complex than positive thinking. It is usually given in 50-minute sessions over 10–15 weeks.

Cognitive behavioural therapy (CBT) refers to the pragmatic combination of concepts and techniques from cognitive and behaviour therapies, common in clinical practice.

Counselling covers a wide range of skills and techniques. Counsellors may, for example, use cognitive or behavioural techniques. In the main, however, it provides a supportive and non-judgemental atmosphere for people to talk over their problems and explore more satisfactory ways of living. Counselling generally deals with specific life situations and is more short-term than analytic psychotherapies — in primary care, it usually lasts from six to 12 sessions. It is generally used for less severe problems. Counselling is often focused, with counsellors or agencies specialising in particular problems, eg relationship problems, rape, bereavement.

Dialectical behaviour therapy (DBT) is a longer-term and intensive cognitive-behavioural treatment devised for borderline personality disorder that teaches patients skills for regulating and accepting emotions and increasing interpersonal effectiveness.

Family therapy sees the problem behaviours of the 'identified patient' as reflecting the generalised dysfunction in family relationships. Therapy therefore focuses on the whole family system. A close and on-going working relationship between the family and therapist offers the best chance of success. However, especially where the family is very dysfunctional, this may be hard to achieve.

Interpersonal therapy (IPT) is a structured, supportive therapy linking recent interpersonal events to mood or other problems and paying systematic attention to current personal relationships, life transitions, role conflicts and losses. Experienced therapists carry out treatment over 10–15 sessions.

Problem-solving therapy systematically teaches generic skills in active problem-solving, helping individuals to clarify and formulate their life difficulties and apply principles of problem-solving to reduce stress and enhance self-efficacy. Self-management is a key goal, with the clinician adopting the role of teacher or guide.

Psychoanalytic psychotherapy is a longer-term process (usually 1 year or more) of allowing unconscious conflicts the opportunity to be re-enacted in the relationship with the therapist and, through interpretation, worked through in a developmental process.

Systemic therapy aims to facilitate personal and interpersonal resources within networks that the patient is involved with — for an adolescent, this may be the family, school and peer environments. The therapist may involve other professionals working with the individual or family. Therapists actively intervene to enable people to decide where change would be desirable and to facilitate the process of establishing new, more fulfilling patterns of interaction.

Therapeutic community refers to a residential treatment in which patients learn to understand their problems and to change through their interactions with other patients and staff throughout the 24 hours of community life.

Mental-health professionals

Psychiatrists are doctors who have specialised in mental health and who work both in hospitals and, increasingly, in the community. They are responsible for diagnosis, the general mental health and physical care of patients, including medication, and have specific responsibilities in the implementation of the Mental Health Act. Some have further specialist training in areas such as the psychiatry of old age or psychotherapy.

- **Forensic psychiatrists** have particular expertise in people with mental illness and personality disorders who come into contact with the criminal justice system. They are more experienced than general psychiatrists at risk assessments related to violence and other antisocial behaviours, offending behaviour and personality disorders.

- **Adolescent psychiatrists** specialise in the treatment of children and adolescents. They usually work in teams with community psychiatric nurses (CPNs), clinical psychologists, educational psychologists, psychotherapists and social workers. They frequently work with the whole family as opposed to with individual patients.

- **Learning disability psychiatrists** specialise in work with people with learning disability who may also have a mental disorder. They usually have expertise in epilepsy as well as learning disability. They too work in teams.

Psychiatric nurses or registered mental nurses (RMNs) are the most numerous professionals in mental health. Most of their basic training takes place in hospital.

Community psychiatric nurses (CPNs) are usually registered mental nurses, some of whom have completed the ENB training for community work. They are based in the community and care for people with mental illness in their own homes and communities. Their role can include psychological therapies, long-term support, counselling and administering medication by 'depot' injection.

Psychologists:

- **Clinical psychologists** have a postgraduate qualification in clinical work. They have a key role in assessment and may carry out a wide range of treatments, such as behaviour therapy and cognitive therapy. They may provide training and supervision in this kind of work to other professionals.

- **Forensic psychologists** are Psychology postgraduates whose work involves applying psychological approaches to the assessment, management and reduction of risk. They are not specialists in the psychological management of depression, anxiety or psychotic symptoms, although they may have some training in these areas. Most Prison Service psychologists are forensic psychologists.

Psychotherapists, psychoanalysts and counsellors all offer 'talking treatments'. The methods, intensity of treatment and the time involved varies. Individual or group therapy may be offered. Some psychotherapists are also psychiatrists, psychologists or nurses. Primary-care counsellors offer a brief, focused intervention across a wide spectrum of mild-to-moderate disorders.

Occupational therapists (OTs) work in hospital and in the community. Their role is to help people develop confidence and skills in daily living by using a variety of techniques such as creative therapies and training in practical tasks.

Mental-health social workers have a general qualification in social work and may have specialised later in mental health. They act as care managers in assessing people with severe and complex needs, coordinating and monitoring care plans, and ensuring service users get the services they need: respite care, residential accommodation, supported housing or support from a community care worker. Less frequently, they may also provide formal counselling or psychotherapy.

Approved social workers (ASW) (in Scotland, mental health officers) have undertaken specialist training in mental health and are approved under the Mental Health Act 1983 (in Scotland the Mental Health Act 1984, in Northern Ireland the Mental Health Order 1986) to carry out the following duties: assessments for urgent admission to hospital — approved social work assessments under the Mental Health Act, acting as supervisors under the supervised discharge procedures, acting as social supervisors for mentally disordered offenders subject to Home Office supervision.

Community mental-health teams provide assessment, treatment and care for individuals and groups outside hospitals. They comprise a mix of the general mental-health professionals described above, but not all are represented in every team. Community psychiatric nurses (CPNs) are the most numerous. Most areas have Child and Adolescent Mental Health Teams (CAMs). A smaller number have Adolescent Mental Health Teams.

Learning disability teams (similar to community mental-health teams) provide specialist health- and socialcare services. Multidisciplinary teams usually include community learning-disability nurses, a psychiatrist, a psychologist, a speech and language therapist, a physiotherapist, an occupational therapist and may also include a dietitian.

Day care services aim to provide a number of groups that offer a supportive environment and a safe space to relax in. This helps people build self-esteem and confidence, while giving an opportunity to meet others. Drop-in sessions, sports and activity groups, and outings are all included as part of the day service.

Prison service terms used in this book

This book is meant to be of use to staff from PCTs and Health Authorities whose work involves prisons as well as workers in prisons. These definitions are provided for them. Those new to the world of the Prison Service may find *The Prisons Handbook* by Mark Leech, published annually by Waterside Press (URL: http://www.watersidepress.co.uk), helpful. It contains a wealth of basic information about prisons.

Adjudications are disciplinary hearings carried out by prison governors (also called 'adjudicators') held when a prisoner is accused of a disciplinary offence. Adjudicators have the power to award up to 42 additional days' imprisonment on each finding of guilt.

Board of Visitors is the group of people (all unpaid volunteers) appointed by the Secretary of State to act as an independent watchdog to ensure that the prison is run fairly and in accordance with the prison rules.

CARATS (counselling, assessment, referral, advice and throughcare services) is the Prison Service drug-treatment programme.

Incentives and Earned Privileges System (IEPS) is the behavioural framework that governs the type of 'regime' that a prisoner experiences. Prisoners can earn or lose privileges by good or bad behaviour. There are three levels: basic, standard and enhanced. The privileges include more access to private cash, more or improved visits, enhanced earning schemes, the right to wear one's own clothes, more time out of cell and in-cell television. Where the scheme is not implemented on an individual basis, prisoners with mental and behavioural disorders may be more likely to find themselves on the lower levels.

Offending behaviour programmes are structured psychological courses that aim to reduce re-offending by challenging ways of thinking that may underlie the offending behaviour. Courses may aim to increase the self-control, interpersonal problem-solving, critical reasoning, moral reasoning and social perspective taking of participants.

Segregation. Prisoners can be segregated from other prisoners either for their own protection (OP) or in the interests of 'good order and discipline' (GOAD). GOAD is a management measure that takes out of circulation those prisoners who the governor believes are a threat to the good order of the prison. Prisoners segregated for this reason are often housed in the Segregation Block. Prisoners segregated for OP may be on a special unit (Vulnerable Prisoners Unit) or, sometimes, on the Segregation Block. In addition, on the Segregation Block are prisoners who have been punished for a breach of discipline with a period of 'cellular confinement'.

Sentence planning is the process of needs' assessment and planning of the time in prison (work, training, education, offending behaviour programmes) that takes place for longer-term prisoners.

Throughcare (also known as resettlement) is the process of prerelease planning. Throughcare in the prison may include prison officers, probation officers and voluntary organisations. Probation officers are involved in risk assessments for parole or home-detention curfew, in sentence planning and bail information, as well as in the preparation for the release of prisoners. They can also help prisoners remain in contact with their families during their time in custody.

---

[1]   *Oxford Handbook of Clinical Specialities*. Oxford: Oxford University Press, 1987.
[2]   From the glossary of the *National Confidential Inquiry into Suicide and Homicide by People with Mental Illness*.

Acknowledgements

The *Mental Health Primary Care in Prison* would not have been possible without the advice, support and collaboration of primary-care workers in prisons, researchers, mental-health and legal specialists, policy workers in the Department of Health and the Prison Service, the World Health Organisation and other agencies, prison officers and prisoners. The WHO Collaborating Centre for Research and Training for Mental Health and the Institute of Psychiatry thank the following for their valuable collaboration.

Organisations

The World Health Organisation
The Royal College of General Practitioners
The Royal College of Psychiatrists
The Royal College of Nursing
The Faculty of Public Health Medicine
HM Prison Service, especially the Training and Development Group Health Care Policy Unit, the Health Care Task Force, the Safer Custody Group, Psychology and Probation Unit, the Women's Policy Unit and the Young Offenders' Policy Unit and the Juvenile Operational Policy Group
The Mental Health Branch, Department of Health
The Association of Chief Officers of Probation.

Editorial Board

Dr Paul Armitage, Senior Medical Officer, HMP Dorchester, then HMP Holloway; Dr Sue Bailey, Consultant Adolescent Forensic Psychiatrist, Mental Health Services of Salford NHS Trust; Lindsay Bates, Head of Nursing, Health Task Force, HM Prison Service; William Bingley, Professor of Mental Health Law & Ethics, University of Central Lancashire; Colin Dale, Forensic Nurse Consultant; Dr Mike Farrell, The Addiction Resource Centre, South London & Maudsley NHS Trust; Steve Gannon, MBE — Prison Nurse and representative of the Royal College of Nursing; Professor Kevin Gournay, Professor of Psychiatric Nursing, Institute of Psychiatry; Mr Alan Hornett, Health Care Officer, HMP Belmarsh; Professor John Gunn, Professor of Forensic Psychiatry, Institute of Psychiatry and representative of the Royal College of Psychiatry; Dr Cliff Howells, Medical Director, Health Task Force, HM Prison Service; Dr G O Ivbijaro, Representative of the Royal College of General Practitioners; Dr John MacInnes, Senior Medical Officer, HMP Aylesbury; Stuart McPhillips, representative of the Association of Chief Officers of Probation; Professor Rachel Jenkins, Director, WHO Collaborating Centre, Institute of Psychiatry; Dr Peter Misch, Department of Adolescent Mental Health, South London & Maudsley NHS Trust; Dr David Ndegwa, South London and Maudsley NHS Trust; Dr Janet Parrot, Clinical Director, Bracton Centre, Oxleas NHS Trust; Jo Paton, WHO Collaborating Centre, Institute of Psychiatry; Dr Mary Piper, Health Policy Unit, HM Prison Service; Ms Ingrid Posen, Head Safer Custody Group, HM Prison Service; Dr Harry Rutter, Representative of the Faculty of Public Health Medicine; Graeme Sandell, Head of Mental Health, NACRO; Revd Peter Stell, Chaplain, HMP Grendon Underwood & Spring Hill; Caroline Stewart, Women's Policy Unit, HM Prison Service; Professor Graeme Towl, Head of Psychology and

351

Probation, HM Prison Service; Professor Andre Tylee, Professor of Primary Mental Health Care, Institute of Psychiatry; Dr John Reed, Medical Director, HM Prison Service Inspectorate; Dr Wolfgang Rutz, Mental Health Unit, Regional Office for Europe, WHO; Mr David Waplington, Juvenile Operational Policy Group, HM Prison Service; Mr Andy Weir, Clinical Director of Healthcare, HMP Brixton; Dr Ellen Wilkinson, Consultant Psychiatrist, Truro, Cornwall; Dr Bedirhan Ustun, WHO.

Primary authors and specialist advisors

Adolescent Conduct Disorder, Paton J, Maden A (authors), Bailey S, Misch P (specialist advisors).

Assessing and Managing People at Risk of Suicide, adapted by Paton J from Andrew G, Jenkins R (eds). *Management of Mental Disorders* (1999), Gunn J (specialist advisor).

Assessment & Management Following an Act of Self-harm, Paton J, Crowe M, Bunclark J.

Attention Deficit/Hyperactivity Disorder, Gaskin C, Paton J (authors), Bailey S, Toone B, Misch P (specialist advisors).

Child Protection. Paton J, Hancock M (authors), Gabbidon P, Poulney P (specialist advisors).

Comorbidity of Mental Illness and Substance Misuse, Farrell M, Palmer J, Paton J, Gardiner P.

Dirty Protests and Mental Disorder, Ndegwa D.

Domestic Violence, Paton J, Means S.

Emergency Management of Poisoning/Overdoses, Wiseman H, Butler J, colleagues in the Medical Toxicology Unit, Guys & St Thomas' Hospital, London.

Emergency Treatment Without Consent Under Common Law, Ndegwa D, Bingley W, Snow G.

Emotional Disorders in Young People, Jasper A, Paton J (authors), Bailey S, Misch P (specialist advisors).

Ethical Issues, Ndegwa D, Bingley W, Paton J, McInnes J, Misch P (authors), Gadd E, Snow G, Wright K (specialist advisors).

Food Refusal and Mental Disorder, Cummings I, Parrot J, Paton J, Bingley W, McInnes J (authors), Gadd E, Wright K (specialist advisors).

General Issues in Young People, Paton J, Misch P.

Helping Victims of Sexual Assault, Paton J, Mezey G (authors), Norton K (specialist advisor).

Learning Disability, O'Brien G, Milne E, Thornton P, English G, Paton J (authors), McInnes J (specialist advisor).

Managing Aggression and Violence, adapted by Paton J, Dale C from Andrew G, Jenkins R (eds). *Management of Mental Disorders* (1999).

Managing the Interface with the NHS and Other Agencies, Wilkinson E, Ndegwa D, Paton J (authors), Armitage P, Telfer J, Maden A (specialist advisors).

Medications Used for Mental Health Problems, adapted by Paton J (author), Lader M, Taylor D, Reuben J (specialist advisors).

Problems with the Mother and Baby Relationship, McGauley G, Hughes P, Paton J.

Nursing a Patient with a Severe Psychotic Illness, Paton J, Noakes J.

Observing a Patient at Risk of Suicide, Dale C (author), Gannon S (specialist advisor).

Offending Behaviour Programmes, Paton J (author), Mann R, Rhodes L (specialist advisors).

Personality Disorder, Paton J (author), Blumenthal S, Cummings I, Moran P, Norton K, Telfer J (specialist advisors).

Postnatal Depressive Disorder, McGauley G, Cantwell R, Paton J (authors), Marks M, Seneviratne T, Taylor D (specialist advisors).

352

Postnatal Psychosis, Cantwell R, Paton J, McGauley G (authors), Marks M, Seneviratne T (specialist advisors).
Prevalence of Mental Disorders, Paton J (author), Bailey S, Jenkins R, Maden T (specialist advisors).
Prisoners from Different Ethnic and Cultural Groups, Paton J, Ndegwa N (authors), Aciemovic A, Baff S, Turner J (specialist advisors).
Prisoners with Complex Presentations and Very Difficult Behaviours, Ndegwa D.
Problems in the Mother–Baby Relationship, McGauley Gill, Hughes P, Paton J.
Psychosis in Young People, Paton J, Byrne P (authors), Misch P (specialist advisor).
Responding to People Who Disclose That They were Abused as Children, Paton J, Hancock M (authors), Feigenbaum J, Mezey G, Norton K (specialist advisors).
Use of the Mental Health Act England and Wales, Paton J, Wilkinson E; Bingley W.
Working with Voluntary and Community Agencies, Paton J.
The Guidelines on Specific Mental Disorders, adapted for the prison situation by Paton J, Wilkinson E, Jenkins R with the help of Clarke A, Dagger S, Dulson D, Palmer J, Walker N.
The Directory of Voluntary and Community Agencies, compiled by Paton R.
Further Reading and Websites and *Training Resources*, compiled by Paton Jenny.

Information for prisoners and prison officers

Coping with Anxiety, adapted for prisoners by Hards S.
Coping with Depression, adapted for prisoners by Patmore C.
Personality (Behavioural) Disorders, Paton J, Harrison M.
Drug Use and Mental-health Problems, Paton J, Palmer J, Marteau D.
Getting a Good Night's Sleep, adapted for prisoners by Patmore C.
Harm Minimisation Advice to Drug Users, adapted by Brewin L, Dual Diagnosis Trainer, the Institute of Psychiatry.
Suicide Prevention, Paton J, Snow L.
Learning Disability, adapted by Paton J.
Mothers and Babies: the Psychological Issues, McGauley G, Hughes P, Paton J.
Immediate Management on Discovery of an Incident of Self-harm, adapted Paton J.
Traumatic Stress: Learning to Cope, adapted by Hards S.
Working with a Prisoner with Severe Mental Illness, Paton J, Noakes J.
Understanding Self-injury, Snow L, Paton J.

Commenters or providers of material

Mike Armstrong, Principal Officer, HMP Low Newton; Dr MK Bradley, HMP Exeter; Dr Claire Diamond, Adolescent Psychiatrist; Keith Green, Suicide and Self Injury Project, 42nd Street; Kevin Gournay, Professor of Psychiatric Nursing, Institute of Psychiatry; Marc Harrison, Head of Health Training, HM Prison Service; David Hillier, Prison Health Policy Unit; Dr Cliff Howells, Medical Director, Prison Health Task Force; Dr Dilys Jones, Home Office; Carol Kellas; Dr Graham Martin, Head of Learning Disabilities, RCG; Dr John MacInnes, HMP Aylesbury; Dr Mark Morris, Director of Therapy, HMP Grendon Underwood; Albert Persaud, public health specialist; Dr Mary Piper, Health Policy Unit, HM Prison Service; Dr Christina Pourgourdes; Dr Roger Ralli, PMO, HMYOI; Glen Parva; Simon Reeve, Health Policy Unit, HM Prison Service; John Reuben, Principal Pharmacist, HMP Norwich; Paul Rogers, Forensic Nurse; John Roughton, York Social Services; Liz Ryan, Prison Health Task Force; Debbie Sharp, Professor of Primary Care, University of Bristol; Dr Jenny Shaw, University of Manchester; Nick Snowden, Juvenile Operational Management Group, HM Prison Service; Caroline Stewart, Women's Policy Unit,

HM Prison Service; Dee Taylor, Family Therapist, HMYOI Feltham; David Taylor, Chief Pharmacist, South London & Maudsley NHS Trust; Graeme Towl, Head of Psychology and Probation, HM Prison Service; Andre Tylee, Professor of Primary Mental Health Care, Institute of Psychiatry; Lynne Wibberley, Prison Service Health Policy Unit; Anita Wilson, Ethnologist, Trust for the Study of Adolescence; Guy Woollven, HM Prison Service.

Members of consensus groups

Dr Paul Armitage, SMO, HMP Holloway; Dr Sue Bailey, Adolescent Forensic Psychiatrist; William Bingley, Professor of Mental Health Law and Ethics; Marion Bullivant, Criminal Justice Mental Health Liaison Service, Liverpool; Jennifer Butler, Medical Toxicology Unit; Dr Clark, Senior Medical Officer, HMP Frankland; Dr David Crighton, Senior Principal Psychologist, Kent, Surrey and Sussex Area; Dr Michael Crowe, Crisis Recovery Unit, South London & Maudsley Hospital; Dr Ian Cummings, Bracton Centre, Oxleas NHS Trust and HMP Belmarsh; Colin Dale, Forensic Nurse Consultant; Sue Dagger, Health Care Manager, HMP Long Lartin; Dr Claire Diamond, Adolescent Forensic Psychiatrist; Dr Mike Farrell, Addiction Centre, South London and Maudsley NHS Trust; Dr Claire Gaskin, Adolescent Forensic Psychiatrist; Dr Steven Geoffreys, General Practitioner, formerly of HMYOI Feltham; Kevin Gournay, Professor of Psychiatric Nursing, Institute of Psychiatry; Keith Green, Suicide and Self Harm Project, 42nd Street; John Gunn, Professor of Forensic Psychiatry, Institute of Psychiatry; Edwin Gwenzie, Department of Psychiatric Nursing, Institute of Psychiatry; Professor Keith Hawton, Suicide Research Centre, University of Oxford; Gary Hogman, National Schizophrenia Fellowship; Alan Hornett, Health Care Officer, HMP Belmarsh; Dr Gabriel Ivbijaro, RCGP; Professor Rachel Jenkins, Director WHO Collaborating Centre, Institute of Psychiatry; Dr Peter Kent, Senior Medical Officer HMP Bristol; Malcolm Lader, Professor of Psychopharmacology, Institute of Psychiatry; Sara Lewis, Revolving Doors; Sarah Mackereth, Probation Officer and researcher; Juliet Lyon, Director, Prison Reform Trust; Tony Maden, Professor of Forensic Psychiatry, Ealing, Hammersmith & Fulham NHS Trust; Sylvie Means, WHO; Jenni McCarthy, The Samaritans; Dr John McInnes, SMO, HMP Aylesbury; Stewart McPhillips, Association of Chief Officers of Probation; Dr Peter Misch, Adolescent Forensic Psychiatrist; Dr Mark Morris, Director of Therapy, HMP Grendon Underwood; Dr David Ndegwa, Consultant Forensic Psychiatrist Maudsley NHS Trust; Robert Newman, Youth Justice Board; Clem Norman, Governor, HMP & YOI Reading; Anne Norton, HMP & YOI New Hall; Dr John O'Grady, Chair Independent Prison Review Group; Jan Palmer, Detoxification Manager, HMP Holloway; Dr Janet Parrot, Clinical Director, Bracton Centre, Oxleas NHS Trust; Jo Paton, WHO Collaborating Centre, Institute of Psychiatry; Louise Pembroke, National Self Harm Network; Jan Picken, Primary Care Manager, HMP Belmarsh; Dr Mary Piper, Prison Service Health Policy Group; Ingrid Posen, Head of Safer Custody Group, HM Prison Service; Dr Roger Ralli, Senior Medical Officer, HMP Glen Parva; Dr John Reed, Prison Service Inspectorate, John Reubens, Pharmacist, Prison Health Task Force; Dr Harry Rutter, Faculty of Public Health Medicine; Graeme Sandell, NACRO; Sharon Scottorn, HMP Glen Parva; Dr Jenny Shaw, University of Manchester; Andy Smith, Mental Aftercare Association; Graeme Snow, Prison Service Health Policy Unit; Louisa Snow, researcher; Dylan Southern, Department of Psychiatric Nursing, Institute of Psychiatry; Caroline Stewart, Women's Policy Unit, HM Prison Service; Dee Taylor, Psychotherapist, HM YOI Feltham; Professor Graeme Towl, Head of Psychology and Probation, HM Prison Service; Dr Glyn Volans, Director, Medical Toxicology Unit;

Dr Walker, Forensic Psychiatric Service, Nottingham, until recently SMO at HMP Manchester; David Waplington, Area Manager; Andy Weir; Dr Ellen Wilkinson, Consultant Psychiatrist; Anita Wilson, Trust for the Study of Adolescence; Steve Wright, Department of Psychiatric Nursing, Institute of Psychiatry.

Prison Service healthcare staff

We are grateful to the 46 prison doctors, nurses and healthcare officers who replied to our two surveys and particularly to the following who sent comments or material: Dr Paul Armitage, SMO, HMP Dorchester; Dr A D Clarke, SMO, HMP Frankland; Kevin Corcoran, Health Care Manager, HMP Woodhill; Sue Dagger, In-patient Manager, HMP Long Lartin; P O Davis, Health Care Manager, HMP Littlehay; Stephanie Dulson, Head of Health Care, HMP Styal; Ms A Farrell, HMP Cookham Wood; Graham Faulkner, Charge Nurse, HMP Brockhill; Dr Garside, HMP Doncaster; Chris McCabe, Health Care Manager, HMP Altcourse; Kenneth McGeachie, HMP Glenochil; Dr R Jones, HMP Swansea; T Kavenagh, HCO, Bedford; Anne Norton, Health Care Manager, HMP New Hall; Jan Picken, Primary Care Nurse, HMP Belmarsh; Simon Rogers, HMP Parc; Dr N D Walker, Clinical Director, HMP Manchester; Andy Weir, Clinical Director, HMP Brixton; Dr Brian Whiting, HMP Canterbury; Keith Wilson, Health Care Manager, HMP Pentonville.

Financial support

We are grateful to the following for their help. The NHS Forensic Mental Health R&D Programme for funding the development of the guide. Marc Harrison, Head of Health Training, Training and Development Group, HM Prison Service, for funding the cost of copies for Prison Service staff. The Department of Health for funding the cost of copies for prison leads in Primary Care Trusts. The Health Services Research Directorate, Institute of Psychiatry, King's College London, for support in kind.

Other supporters

Dr Joe Neary, Head of Clinical Programmes, Royal College of General Practitioners; Kenny McGeachie, Head of Health Care, HMP Glenochil and a representative of the Scottish Prison Service; Dr Alan Mitchell, Medical Director, Scottish Prison Service; Sally Newton, Northern Ireland Prison Service.

Editorial

Editing was done by Jo Paton and Rachel Jenkins with help from Samantha Maingay, Jane Penn and Harry Rutter.

Administrative help

Julie Smith, Jenny Paton and Richard Paton.

Managing Editor

Jo Paton and Professor Rachel Jenkins.

Permissions

We are grateful to the following for permission to use or adapt their material: Addiction Centre, Institute of Psychiatry, King's College, London (SADQ, SODQ).

HM Prison Service, *Management of an Inmate at Risk of Suicide* — checklist for Prison Officers.

Home Office, leaflet on *Domestic Violence*.

Mentality, *Stress and Stress Reactions in Refugees*.

National Association for the Care and Rehabilitation of Offenders, *Just Imprisoned*.

North East London Mental Health NHS Trust, *Stress and Stress Reactions for Refugees*).

Nottingham Alcohol and Drug Team, *Harm Reduction* leaflet, adapted, with permission, by Liz Brewer, Dual Diagnosis Trainer, Institute of Psychiatry, from: *Problem Drug Use: A Guide to Management in General Practice*.

Royal College of Psychiatrists, *Brief Risk Indicator Check List*.

Scottish Prison Service, *Nurse Initial Assessment Form, Example of Communication Sharing Proforma*.

Treatment Protocol Project, Sydney, WHO Collaborating Centre for Mental Health and Substance Misuse (Permission to adapt *Managing Aggression and Violence* and to include an MSE Form, drug-use diary, early warning signs form, food and behaviour diary.)

WHO (Regional Office for Europe) Health in Prisons Project (Health promotion checklist for managers taken from *Mental Health Promotion in Prisons*.)

Interactive summary cards

The six pages that follow contain summaries of information about the six disorders most common in primary care.

These are designed to be used interactively within the consultation, to help the practitioner explain key features of the disorder to the patient and enter into discussion about a possible management plan. They are also contained on the disk and can be printed out and mounted on either side of a piece of A4 card for ease of use.

Mental health in primary care
Alcohol problems

There is one unit of alcohol in:
½ pint of ordinary strength beer, lager or cider
¼ pint of extra strength beer, lager or cider
1 small glass of white (8 or 9% ABV) wine
⅔ small glass of red (11 or 12% ABV) wine
1 single measure of spirits (30 ml)

Common symptoms

'High-risk' drinking:

Men
More than three units
alcohol/day
(21 units/week)

Women
More than two units
alcohol/day
(14 units/week)

**Many have no
symptoms but
are at risk**

Psychological:
→ Poor concentration
→ Sleep problems
→ Less able to think
   clearly
→ Depression
→ Anxiety/stress

Physical:
→ Hangovers/blackouts
→ Injuries
→ Tiredness/lack
   of energy
→ Weight gain
→ Poor coordination
→ High blood pressure
→ Impotence
→ Vomiting/nausea
→ Gastritis/diarrhoea
→ Liver disease
→ Brain damage

→ Difficulties and arguments with family/friends
→ Difficulties performing at work/home
→ Withdrawal from friends and social activities
→ Legal problems.

Alcohol problems are treatable
Alcohol problems *do not* mean weakness
Alcohol problems *do not* mean you are a bad person
Alcohol problems *do* mean that you have a medical problem or a lifestyle problem.

What treatments can help?
Both therapies are most often needed:

Supportive therapy:
→ to reduce drinking
→ to stop drinking
→ for stress
→ for prevention of life problems
→ for education of the family members
   for support.

Medication:
→ for moderate to severe withdrawal
→ for physical problems
→ consider for relapse prevention.

Set goals for post-release: acceptable levels of drinking

Who?	**How many drinks?**	**How often?**
Men	No more than three units	Each day (only for five days/week)
Women	No more than two units	Each day (only for five days/week)

Have two non-alcohol drinking days/week.

Keep in mind: the less the person drinks, the better it is.

> ➡ Pregnancy
> ➡ Physical alcohol dependence
> ➡ Physical problems made worse by drinking
> ➡ Driving, biking
> ➡ Operating machinery
> ➡ Exercising (swimming, jogging, etc.)

→ Recommendation is not to drink

Determine action: how to reach target levels

➡ Keep track of your alcohol consumption

➡ Turn to family and/or friends for support

➡ Have one or more non-alcoholic drinks before each drink

➡ Delay the time of day that you drink

➡ Take smaller sips.

➡ Engage in alternative activities at times that you would normally drink (eg when you are feeling bored or stressed)

➡ Switch to low alcoholic drinks

➡ Decide on non-drinking days (2 days or more per week).

➡ Eat before starting to drink

➡ Join a support group

➡ Quench your thirst with non-alcoholic drinks

➡ Avoid or reduce time spent with heavy-drinking friends

➡ Avoid bars, cafes or former drinking places.

Review progress: are you keeping on track?

Questions to ask:

➡ Am I keeping to my goals?

➡ What are the difficult times?

➡ Am I losing motivation?

➡ Do I need more help?

Progress tips:

➡ Every week, record how much you drink over the week

➡ Avoid these difficult situations or plan activities to help you cope with them

➡ Think back to your original reasons for cutting down or stopping

➡ Come back for help, talk to family and friends.

Mental health in primary care
Anxiety

Common symptoms

Psychological:
→ Tension
→ Worry
→ Panic
→ Feelings of unreality

→ Fear of going crazy
→ Fear of dying
→ Fear of losing control

Physical:
→ Trembling
→ Sweating
→ Heart pounding
→ Light headedness
→ Dizziness

→ Muscle tension
→ Nausea
→ Breathlessness
→ Numbness
→ Stomach pains
→ Tingling sensation

Disruptive to work, social or family life

Anxiety disorders are common and treatable
Anxiety *does not* mean weakness
Anxiety *does not* mean losing the mind
Anxiety *does not* mean personality problems
Severe anxiety *does* mean a disorder which requires treatment.

Common forms of anxiety

Generalized anxiety disorder:
→ persistent/ excessive worry
→ physical symptoms.

Panic disorder:
→ sudden intense fear
→ physical symptoms
→ psychological symptoms.

Social phobia:
→ Fear/avoidance social situations
→ fear of being criticized
→ physical symptoms
→ psychological symptoms.

Agoraphobia:
→ Fear/avoidance of situations where escape is difficult
→ leaving familiar places alone
→ physical symptoms
→ psychological symptoms.

What treatments can help?
Both therapies are most often needed:

Supportive therapy for:
→ slow breathing/relaxation
→ exposure to feared situations
→ realistic/positive thinking
→ problem-solving.

Medication:
→ for severe anxiety
→ for panic attacks.

About medication

Short term
➡ use for severe anxiety
➡ can be addictive and ineffective when used in the long term.

Side-effects
➡ are important to report

Counselling
➡ (emotional support and problem-solving) is always recommended with medication.

Ongoing review
➡ of medication use is recommended.

Slow breathing to reduce physical symptoms of anxiety

➡ Breathe in for three seconds and out for three seconds, and pause for three seconds before breathing in again.
➡ Practise 10 minutes morning or night (five minutes is better than nothing).
➡ Use before and during situations that make you anxious.
➡ Regularly check and slow down breathing throughout the day.

Change attitudes and ways of thinking

'My chest is hurting and I can't breathe, I must be having a heart attack.'

Instead:

'I am having a panic attack, I should slow my breathing down and I will feel better.'

'I hope they don't ask me a question, I won't know what to say.'

Instead:

'Whatever I say will be OK, I am not being judged. Others are not being judged, why should I be?'

'My partner has not called as planned. Something terrible must have happened.'

Instead:

'They might not have been able to get to a phone. It is very unlikely that something terrible has happened.'

Exposure to overcome anxiety and avoidance

Easy stage ➡ **Moderate stage** ➡ **Hard stage**
(eg walking on own)   (eg lunch with a friend)   (eg shopping with a friend)

➡ Use slow breathing to control anxiety
➡ Do not move to the next stage until anxiety decreases to an acceptable level.

Mental health in primary care
Chronic tiredness

Common symptoms

Compared with previous level of energy, and compared to people known to you:

Tired all the time   **Tire easily**   **Tired despite rest**

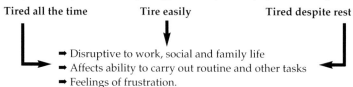

➡ Disruptive to work, social and family life
➡ Affects ability to carry out routine and other tasks
➡ Feelings of frustration.

Chronic Fatigue Syndrome is a much rarer condition, diagnosed when substantial physical and mental fatigue lasts longer than six months and there are no significant findings on physical or laboratory investigation.

Common triggers

Psychological triggers:		Physical triggers:		Medication:
➡ Depression	➡ Doing too much activity	➡ Anaemia	➡ Thyroid disorder	➡ Steroids
➡ Stress		➡ Bronchitis		➡ Antihistamines.
➡ Worry		➡ Asthma	➡ Influenza	
➡ Anxiety.	➡ Doing too little activity.	➡ Diabetes	➡ Alcohol/ drug use	
		➡ Arthritis.	➡ Bacterial, viral and other infections.	

What treatments can help?
Both therapies are most often needed:

Supportive therapy for:
➡ depression
➡ worry/anxiety
➡ stress/life problems
➡ lifestyle change
➡ level of physical activity.

Medication:
➡ for other mental or physical disorders
➡ anti-depressants are sometimes useful
➡ there are no effective medications specific to fatigue and the main treatment follows psychological lines.

Behavioural strategies

- ➡ Examine how well you are sleeping.
- ➡ Have a brief rest period of about 2 weeks, in which there are no extensive activities.
- ➡ After the period of brief rest, gradually return to your usual activities.
- ➡ Plan pleasant/enjoyable activities into your week.
- ➡ Gradually build up a regular exercise routine.
- ➡ Do not push yourself too hard; remember to build up all activities gradually and steadily.
- ➡ Try to have regular meals during the day.
- ➡ Try to keep to a healthy diet.
- ➡ Use relaxation techniques, for example, slow breathing.

Slow breathing for relaxation

- ➡ Breathe in for three seconds
- ➡ Breathe out for three seconds
- ➡ Pause for three seconds before breathing in again
- ➡ Practise for 10 minutes at night (five minutes is better than nothing).

Increase level of physical activity

A little activity one or two times a week (eg walking)

Inactive

Daily activities — not much effort (eg fast walking, shopping, cleaning)

Some activity

Activity that makes you out of breath for 20 minutes or more, three to five times a week (eg jogging)

Active

Mental health in primary care
Depression

Common symptoms

Mood and motivation:
- ➡ Continuous low mood
- ➡ Loss of interest or pleasure
- ➡ Hopelessness
- ➡ Helplessness
- ➡ Worthlessness

Psychological:
- ➡ Guilt/negative attitude to self
- ➡ Poor concentration/ memory
- ➡ Thoughts of death or suicide
- ➡ Tearfulness

Physical:
- ➡ Slowing down or agitation
- ➡ Tiredness/lack of energy
- ➡ Sleep problems
- ➡ Disturbed appetite (weight loss/increase)

- ➡ Difficulties carrying out routine activities
- ➡ Difficulties performing at work
- ➡ Difficulties with home life
- ➡ Withdrawal from friends and social activities.

Depression is common and treatable
- ➡ Depression *does not* mean weakness
- ➡ Depression *does not* mean laziness
- ➡ Depression *does mean* that you have a medical disorder which requires treatment.

Common triggers

Psychological:
Major life events, eg
- ➡ Recent bereavement
- ➡ Relationship problems
- ➡ Imprisonment
- ➡ Bullying
- ➡ Bad visit
- ➡ Parole refused

Other:
- ➡ Family history of depression
- ➡ Childbirth
- ➡ Menopause
- ➡ Seasonal changes
- ➡ Chronic medical conditions
- ➡ Alcohol and substance use disorders.

Illness:
- ➡ Infectious diseases
- ➡ Influenza
- ➡ Hepatitis.

Medication:
- ➡ Antihypertensives
- ➡ H2 blockers
- ➡ Oral contraceptives
- ➡ Corticosteroids.

What treatments can help?

Both therapies are most often needed:

Supportive therapy for:
- ➡ stress/life problems
- ➡ patterns of negative thinking
- ➡ prevention of further episode.

Medication:
- ➡ for depressed mood or loss of interest/ pleasure for two or more weeks and at least four of the symptoms mentioned earlier
- ➡ for little response to supportive therapy (counselling)
- ➡ for recurrent depression
- ➡ for a family history of depression.

Depression

About medication

Effective
Usually works faster than other methods.
Treatment plan
must be strictly adhered to.
Drugs
➡ are not addictive
➡ interact in a harmful way with alcohol
➡ improvement takes time, generally three weeks for a response
➡ do not take in combination with St John's wort.

Side-effects
must be reported, but generally start improving within 7–10 days.
Progress
➡ same medication should continue unless a different decision is taken by the doctor
➡ medication should not be discontinued without doctor's knowledge
➡ in case a drug is not effective, another drug may be tried.

Time period
Medication to be continued at least four to six months after initial improvement.
Ongoing review
is necessary over the next few months.

Increase time spent on enjoyable activities

➡ Set small achievable, daily goals for doing pleasant activities
➡ Plan time for activities and increase the amount of time spent on these each week
➡ Plan things to look forward to in future
➡ Keep busy even when it is hard to feel motivated
➡ Try to be with other people/friends

Problem-solving plan

Discuss
problems with partner/family members, trusted friend or counsellor.
Distance
yourself to look at problems as though you were an observer.

Options
Work out possible solutions to solve the problems.
Pros and cons
Examine advantages and disadvantages of each option.

Set a time frame
to examine and resolve problems.
Make an action plan
for working through the problems over a period of time.
Review
Progress made in solving problems.

Change attitudes and way of thinking

'I will always feel this way; things will never change.'

Instead: 'These feelings are temporary. With treatment, things will look better in a few weeks.'

'It's all my fault. I do not seem to be able to do anything right.'

Instead: 'These are negative thoughts that are the result of depression. What evidence for this do I really have?'

Mental health in primary care
Sleep problems

Common symptoms

➡ Difficulty falling asleep
➡ Frequent awakening

➡ Early morning awakening
➡ Restless or unrefreshing sleep

 ➡ Difficulties at work and in social and family life
➡ Makes it difficult to carry out routine or desired tasks.

Common causes

Psychological:	Physical: Medical problems:	Lifestyle:	Environmental:
➡ Depression	➡ Overweight	➡ Too hot or too cold	➡ Noise
➡ Anxiety	➡ Heart failure	➡ Tea, coffee and	➡ Pollution
➡ Worries	➡ Nose, throat and	alcohol	➡ Lack of
➡ Stress.	lung disease	➡ Heavy meal before	privacy
	➡ Sleep apnoea	sleep	➡ Over-
	➡ Narcolepsy	➡ Daytime naps	crowding.
	➡ Pains.	➡ Irregular sleep	
	Medications:	schedule.	
	➡ Steroids		
	➡ Decongestants		
	➡ Others.		

What treatments can help?

Supportive therapy is the preferred treatment

Supportive therapy for:
➡ stress/life problems
➡ depression
➡ worry
➡ changes in lifestyle and sleep habits.

Medication:
➡ for temporary sleep problems
➡ for short term use in chronic problems
to break sleep cycle.

Sleep problems

About medication

Short term
➡ use for short period of time.

Long-term
➡ when used in the long term, there may be difficulties stopping, leading to dependence.

Side-effects
➡ are important to report.

Harmful
➡ when alcohol and other drugs are used.

Ongoing review
➡ of medication use is recommended.

Lifestyle change strategies

➡ Try ways of reducing noise and light at night. Ask if foam ear plugs or cloth eye shades are allowed.

➡ Try to cut down on coffee drinking and smoking, especially in the evenings.

➡ Avoid daytime naps even if you are bored or have not slept the night before.

➡ Be as active as you can during the day – go to work, education or gym if you can. Ask the PE Instructor for exercises you can do in your cell.

➡ Have a regular relaxation period before bed. Try reading or listening to music.

➡ Don't lie in bed trying to sleep. If possible, get up and read, listen to the radio or tape-recorder, using headphones, until you feel sleepy.

➡ Use relaxation techniques, for example, slow breathing.

Slow breathing for relaxation

➡ Breathe in for three seconds
➡ Breathe out for three seconds
➡ Pause for three seconds before breathing in again
➡ Practise for 10 minutes at night (five minutes is better than nothing).

More evaluation may be needed:
➡ if someone stops breathing during sleep (sleep apnoea)
➡ if there is a daytime sleepiness without possible explanation.

Mental health in primary care
Unexplained somatic complaints

Common, unexplained physical problems

- Headaches
- Chest pains
- Difficulty in breathing
- Difficulty in swallowing

- Nausea
- Vomiting
- Abdominal pain
- Lower back pain

- Skin rashes
- Frequent urination
- Diarrhoea
- Skin and muscle discomfort.

Associated worries and concerns

- Associated symptoms and problems
- Beliefs (about what is causing the symptoms)
- Fear (of what might happen).

Physical symptoms are real

A vicious circle can develop:
- Emotional stress can cause physical symptoms or make them worse.
- Physical symptoms can lead to more emotional stress.
- Emotional stress can make physical symptoms worse.

Headaches
Difficulty in swallowing
Chest pain/difficulty in breathing   ➡
Abdominal pain/nausea/vomiting
Frequent urination/diarrhoea/impotence
Skin rashes

may all be
caused or made worse
by stress, anxiety
worry, anger, depression.

What treatments can help?

Supportive treatment most often needed:

- Effective reassurance, after history and detailed physical examination.
- Management of stress/life problems.
- Treatment of associated depression, anxiety, alcohol problems.
- Learning to relax.
- Avoiding patterns of negative thinking.
- Increasing levels of physical activity.
- Increasing positive/pleasurable activities.

Unexplained somatic complaints

Useful strategies

Reassurance
➡ Stress often produces physical symptoms or makes them worse.
➡ There are no signs of serious illness.
➡ You can benefit from learning strategies to reduce the impact of your symptoms.

Slow breathing to reduce common physical symptoms
(eg muscle tension, hot and cold flushes, headaches, chest tightness)
➡ Breathe in for three seconds and out for three seconds and pause for three second: before breathing in again.
➡ Practise 10 minutes morning or night (five minutes is better than nothing).
➡ Use before and during situations that make you anxious.
➡ Regularly check and slow down breathing throughout the day.

Change attitudes and way of thinking

'I can't understand why the tests are negative. I feel the pain; it is probably something really unusual that I have.'

Instead: 'The pain is real, but I've been checked out physically and I have had all the relevant tests. Many other things, such as worry and stress, can cause these pains.'

'Maybe my doctor has missed something. I should try another doctor or better still a specialist instead.'

Instead: 'It is very unlikely that these doctors have missed something. It is unlikely that a specialist would say anything different. Maybe I should examine whether stress, tension, or my lifestyle is contributing to the pain.'

'Why won't this pain go away. I'm not feeling well; I've probably got cancer.'

Instead: 'This is not the first time that I've thought that there was *something* terribly *wrong* and *in fact* nothing serious developed. I should learn to relax and focus my thoughts on other things to distract myself from the pains.'

Increase level of physical activity

A little activity one or two times a week (eg walking)	**Daily activities —** not much effort (eg fast walking, shopping, cleaning)	**Activity that makes** you out of breath for 20 minutes or more, three to five times a week (eg jogging)
Inactive	**Some activity**	**Active**

Stress reactions for detainees

Leaflets in other languages, including English, can be found on the disks given at the back of this book.

ARABIC

- سرعة البكاء و العصبية
- تجنب الآخرين و الخطر ء على

التأثير على علاقاتك بالآخرين

- فقد ان الرغبة في التعامل مع الناس
- الجدل و الاختلاف بين الزوج والزوجة

إذا كنت تعاني من الأعراض التي ترتبط بالصعوبات في بعض هذه الأعراض التي ترتبط بالضغط النفسي قد تتناول في نفس الوقت و لكن هذا لا يعني ان كل في نفس الوقت و لكن هذا لا يعني ان كل فرد الأفراد يعانون من نفس الأعراض التي تركب من شخص لآخر. و قد تجد فيها ان سلوكك و احساسك قد تغيرت من الأعراض المذكورة في هذه

ما الذي يمكنك فعله عند التعرض للضغط النفسي

إذا كنت تعاني من الأعراض المذكورة في هذه فربما لأنك تمر بشيء طبيعي لظروف غير طبيعية أن لا تشعر بشيء طبيعي لظروف غير طبيعية تمر بها و لكنه و في كثير من الأحيان يتلاشى بمرور الزمن و لا يعني ذلك بأنك أصبحت مجنونا.

قد تجد ان التحداك و انشغالك في الأعمال المفيدة بخبير ما.

إذا ما تشعر به شيء طبيعي لظروف غير طبيعية قريبا لأنك تمر بشيء طبيعي و الحط عند الأعراض المذكورة في هذه النشرة كليا و في بعض

- و إذا كان هناك من تعرف قد ترغب في بعض الأعراض و كيف تؤثر في تأثيرات الضغط النفسي، يمكنك تؤثر في شعور و تصرفاته.
- يمكنك مساعدة الآخرين الذين يعانون من الضغط النفسي بتوصيل هذه المشكلة.

كيف التعامل مع الآخرين الذين يعانون من الضغط النفسي بتوصيل كل الآراء الجيدة من الاتصال بجمعيات حياتك التي تنتمي إليها أو بطبيبك العائلي

- فإذا وجدت أن هذه التأثيرات قوية جدا أو استمرت لمدة أشهر قد ترغب حينها اطلب المساعدة.

للمزيد من المساعدة يمكنك مساعدته أو يمكنك الاتصال بجمعيات حياتك التي تنتمي إليها أو بطبيبك العائلي

لمواصلة النشاطات المختلفة والمفيدة هي طريقة للإحساس بالتحسن و الجيدة توفير الحلول العملية لك للإحساس بالتحسن و معرفتك بكل الخدمات التي تساعدك في توفير الحلول العملية.

و يمكنك أيضا الاتصال بجمعيات و منظمات جاليتك لتوجيهك و ارشادك للخدمات المتوفرة و يمكن أيضا أن ترشدك قد تكون قادرة مفيدة و يمكن أيضا بالمعلومات الخاصة بذلك.

قد تنظم هذه الجمعيات و الدراسة في المشاكل العملية أيضا على اسداء التدريب و الدراسة في المشاكل العملية.

الضغط النفسي و الأعراض المتعلقة بذلك

معلومات للاجئين

Reproduced with kind permission from Forest Healthcare NHS Trust, and supported by Redbridge & Waltham Forest Health Authority and Leytonstone Life Government Challenge Fund. Developed by Refugee Support Project, Forest Healthcare NHS Trust.

Translated by Dr N. Fathi and D. Zitouni Algerian Education Project

كل ما يتعلق بالضغط النفسي و الأعراض الخاصة بك

مقدمة

كل ما تشعر به داخل عقلك و جسدك يتأثر بالظروف التي تمر فيها عندما تتغير تلك الظروف يتغير معي شعورك و أحاسيسك و مثال ذلك حين يصبح الجو حار بما جسمك في قرر ذلك حين تزداد خفقات قلبك فالتغير في المرق و حينما يتأثر المجهد القاسية تؤثر على عقلك و جسدك و طرق تفكيرك أو شخص تزداد خفقات قلبك فالتغير في عقلك و جسدك و هذا ما يعرف بالضغط النفسي

أسباب الضغط النفسي

عندما تتغير حياتك بصورة جيدة سوف تشعر بالسعادة و الرضا. و ما تحسه داخل عقلك و جسمك و طرق تفكيرك

أحاسيسك النفسية اختلفت.

و ينتج ذلك للأسباب التالية:

القلق

- لأنك اضطررت للرجل دون عائلتك و
- لأنك اضطررت للرجل دون عائلتك و الأصدقاء بسبب

الاعتقال أو القلق

- من تخبر
- القلق أفراد من الأسرة أو الأصدقاء أو

يوصف الأعراض التالية.

الحزن، الكأبة، الإحباط

- الإحساس بالخجل

ما هي مؤثرات الضغط النفسي عليك

بالطرق التي يمر فيها شخص عائد من الضغط النفسي

تأثيره على العقل

- الاضطرار للقيام بأعمال لا ترغب في القيام بها
- عدم القدرة على تغيير ظروفك المعيشية
- الاضطرار للعيش في غير وطنك

الحزن

- لمجرد معرفة ما ينطوي عليه المستقبل

عدم الأمان

- إذا كنت حياتك في ظروف غير آمنة
- القلق على إمكانية البقاء في هذا البلد
- القلق على حالتك المالية في بلد

العنف

- تعرضك للتهديد أو الإيذاء أو التعذيب
- التعرض للتعذيب أو الاعتداء الجنسي
- التعرض لمشاهدة أو المعاملة القاسية و الإهانة
- أفراد الأسرة أو الأصدقاء خاصة من
- تعرضك لمشاهدة قتل الآخرين

التأثير على السلوك و قلة النشاط

- تغيير في السلوك الجنسي

التأثير على الجسم

- اضطرابات في النوم
- أحلام مزعجة (كوابيس)
- الإحساس بالتعب و الإرهاق
- الألم في البطن
- الإسهال
- ضعف الشهية
- خفقان القلب
- الدوران
- الإحساس برعشات أو رخفة في الجسم
- صعوبة في التنفس
- الألم و أوجاع في الجسم

- مشتركة
- الإحساس بأن الأحداث السابقة السابقة سيحدث مرة أخرى (أو أنها ستتكرر)
- التفكير الرجعية في الحياة السابقة بصورة
- فقدان الرغبة في الحياة
- ضعف المعنوية و سرعة الانفعال
- التوتر
- سرعة الغضب
- القلق

373

فشار های روحی و تأثیرات ان

اطلاعات برای پناهندگان

فشار های روحی و تأثیرات ان

مقدمه

احساسات روحی و جسمی حالزار محیط زندگی شماست. وقتی شرایط زندگی تغییر میکند روی احساسات تأثیر میگذارد. بعضی حال کرمیدیزان باعث غرق کردن میشود و بعضی شرایط شریدن قلب روحی و جسمی شخص را اداز میدهد و باعث فشارهای روحی میشود.

عواملی که باعث "فشار روحی" میشوند:

وقتی زندگی در وفق مراد است. شما احساس خوشحالی و راحتی میکنید اما وقتی شرایط مناسب نیست و دیگر شرایط ناسازگار خواهید داشت. ناسازگارانده همید احساس دیگری میشود. دلایلی که باعث تغییر احساسات میشود:

از دست دادن:

• مجبور به ترک خانه و منطقات شدن

از دست دادن اعضای خانواده و دوستان شدن

فشنونت

• مورد بی بودن از کره در رفتن

• مورد تهدید. صدمه و شکنجه قرار گرفتن

• شاهد قتل و خشونت نسبت به اعضای خانواده و دوستان

بودن

• مورد اذاب ظلم گذشته

• ترس از تکرار حوادث یا گذشته

تأثیر فشار روحی روی افکار:

• خشمگین کریه، پایس

• خجل بردن

• نگرانی

• زود عصبانی شدن

• عصبی بودن و از کره در رفتن

• عدم تمرکز

• بی علاقگی به ادامه زندگی

• ترس از دکار حوادث یا گذشته

تأثیر فشار روحی دارد که میزند اثر انکار نویسهد کرده اند:

• مجبور به ماندن در جایی که شما نیست

• نداشتن اختیار برای تغییر شرایط ایجام دهد

شما این انکار نویسهد
"روی شما" :

• شاهدان دیگران بخصوص اعضای خانواده و یا دوستان

عدم اعتبار:

• در شرایط تا امن سفر کردن

• نگرانی در مورد اجاره الاست درای کشور

• اضطراب در مورد مسایل مالی ومسکن

عدم / اخیار:

• مجبور به ماندن در جایی که خانه شما نیست

• مجبور شدن به کارهایی که نمی خواهید ایجام دهد

تاثیر فشار روحی روی جسم؟

- بیخوابی
- کابوس
- خستگی و کرختی
- درد جسمانی
- گرفتگی عضلات
- تپش قلب
- تنگی نفس
- حالت تهوع
- اسهال
- رنگ پریدگی
- تعریق

تاثیر فشار روحی روی رفتار:

- تغییر در تمایلات جنسی
- عدم تحرک و بیقراری
- زیاده روی در مصرف الکل و مواد مخدر

اگر تحت تاثیر فشار روحی مسئله ممکن است این مشکلات را درگیری بهم اوائل، خشونت بین زن و شوهر بیماری سبب به آنها یا اجتماعی

پناهگان تماس بگیرید.

اگر تاثیر فشار روحی روی رفتار یا سازمان حمایت از مدت طولانی شما را ازار داد موارد یا سازمان حمایت از

تحصیلی، اموزشی و مشاوره برای حل جنبه مشکلات یا اگر تاثیر فشار روحی روی حل ماهیا ارائه بهداشتی و برای

جوانب و کارنهای ایرانی یا احتمال زیاد سرویس خدمت دارند تماس بگیرید.

سعی کنید اطلاعات کاملی از این موارد سازمانهای خدماتی که برای کمک به جوانب مشکلاتی تاسیس شده اند بدست اورید با

بیشتر مراحل یا مورد زمان کم میشود وجود جوانب احساساتی دارد این نیست که از دست دارم؟

اگر مشغول به جوانب شوید فشارهای روحی کمترشما را ازار خواهد داد. تحرک و فعالیت یکی از راه های موردی است.

در شرایط غیر عادی جوانب عادی است و در

این ممکن است دلایل دلمداری ما و مشکلاتی باشد که در گذشته برایمان اتفاق افتاده باشد.

تجربه کنید که رابطه سالم با مشکلات زندگی دارند. ممکن است تصورات کلی در رفتار و احساسات بوجود بیاید. هر چند که به این مشکلات در یک نفر برد نمی کنند زیرا اشخاص

اگر به طرف بدانسب های منفی شدن حال یا کشته باشد که شما را راج میبرد.

زمانی که تحت فشار روحی هستید چه باید بکنید؟ زمانی که تحت فشار روحی هستید چه باید بکنید عکس العمل های منفی نشان خواهد داد.

پناهگان معرفی کنید.

اگر کسی را می شناسید که از این ناراحتی رنج میبرد موارد یا موارد فشارهای روحی را برای او توضیح دهید. شما موارد یا حل درمان های بکارد و از این راه با او کمک کنید.

برای کمک و حل مشکلاتی که در اینجا ذکرشده موارد یا جوانب و کارنهای ایرانی یا دکتر (GP) تماس بگیرید تا شما را یا سازمان حمایت از

375

உள உடல் உளைச்சலும் (Stress) அதன் விளைவுகளும்

அகதிகளுக்கான தகவல்கள்

Reproduced with kind permission from Forest Healthcare NHS Trust, and supported by Redbridge & Waltham Forest Health Authority and Leytonstone Life Government Challenge Fund. Developed by the Refugee Support Project, Forest Healthcare NHS Trust

தகிலாலயை விரும்பகரும்,

உள உடல் உழைச்சல், மற்றவர்களுடன் இருக்கும் தொடர்புகளில் ஏற்படுத்தும் விளைவு

* மற்றவர்களிடம் அக்கறை இல்லாமல், கணைவை மனைவபியிடையே வாக்குவாதங்கள், விளைசக்கபபாடிய்ளளவம், மனப்புவை உணர்முற்ற இ்ணடுகலும்,

* நீங்கள் உள உடல் உழைச்சலுக்கு உள்ளனாவனால், உங்களுடன வாழ்க்கையில் ஏற்படும் கஸ்டங்களோடு தொடர்புடை்ய பேற்குத்துயலைகளில் சிலவற்றை அலுபயைப்பீர்கள். உங்களுடைய நிடத்கைகலிலும் உணர்வுகளிழும் ஒ்லசகவந்தில் மாற்றங்கள் ஏற்படுதலிருக்த காரணிர்கள். எப்படியாயினும், எல்லோரும் மேல் குறிப்பிட்ட அனைதுதயம் வேளவ்வறு விதமாக இந்த உள உடல் உழைச்சலை வெளிக்காடுனேர்.

உள உடல் உழைச்சலுக்கு உன்னாலும்போது உங்களால் என்ன செய்ய முடியும்?

இந்தப் பிரகத்தில் கூறபட்டுள்ளவற்றில் ஏதாவது வகைகளில் நீங்கள் பாதிக்கப்படுவதாக உணரந்தால்:

* கடந்த காலத்திலோ அல்லது இன்னௌ உங்களுக்கு ஏற்பட்ட தகுதில்டம் இ்தற்குக் காலனைனாக இருப்புடியை உணர்ந்திதனை அனாந்தாயா இநதியில் உங்களுக்கு ஏற்றும். காலப்பொக்கிற பலருக்கு இந்த உணர்ச்சி குணடிகும். அறிகுறியல் உங்கள் "முதலை பாதிக்கப்படுகிறது" எனற அர்த்தமில்லை.

* நீங்கள் எதிவாவது புருவமாயாக ஈடுபட்டிருக்கும் போது, இந்த உள உடல் உழைச்சல் உங்களை அதிகம் பாதிப்பதாக உணரமாடைர்கள். உங்களைச்

---

* கறுகறும்பாகக் கொள்வது, நீங்கள் நல்ல நிடலவமில இ்ருப்பதாக உணரச்செய்ய நல்ல வழி. உங்களுக்கு என்ன பிரச்சனைகளுக்கு உதவக்கடிய எவ்வனச் செயலகள் பற்றியும் நிசையமாக அறிந்து கொள்வகளுக்கான பற்றிய செயலகள் அதிகள் சார்க்ணதச் செர்ந்த குழுக்கள் அதிகம்.

* அறிமதிருப்பார்கள். இலவய பற்றிய மேலதிக விபரங்களை அவர்களிடம் பேறலாம்.

* நீங்கள் எழுகதைச் செர்ந்த அலைமப்புக்கள் இலவய பற்றிய திகழ்மிகலனை ஆரம்பிக்க்கை்கம். அலையைவரவும், உங்களுக்கு ஏற்ற தொழிலில் பயிற்சிபெற்றியோ கல்வி மற்றும் நல முறையா பிரச்சினைகள் பற்றியோ அவர்கள் உங்களுடுக்க ஆலோசனைகள் வழங்குவான்கள்.

* மேல்வு குறிப்பிட்ட பாதிப்புக்கள் கூருதலாக்க காலணால்ட்டேன், அல்லது அவைது பல மாதங்களாக்கத் தொடர்ந்து இருந்தக்போ நீங்கள் நிச்சயம் நித்தவை வியரிப்பனிர்கள்.

* உங்களுக்குக் தெரிந்த யாரவேனது உள உடல் உழைச்சலினார் கவலைப்பட்டனால், நீங்கள் அவர்களுக்கு இலவை பற்றி விளக்குவும் அவர்களுக்கு வேறும்பினாக செய்யுப்டல்லும் உதவலாம், உள உடல் உழைச்சலனா பாதிக்கப பட்டவர்களுக்கு அதிகிக்குக்கு விடடா, எது பற்றி உங்களுடைய முனைனா நலம் உதவ முடியும்.

இந்த வெளிபிட்டிடல் ஆராயப்பட்ட பிரச்சலைகவை பற்றிய இயலவுதரிக உடுவதகளுக்கு உங்கள் சமுதைதொடவரி்களின் அலைம்பபடிய்க்களுட்போ இருப்ப வையுப்பரீயி்போ உதவாநிர்கள்.

TAMIL

உள உடல் உறுத்தலும் அதன் விளைவுகளும்

முன்னுரை

உங்கள் உள்ளத்திலும் உடலிலும் ஏற்படும் உணர்ச்சி தீங்கள் உங்கள் வாழும் ஆழ்வாற் பாதிக்கப்படுகிறது. தீங்கள் வாழும் ஆழல் மாறும்போது, உங்கள் உணர்வுகளும் மாற்றம் ஏற்படலாம். உ, தாரணமாக, காலநிலை வெப்பமாக இருந்தால் உங்கள் தேகத்தில் இருந்து வியர்வை சிந்தலாம். தீங்கள் பயம்/அழுத்தமாக இருக்கும்போது உங்கள் உடல் பயபுறுத்தும்போதோ உங்கள் இதயத்துடிப்பு அதிகரிக்கலாம்.

கெட்ட அனுபவங்களுக்கும் எத்தொகையற்ற வாழ்க்கை நிலைகளுக்கும் உங்கள் உள உணர்வுகளிற் பாதிப்பை ஏற்படுத்தலாம். இவ்வாறான நிலை ஏற்படும்போது, தீங்கள் உள உணர்ச்சி உறுத்தலுக்கு உட்படுகின்றீர்கள்.

உள உடல் உறுத்தல் எதனால் ஏற்படுகின்றது?

உங்கள் வாழ்க்கை சுமுகமாக ஒழுகும்போது தீங்கள், எத்தொகையுமாகவும் நிம்மதியாகவும் இருப்பீர்கள். தீங்கழ்வுகள் சிரமமான நிலை பொறுவிட்டால் அல்லது உங்களில் நல பேறுதேள்கி தீங்கள் கவலைப்பட்டால் உங்களில் விழிதியாகவான உணர்வுகள் உணர்வாகவும் தீங்கள் கவலைப்பீர்கள். பின்வரும் தீங்குகளைல் இருக்க உணர்ாகலாம்:

இழப்பு

* உங்கள் விட்டை உயும் உடமைகளையும் விட்டு, பலவந்தமாக வெளியேற்றப்படோவோ ஏற்படுவோவா.
* உங்கள் குடும்பத்தினரையோ தீங்கள் தெரிப்பவர்களையோ விட்டு, பழிந்தமாக வெளியேறவோ ஏற்படுவோவது.
* சுகாதி அல்லது வேலை காரணமாக உங்கள் குடும்ப உறுப்பினர்களை நடமர்ிங்களை இருக்க தெரிந்தும் போவது.

வன்முறை

* பயமுறுத்தப்பட்டால், தாக்கப்பட்டால் அல்லது சித்திரவதை செய்யப்பட்டால்,
* பாலியல் வன்முறைக்கு உள்ளாக்கப்பட்டால் அல்லது கேட்க்கப்பட்டால்,
* மற்றவர்களோ, குடும்பத்த, குடும்ப உறுப்பினர்களையோ நண்பர்களையோ கொடுரமாக நடத்துவட்டதையோ பார்த்தால்,
* மற்றவர்களோ, குடும்பத்தை உறுப்பினர்களையோ நண்பர்களையோ கொலைசெய்யப்பட்டதை நட பார்த்தால்.

பாதுகாப்பின்மை

* பாதுகாப்பில்லாத தழ்நிலையிற் பயணத்தை மேற் கொண்டால்,
* இந்திய ராப்பிற் தொடர்ந்து தீங்கள் தங்கள்காலில் எங்கடயாரற்ற கவலை கொள்ளல்,
* பணமில்லை எனவோ வேறோவில் வாழ்வில்லை எனவோ கவலைகொண்டால்,
* எதிர்காலம் எப்படி அமையுமோ எள்பது பற்றி தெரியாமையினைால்.

உளவியல்/வன்முறை

* அனைய இடத்தில் வசிக்க நேரும்போழுது.
* உங்கள் வாழ்க்கைக நிலைகளை உங்களால் மாற்ற முடியாமையிரக்கும் பொழுது.
* தீங்கள் வாழ்க்கையிருப்பாக ஒண்பமாக பலவந்தமாக செய்ய லைப்படுகின்றது.

உள உடல் உறுத்தல் உங்களை எத்தனைய தாக்குவதை உங்களில் ஏற்படுத்தும்?

உள உடல் உறுத்தலினால் பாதிக்கப்பட்டஸ்கள் சிலவேளைகளில் பின்வருபவைற்றில் சில தாக்கங்கள் இருப்பதைக் சொல்லுவார்கள்:

உள உறுத்தலின் விளைவுகள்:

* அங்கக்ம், அழுகை, விசேசி.
* தன் நிலைமையலை எனக்கணி வெட்கப்படல்,
* கவலைலயப்படுதல்.
* இலகுவில் கோபடையுதல்,
* நம்பிக்கமாப்பியும் முறுகாமயும்,
* கவலை செழ்த்தி முடியாமை,
* வாழ்க்கையில் விருப்பமில்லாமை.
* உங்களுக்கு முன்பு நடக்குிந்ஸ்றுப்பற்ற மீண்டும் மீண்டும் சிந்தித்தல்,
* முன்பு ஏற்பட்ட கொடிய சம்பவம் ஒன்று மீண்டும் ஏற்படுவது போனற உணர்வு,

உடல் உறுத்தலின் விளைவுகள்

* நித்திரையின்மை.
* கெட்ட கனவுகள்,
* கவலையும் சோர்வும்,
* உடல் உணர்வு வலியும்,
* தசையிடம்பு,
* இதயம் படபடப்,
* உணரவில் விருப்பக்குறைவு,
* வாழ்த்து எடுப்பது போனற உணர்வு,
* வயிற்றுநொ தேர்,
* வயிற்றுவலை,
* மூச்செடிப்பிற் பிரச்சிவை,
* தலைசுற்றுறு.
* கடுப்பங்கத் புடியாக உடல் நடுக்கள்,
* பாலியலை வாழ்க்கையில் ஏற்படும் மாற்றம்

உள உடல் உறுத்தலினால் நடத்தையிலை ஏற்படும் விளைவுகள்

* உறானத்தினையையும் மந்தத்தினையயும்.
* விலைகளில் சிரத்த்தைக்குன்னாத்ல்.
* வழுவுக்கு பேறாக, ஆதுரவைன்மையயும்,
* மதுசாரத்தைவும்/போமதைவம்யோ அதிகமாசும்.
* மற்றவர்களைக் காணுவலைக்க தவிர்த்திக்கமும்

STRES & STRESİN ETKİLERİ

Göçmenler İçin Bilgiler

kuruluşları bu yardım konularını bilebilir ve size daha detaylı bilgileri ayrıntılarıyla birlikte verebilir.

- Toplum kuruluşları çeşitli etkinlikler düzenleyebilir, eğitim yada yeni bir meslek edinmeyle ilgili olarak detaylı bilgiler verebilir. Yine ayrıca pratik problemleriniz için size danışmanlık yapabilir.

- Eğer üzerinizdeki stresin yol açtığı etkilerin çok şiddetli olduğunu yada birkaç ay boyunca sürdüğünü hissediyorsanız, bu durumda sizin yardıma ihtiyacınız vardır.

- Eğer çektiği stresin etkilerinden dolayı endişeli başka insanlar tanıyorsanız, onlara stresin etkilerini ve nasıl davranarak daha iyi şeyler hissedebileceklerini anlatarak yardım edebilirsiniz. Yine başka stres çeken insanlara kendi problemlerinizle nasıl uğraştığınızı ve bu konulardaki tecrübelerinizi anlatarak da yardımcı olabilirsiniz.

Bu konularla ilgili olarak bu broşürde anlatılan zorluklarla ilişkin daha detaylı bilgi almak için Toplum Merkezlerine yada Mahalle Doktorunuza gidebilirsiniz.

TURKISH

Reproduced with kind permission from Forest Healthcare NHS Trust, and supported by Redbridge & Waltham Forest Health Authority and Leytonstone Life Government Challenge Fund. Developed by the Refugee Support Project, Forest Healthcare NHS Trust

Başka İnsanlarla Olan İlişkilerde Stresin Yol Açtığı Etkiler

- Başka insanlara olan ilginin azalması.
- Tartışma, itiraz etme, eşler arasındaki şiddet.

Eğer stres probleminiz varsa yukarıda sıraladığımız etkenlerin bazılarının sizin yaşamınızı da etkilediğini ve bu konuda zorluklar çekiyor olduğunuzu görebilirsiniz. Bununla birlikte yine aynı süre döneminde davranışlarınızın ve duyumlarınızın da değiştiğini anlayabilirsiniz. Fakat her insanın aynı etkileri yaşaması söz konusu olmayabilir, bazı insanlar bunları farklı biçimlerde yaşayabilir.

EĞER STRES PROBLEMİNİZ VARSA NELER YAPABİLİRSİNİZ

Bu broşürde anlatılanların herhangi birinden dolayı kendinizi iyi hissetmiyorsanız ;

- Kendinizi iyi hissetmemeniz geçmişte yaşadığınız herhangi bir talihsizlikten dolayı olabilir.

- Anormal bir koşulda yaşıyor olduğunuzda kendinizi kötü hissetmeniz gayet normaldir ve bir çok durumda olduğu gibi istek ve arzularınız zamana bağlı olarak azalır. Fakat bunlar bir gün dayanamayıp çılgına anlamına gelmemektedir.

- Kendinizi birşeylerle meşgul ettiğinizde stresin sizi daha az etkilediğini görebilirsiniz. Kendinize çeşitli meşkuliyetler bulmanız daha iyi hissetmeniz için güzel bir yoldur.

- Bazı pratik problemlerinizle ilgili olarak alabileceğiniz tüm yardımları kullanabildiğinize emin olunuz. Bağlı olduğunuz toplum

STRESLE İLGİLİ BİLGİLER VE STRESİN ETKİLERİ

GİRİŞ

Günlük hayatımızda yaşadığımız koşullar bedenimizde ve kafamızda neler hissettiğimizi ve nasıl hissettiğimizi direk olarak belirlemektedir. Yaşadığımız şeyler değiştiğinde doğal olarak hissettiklerimizde değişecektir. Örneğin eğer hava çok sıcak ise terlemeğe başlarız. Yine herhangi bir şekilde korkar yada biri tarafından korkutulursanız kalbiniz daha hızlı atmaya başlar.

Kötü deneyimler yada hoş olmayan yaşam koşulları bedenimizde ve kafamızda hissettiklerimizi etkilemekte ve bizleri rahatsız etmektedir. Eğer böyle şeyler yaşıyor iseniz STRES çekiyorsunuz demektir.

STRESE NELER YOL AÇAR

Yaşamınızdaki her şey iyi gidiyorsa kendinizi mutlu ve huzurlu hissedersiniz. Fakat yaşamınızdaki şeyler iyi gitmiyor yada birşeylerin iyi gitmediği konusunda endişe duyuyor iseniz, doğal olarak artık farklı şeyler hissettiğinizi anlayabilirsiniz.

Bunlar şu aşağıda sıraladığımız nedenlerden dolayı meydana gelmektedir ;

Kaybetme

· Evinizden ayrılmaya yada birşeyleri geride bırakmaya zorlandığınız durumlarda.
· Ailenizden yada sevdiklerinizden ayrılmaya zorlandığınız durumlarda.
· Aile bireylerden birini kaybettiğiniz yada bir arkadaşınızın tutuklandığı yada öldürüldüğünü duyduğunuz durumlarda.

Şiddet

· Tehdit edildiğiniz, yaralandığınız yada işkence gördüğünüz durumlarda.
· Cinsel tacize uğrama yada bu konularda korkutulduğunuz hallerde.
· Özel olarak aile üyelerinizden birine yada bir arkadaşınıza olduğu gibi, birilerine çok kötü ve acımasız davranıldığı durumlarda.
· Özel olarak aile üyelerinizden birinin yada bir arkadaşınızın uğradığı gibi birilerinin öldürüldüğü durumlarda.

Güvensizlik

· Güvenli olmayan koşullarda yolculuk yaptığınız durumda.
· Bir ülkede kalıp kalmayacağınız konusunda endişeleriniz olduğu durumlarda.
· Başka bir yerde yaşama yada ekonomik koşullarınızın zorluğu konularında endişelerinizin olduğu durumlarda.
· Geleceğin sizin için neler getireceğini bilemediğiniz durumlarda.

Güçsüzlük

· Kendinize ait olmayan bir evde yaşıyor olma zorunda kaldığınız durumlarda.
· Yaşam koşullarınızı değiştirme olanaklarına sahip olamadığınız durumlarda.
· Yapmak istemediğiniz şeyleri yapıyor olmak zorunda bırakıldığınız durumlarda.

STRESİN ÜZERİNİZDE BIRAKTIĞI ETKİLER NELERDİR

Stres sorunu olan insanlarda zaman zaman aşşağıda yazılı olan belirtiler görülmektedir ;

· Ağlamak, sürekli üzintülü ve çaresizlik içinde hissetmek.
· Utanma duygusu hissetmek.

· Endişeli olmak.
· Çabuk sinirlenmek.
· Sinirli ve sürekli bir kızgınlık halinde görünmek.
· Dikkatini belli bir şeye yöneltmemek.
· Yaşama olan ilginin azalması.
· Sürekli size ne olduğu konusunda kendinizi sorgulamak ve düşünmek.
· Sürekli daha önce yaşamınızda var olan kötü şeylerin devam ediyor olduğunu hissetmek.

Stresin İnsan Vucudunda Ortaya Çıkardıkları ;

· Uyuyamama problemi.
* Kabus görmeler.
* Yorgunluk ve bitkinlik.
* Vucut ağrıları ve acıları.
* Vucut kaslarının gergin bir halde olması.
* Kalp çarpıntıları.
* İştahsızlık.
· Hasta gibi hissetmek.
* Karın ağrıları.
· İshal şikayetleri.
· Nefes alma güçlüğü.
· Baş dönmesi.
* Kontrol edilemeyen vucut titremeleri.
* Cinsel yaşamdaki belirgin değişimler.

Stresin Davranışlarımız Üzerindeki Etkileri ;

* Hareketliliğin azalması, uyuşukluk ve bitkinlik hali.
· Çabuk sinirlenmek ve kızmak.
* Sürekli çalışmak ve yorgun hissetmemek.
* İçki yada uyuşturucuları fazla kullanmak.
* Diğer insanlarla fazla ilgilenmemek ve kendi kabuğuna çekilmek.